Fourth Edition

Manual of Psychiatric Nursing Care Plans

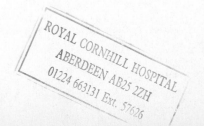

Fourth Edition

Manual of Psychiatric Nursing Care Plans

Judith M. Schultz, R.N., M.S.

Program Director
Diabetes Treatment Center
Sequoia Hospital
Redwood City, California

Sheila Dark Videbeck, R.N., M.S.

Assistant Professor
Nursing Department
Edgewood College
Madison, Wisconsin

J. B. Lippincott Company Philadelphia

Acquisitions Editor: Margaret Belcher
Sponsoring Editor: Ellen M. Campbell
Project Editor: Jim Slade
Indexer: Victoria Boyle
Design Coordinator: Kathy Kelley-Luedtke
Interior Designer: Susan Hess Blaker
Cover Designer: Jerry Cable
Production Manager: Helen Ewan
Production Coordinator: Nannette Winski
Compositor: Compset Inc.
Printer/Binder: Courier Book Company/Kendallville

Fourth Edition

6 5 4 3 2 1

Library of Congress Cataloging-in-Publication Data

Schultz, Judith M.
    Manual of psychiatric nursing care plans / Judith M. Shultz,
Sheila Dark Videbeck. — 4th ed.
        p.   cm.
    Includes bibliographical references and index.
    ISBN 0-397-55067-7
    1. Psychiatric nursing—Handbooks, manuals, etc.   2. Nursing care
plans—Handbooks, manuals, etc.   I. Videbeck, Sheila Dark.
II. Title.
    [DNLM: 1. Psychiatric Nursing—handbooks.   2. Patient Care
Planning—handbooks.   WY 39 S389m 1994]
RC440.S3317   1994
610.73'68—dc20
DNLM/DLC   93-5627
for Library of Congress   CIP

Any procedure or practice described in this book should be applied by the health care practitioner under appropriate supervision in accordance with professional standards of care used with regard to the
unique circumstances that apply in each practice situation. Care has been taken to confirm the accuracy
of information presented and to describe generally accepted practices. However, the authors, editors,
and publisher cannot accept any responsibility for errors or omissions or for any consequences from
application of the information in this book and make no warranty, express or implied, with respect to
the contents of the book.

Every effort has been made to ensure drug selections and dosages are in accordance with current recommendations and practice. Because of ongoing research, changes in government regulations, and the
constant flow of information on drug therapy, reactions, and interactions, the reader is cautioned to
check the package insert for each drug for indications, dosages, warnings, and precautions, particularly
if the drug is new or infrequently used.

Preface

The widespread use of the first three editions of this *Manual* and the gradual proliferation of other, similar books continue to support our belief in the need for a practical guide to nursing care planning for clients with emotional or psychiatric problems. The *Manual of Psychiatric Nursing Care Plans* was written as a reference manual to be used to facilitate implementation of the nursing process, particularly in the mental health setting. Because each client is an individual, he or she needs a plan of nursing care specifically tailored to his or her own needs, problems, and circumstances. The care plans in this *Manual* do not replace the nurses' skills in assessment, formulation of specific nursing diagnoses, expected outcomes, nursing interventions, and evaluation of nursing care. Rather, these plans cover a range of emotional and behavioral problems that may be encountered and a variety of approaches that may be employed. This information is meant to be adapted and used appropriately in planning nursing care for each client.

The *Manual*, therefore, is a learning tool and a reference book that presents information, concepts, and principles in a simple and clear format so that it can be used in a variety of settings and situations. Because the *Manual* offers practical suggestions for particular situations and can be adapted to the care of any client, it is helpful in both academic and clinical settings.

Each care plan in the fourth edition has been rewritten to provide a focus on the nursing diagnosis as the basis for nursing care planning. The *Manual* retains its behavioral organization, however, and remains easy to use and apply to individual clients based on behaviors assessed by the nurse. Within each care plan in the fourth edition, however, the nursing process is driven by the formulation of nursing diagnoses and a subsequent written plan of care, including defining characteristics, related factors (or risk factors for high risk diagnoses), expected outcomes, and nursing interventions, with a rationale given for each intervention. One or more nursing diagnosis that may be pertinent to a client with the particular behavior or problem is used to develop a plan of care (for each of the diagnoses addressed in the behaviorally based Care Plan), and several other nursing diagnoses are suggested as possibly relevant to a client in that situation. The authors have used the nursing diagnoses approved by the North American Nursing Diagnosis Association (NANDA).

Two additional Care Plans have been included in the General Care Plan section of this edition of the *Manual*: Noncompliance and Knowledge Deficit. Although these plans are based primarily on the corresponding nursing diagnosis, they present each situation in a more general way in addition to developing a care plan from the nursing diagnosis itself. In addition, new information has been integrated throughout the *Manual*, and all material was reviewed and revised according to current nursing knowledge and practice.

The *Manual of Psychiatric Nursing Care Plans*, in its fourth edition, continues to effectively address the need for skills education in psychiatric–mental health nursing. The *Manual* complements the more theoretic general psychiatric nursing texts and provides a solid clinical orientation for the student learning to use the nursing process in the clinical psychiatric setting. Too often, students feel ill-prepared for the clinical psychiatric experience, and their anxiety interferes with both their learning and their appreciation of psychiatric nursing. The *Manual* can help to lessen this anxiety by using the nursing process in conjunction with suggestions for specific interventions and rationale that address particular behaviors, giving the student a sound basis on which to build clinical skills.

We feel that the *Manual* is ideal as a handbook in both mental health and general medical units for use in developing individual care plans and in helping new staff members by offering clear and specific approaches to various problems. It also can be used by nonprofessional health care staff members and nonnursing staff members and can be especially helpful in the general medical or continuing care facility, where staff members may encounter these kinds of behaviors infrequently and may have less formal education and less confidence in dealing with clients who are experiencing emotional difficulties.

We believe that effective nursing care must begin with a holistic view of each client, whose life is composed of a particular complex of physical, emotional, spiritual, interpersonal, socioeconomic, and environmental factors. We sincerely hope the *Manual of Psychiatric Nursing Care Plans*, in its fourth edition, continues to contribute to the delivery of nonjudgmental, holistic care and to the development of sound knowledge and skills in students, all solidly based in a sound nursing framework.

We wish to express our appreciation to all of the people we have encountered in our professional lives who have helped our own learning and growth and enabled us to write this *Manual* in its four editions. We are truly grateful for the opportunity to know and work with them and to benefit from their work. Finally, we offer our heartfelt thanks to all those in our personal lives who have been supportive of us and of this work over these four editions and more than 17 years!

J.M.S. & S.D.V.

Contents

Part 1

Using the Manual

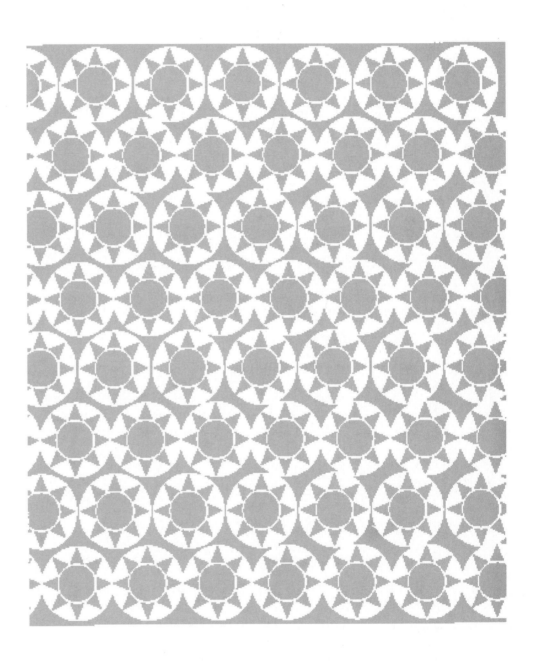

Schultz JM, Videbeck SD: MANUAL OF
PSYCHIATRIC NURSING CARE PLANS, 4th ed.
© 1994 J. B. Lippincott Company.

The *Manual of Psychiatric Nursing Care Plans* is designed to be used in both educational and clinical nursing situations. Because the care plans are organized according to the basic elements of the nursing process within each nursing diagnosis addressed, the *Manual* can effectively complement virtually any psychiatric nursing text and can be used within any theoretic framework. Because the plans are based on client behaviors and are oriented toward clinical problems, the *Manual* is appropriate for both undergraduate and graduate levels of nursing education.

In the clinical realm, the *Manual* is useful in any nursing setting. The *Manual* can be used to help formulate individual nursing care plans in both inpatient and outpatient situations; in psychiatric settings, including residential and acute care units, locked and open units, and with adolescent and adult client populations; in community-based programs, including individual and group situations; in general medical settings, for work with clients who have psychiatric diagnoses and those who may not have such a diagnosis but whose behavior or problems are addressed in the *Manual*; and in skilled nursing facilities and long-term residential, day treatment, and outpatient settings.

Nursing Students and Instructors

Development of Psychiatric Nursing Skills in Students

For a student, the development of nursing skills and comfort with psychiatric clients is a complex process of integrating knowledge of human development, psychiatric problems, human relationships, self-awareness, behavior and communication techniques, and the nursing process with clinical experiences in psychiatric nursing situations. This process can be fascinating, stimulating, and satisfying for both students and instructors, or both students and instructors may see it as arduous, frustrating, and frightening. We hope that the former is the common experience and that the *Manual* can be used in that process to add to the students' knowledge base, to guide their use of the nursing process, and to suggest ways to interact with clients that result in positive, effective nursing care, increased confidence, and comfort with psychiatric nursing.

Good interaction skills are essential in all types of nursing and enhance the student's nursing care in any setting. In addition, skillful communications enhance the student's (and the nurse's) enjoyment of working with clients and help avoid burnout later in his or her career. Efficient use of the nursing process and skills in writing and using care plans also help avoid burnout by decreasing frustration and repetition and increasing effective communication among the staff.

An important part of psychiatric nursing skill is conscious awareness of interactions, including both verbal and nonverbal components. In psychiatric nursing, interactions are primary tools of intervention. Awareness of these interactions is necessary to ensure *therapeutic*, not social, interactions, and requires thinking on several levels. First, the nurse must be knowledgeable about the client's present behaviors and problems. Second, the interaction should be goal directed: What is the purpose of the interaction in view of the client's nursing diagnosis and expected outcomes? Third, the skills or techniques of communication must be identified and the structure of the interaction planned. Finally, during the interaction itself, the nurse must continually be aware of the responses of the client, evaluate the effectiveness of the interaction, and make changes as indicated.

Techniques for Developing Interaction Skills

Developing interaction skills and awareness can be facilitated by using the *Manual* in classes, group clinical settings, and individual faculty–student interaction in conjunction with various teaching methods. Effective techniques include:

Case studies: presentation of a case (a client encountered in the clinical setting, a hypothetical example, or paradigm case) by the instructor or student. The case may be written, presented by role-playing, or verbally described. Students (individually or in groups) can perform an assessment and write a care plan for the client, using the *Manual* as a resource.

Role-play and feedback in conjunction with a case study or to develop specific communication skills. Interactions with actual clients can be reenacted for identification and evaluation of communication techniques, or the instructor may portray a client with certain behaviors and students can employ various communication skills, and both students and instructors can give feedback regarding the interactions.

Videotaped interactions for case presentations and role-play situations to help the student develop awareness by actually seeing his or her own behavior and seeing the interaction as a whole from a different, "outside observer" perspective. Review of the tape by both the instructor and the student (and in groups, as the students' comfort levels increase) allows feedback, discussion, and identification of alternative techniques.

Written process recordings of brief interactions or portions of interactions can be helpful with or without videotaping. Recalling the interaction in detail sufficient for a written process recording helps the student to develop awareness during the interaction itself and to develop memory skills that will be useful in other types of documentation. Process recordings can include identification of goals, evaluation of the effectiveness of skills and techniques or of the client's responses to a statement or behavior, and ways to change the interaction (that is, if it could be redone), in addition to the recording of actual words and behaviors of the client and the student.

Writing care plans for each client, based on the student's assessment of the client. Prior to an interaction with the client, the instructor can review the plan with the student, and the student can identify expected outcomes, nursing interventions, or interactions he or she will attempt to use, and so forth. Following the interaction, both the care plan and the specific interaction can be evaluated and revised.

Using the Manual in Teaching Psychiatric Nursing

Instructors may find the *Manual* useful in organizing material for teaching classes and for discussion points. The "Basic Concepts" section examines a number of issues germane to the practice of psychiatric nursing and the delivery of nonjudgmental nursing care. Each group of care plans deals with a set of related problems that students may encounter in the psychiatric setting. A small group of students could be responsible for the presentation of one of these topics (eg, loss or chemical dependence) to the entire class, with subsequent discussion of specific behaviors, problems, nursing diagnoses, interventions, and so forth. Study questions and test questions can be formulated based on information found in the "Basic Concepts" section, the introductory paragraphs in each care plan, the assessment data section, or in other sections.

Clinical Nursing Staff

The use of written individual nursing care plans is necessary in any clinical setting for a number of reasons. First, nursing care plans provide a focus for using the nursing process in a deliberate manner with each client. Second, written care plans provide the basis for evaluating the effectiveness of nursing interventions and allow revisions based on actual plans of care, not unspecified or haphazard nursing interven-

tions. Third, written care plans are the only feasible means of effective communication about client care among different members of the nursing staff, who work at different times and who may not be familiar with the client (eg, float, registry, or part-time nurses). Fourth, written care plans provide a central point of information for coordination of care, the identification of goals, and the use of consistent limits, interventions, and so forth, in the nursing care of a given client. Even when only one nurse expects to work with a client over time (eg, in a home health or other community-based setting or private practice), a written plan is the only workable means of maintaining continuity over time. Fifth, nursing standards of care and accreditation standards require that each client have a written plan of care. Finally, the integration of written care plans into the daily routine of the nursing unit allows for efficient care that saves time and avoids burnout in the staff.

However, written care plans are not always done and are often perceived as troublesome, time-consuming, useless, or unrelated to the actual care of the client. This *Manual* was originally conceived to alleviate some of the problems involved in writing care plans that deal with psychiatric problems in clients. Many nurses felt that they had to "reinvent the wheel" each time they sat down to write a care plan for a client whose behavior was in fact similar to the behavior of other clients in their experience, although they recognized differences among individual clients and their needs. The *Manual* was first written to be a sourcebook for writing care plans, to allow nurses to choose the parts of a comprehensive care plan that are appropriate to the needs of a unique person and to adapt and specify those parts according to that person's needs. The *Manual* can be seen as a catalog of possibilities for the care of psychiatric clients, with suggestions of nursing diagnoses, assessment data, expected outcomes, therapeutic aims, and interventions. (We do not mean to suggest, however, that all possibilities are contained in the *Manual*.) It is also meant to be a catalyst for thought about nursing care, as a starting point in planning care for the client. In addition, the *Manual* suggests a structure for using the nursing process in the formulation of care plans and allows the nurse to efficiently address the client's needs.

Strategies for Promoting the Use of Written Care Plans

Even with the *Manual* present as a resource, the nursing staff still may be reluctant to write and use care plans. To encourage the use of written plans, we suggest that nurses identify the barriers to their use and plan and implement strategies to overcome these barriers. In addition, it may be helpful to present the use of written plans in such a way that they can be easily integrated into the existing routine of the nursing staff and seen as positive or beneficial to the staff itself (not only to clients or for other purposes, such as accreditation requirements).

Some possible barriers to the use of written plans and suggested strategies to overcome them are:

Barrier: Not enough time allowed to write care plans.

Strategies: When making nursing assignments, consider writing the nursing care plan as a part of the admission process for a newly admitted client and allot time accordingly. Enlist the support of the nursing administration in recognizing the necessity of allowing time to write nursing care plans when planning staffing needs. Include writing and using care plans in performance review criteria and give positive feedback for nurses' efforts in this area. Nursing supervisors and nursing education personnel also can assist staff nurses in writing plans on a daily basis.

Barrier: Having to "reinvent the wheel" each time a care plan is written.

Strategies: Use the *Manual* as a resource for each client's care plan to suggest assessment parameters, nursing diagnoses, and so forth and as a way to stimulate thinking about the client's care. If your unit has standard protocols for certain situations (eg, behavior modification, detoxification), have these printed in your care plan format with blank lines (____) to accommodate individual parameters or expected outcome criteria as appropriate.

Barrier: Care plans require too much writing, or the format is cumbersome.

Strategies: Streamline care plan forms and design them to be easily used for communication and revision purposes. Write plans in collaboration with other nursing staff, in care planning conferences, or in informal, impromptu sessions. Design systems to address common problems that can be consistently used and adapted to individual needs (eg, levels of suicide precautions). These can be specifically delineated in a unit reference book and briefly noted in the care plan itself (eg, "Suicide precautions: Level 1").

Barrier: No one uses the care plans once they have been written.

Strategies: Integrate care plans as the basic structure for change of shift report, staffings and case conferences, and documentation. For example, review interventions and expected outcomes for current problems as you review clients in report, and revise care plans as clients are reviewed. Base problem-oriented charting on nursing diagnoses in care plans; update care plans while charting on clients.

It may be helpful to hold a series of staff meetings and invite the input of all the nursing staff to identify the particular barriers in place on your nursing unit and to work together as a staff to overcome them.

Additional Benefits of Using Written Care Plans

In addition to overcoming resistance such as that noted, presentation of the benefits of using care plans may be useful. Because the use of written care plans can enhance the consistency and effectiveness of nursing care, it also can increase the satisfaction of the staff and help avoid burnout. The following are among the benefits of using written care plans:

Increased communication among nursing staff and other members of the health care team

Clearly identified expected outcomes and strategies

Decreased repetition (ie, each nursing staff member does not need to independently, albeit informally, assess, diagnose, and identify outcomes and interventions for each client)

Routine evaluation and revision of interventions

Decreased frustration with ineffective intervention strategies: If a nursing intervention is ineffective, it can be revised and a different intervention implemented in a timely manner

Increased consistency in the delivery of nursing care

Increased satisfaction in working with clients as a result of coordinated, consistent nursing care

Efficient, useful structure for change of shift report, staffings or clinical case conferences, and documentation

More complete documentation with decreased preparation time and effort related to quality assurance, utilization review, accreditation, and reimbursement issues.

In addition to presentation of the above points in working with the nursing staff to implement or strengthen the use of care plans, it may be helpful to integrate care plans and their use into other nursing education programs. For example, nursing grand rounds can include a case study presented in terms of the nursing process with that client, including the use of a written care plan as a handout, a visual aid (eg, a slide or an overhead transparency), or an exercise for the participants. Videotaped or role-playing sessions, or both, for nursing orientation programs or to discuss nursing assessment, planning, and intervention also can employ written care plans or portions of plans. In similar ways, the *Manual* can be used as a resource in planning programs such as these or can be used by the participants during the programs. Also, topics covered in the "Basic Concepts" section, groups of care plans, or specific care plans can be used to plan and implement topical in-service presentations, nursing development, or nursing orientation programs. Finally, the format used for the care plans in the *Manual* can be easily adapted to construct nursing care plan forms for use in the clinical setting (eg, delete "Rationale" column, replace with "Outcome Criteria" column).

Using Written Psychiatric Care Plans in Nonpsychiatric Settings

Written care plans to address the emotional or psychiatric needs in the nonpsychiatric setting are especially important. In such settings, certain psychiatric problems are rarely encountered, and the nursing staff may lack the confidence and knowledge to readily deal with these problems. Using the Manual in this situation can help in planning holistic care by providing concrete suggestions for care as well as background information related to the problem per se. Because the care plans are behaviorally based, the Manual can be used effectively without a psychiatric (medical) diagnosis, based on the client's behavior as assessed by the nurse. In addition, the care plans can be used as the basis for a staff review or nursing in-service regarding the problem or behavior soon after it is assessed in the client.

Part 2

Basic Concepts

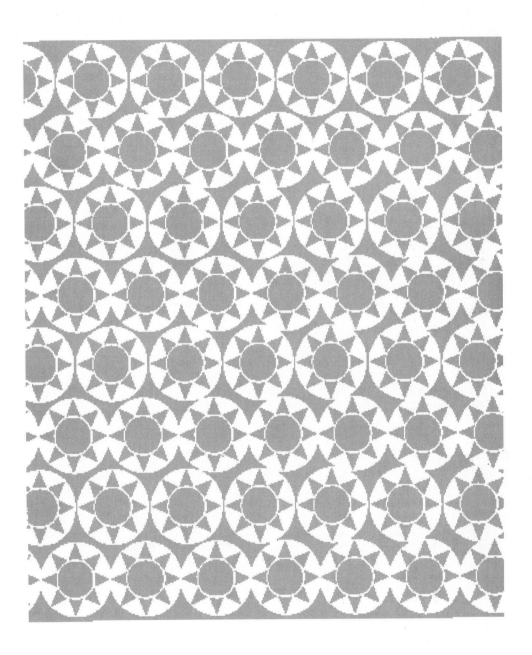

The care plans in this book have been created with certain fundamental concepts in mind. In this section, we will delineate these concepts and beliefs, hoping to stimulate the reader's thinking about these aspects of working with clients.

Fundamental Beliefs

1. A nurse provides only the care the client cannot provide for himself or herself at the time.
2. The client is basically responsible for his or her own feelings, actions, and life (see "Client's Responsibilities" below), although he or she may be limited in ability or need help.
3. The client must be approached by the nurse as a whole person with a unique background and environment and a set of strengths, behaviors, and problems, not as a psychiatrically labeled nonentity to be manipulated.
4. The client is not a passive recipient of care. The nurse and the client work together toward mutually determined and desirable goals or outcomes. The client's active participation in all steps of the nursing process should be encouraged within the limits of the client's present level of functioning (see "Client's Responsibilities").
5. The predominant focus of work with the client is health, not merely the absence or diminution of the disease process. This means that one goal of therapy is the client's eventual independence from the hospital and the staff. If this is impossible, the client should reach his or her optimum level of functioning and independence.
6. Given feedback and the identification of alternative ways to meet needs that are acceptable to the client, he or she will choose to progress toward a healthy lifestyle with more appropriate coping mechanisms.
7. Physical and emotional health are interconnected; therefore, physical health is a desirable goal in the treatment of emotional problems. Nursing care should incorporate this concept and focus on the client's obtaining adequate nutrition, rest, and exercise and the elimination of chemical dependence (including tobacco, caffeine, alcohol, over-the-counter medications, or other drugs) as part of the client's progress toward health.
8. The nurse works with other health professionals (and nonprofessionals) in a multidisciplinary approach; the nurse may function as a team coordinator. The team works within a milieu that is constructed as a therapeutic environment, with the aims of developing a holistic view of the client and providing effective treatment.

Therapeutic Milieu

Purpose and Definition

The therapeutic milieu is an environment that is structured and maintained as an ideal, dynamic setting in which to work with clients. This milieu includes safe physical surroundings, all staff members, and other clients. A therapeutic setting should minimize environmental stress, such as noise and confusion, and physical stress caused by such factors as lack of sleep and substance abuse. Removal of the client from a stressful environment to a therapeutic environment provides a chance for rest and nurturance of self, a time to focus on the development of strengths, and an opportunity to learn to identify alternatives or solutions to problems and to learn about the psychodynamics of those problems. This setting also allows clients to take part in a community in which they can share feelings and experiences and enjoy social interaction and growth as well as therapy. The nurse has a unique opportunity to facilitate (and model) communication and sharing among clients in the creation of a continuing, dynamic, informal group therapy.

A therapeutic milieu is a "safe space," a nonpunitive atmosphere in which caring is a basic factor. In this environment, confrontation may be a positive therapeutic tool that can be tolerated by the client. Nurses and other staff members should be aware of their own roles in this environment, minimizing an authoritarian position (eg, displaying keys as a reminder of status or control) yet maintaining a professional role (see "Nursing Responsibilities and Functions"). Clients are expected to assume responsibility for themselves within the structure of the milieu when they are able to do so. Feedback from other clients and the sharing of tasks or duties facilitate the client's growth.

Maintaining a Safe Environment

One important aspect of a therapeutic environment is the exclusion of objects or circumstances that a client may use to harm himself or herself or others. Although this is especially important in a mental health setting, this should be considered in any health care situation. The nursing staff should follow the facility's policies with regard to prevention of routine safety hazards and supplement these policies as necessary, for example:

Dispose of all needles safely and out of reach of clients.
Restrict or monitor the use of matches and lighters.

Do not allow smoking in bedrooms (clients may be drowsy owing to psychotropic drugs).

Remove mouthwash, cologne, aftershave, and so forth if substance abuse is suspected.

Listed below are the *most restrictive* measures to be used on a unit on which clients who are exhibiting behavior directly threatening or harmful to themselves or others may be present. These measures may be modified based on the assessment of the client's behavior.

Do not use glass containers (eg, ashtrays, drinking glasses, vases, salt and pepper shakers) or have them accessible.

Be sure mirrors, if glass, are securely fastened and not easily broken.

Keep sharp objects (eg, scissors, pocket knives, knitting needles) out of reach of clients and allow their use only with supervision. Use electric shavers when possible (disposable razors are easily broken to access blades).

Identify potential weapons (eg, mop handles, hammers, pool cues, baseball bats) and dangerous equipment (eg, electrical cords, scalpels, pap smear fixative), and keep them out of the clients' reach.

Do not leave cleaning or maintenance carts, which may contain cleaning fluids, bleach, mops, and tools, unattended in client care areas.

Do not leave medicines unattended or unlocked.

Keep keys (to unit door, medicines) on your person at all times.

Be aware of items that are harmful if ingested, for example, mercury manometers or poisonous plants (eg, philodendron).

Immediately on the client's admission to the facility, staff members should search the client and all of the client's belongings and remove potentially dangerous items, such as wire clothes hangers, ropes, belts, safety pins, scissors and other sharp objects, weapons, and medications. Keep these belongings in a designated place inaccessible to the client. Also, search any packages brought in by visitors (it may be necessary to search visitors in certain circumstances). Explain the reason for such rules briefly and do not make exceptions.

The Trust Relationship

One of the keys to a therapeutic environment is the establishment of trust. Not only must the client come to trust the nurse, but the nurse must trust himself or herself as a therapist and must trust in the client's motivation and ability to change. Both the client and the nurse must trust that therapy is desirable and productive. Trust is the foundation of a therapeutic relationship, and consistency and limit-setting are its building blocks. A trust relationship between the nurse and the client creates a space in which they can work together, using the nursing process and their best possible efforts toward attaining the goals they have both identified. See Care Plan 1: Building a Trust Relationship.

Building Self-Esteem

Just as a physically healthy body may be better able to withstand stress, a person with adequate or high self-esteem may be better able to deal with emotional difficulties. Thus, an essential part of a client's care is helping to build the client's self-esteem. Because each client retains the responsibility for his or her own feelings, and one person cannot *make* another person *feel* a certain way, the nurse cannot increase the client's self-esteem directly. Strategies to help build or enhance self-esteem must be individualized and must be built on honesty and on the client's strengths. Some general suggestions are:

Build a trust relationship with the client (see Care Plan 1: Building a Trust Relationship).

Set and maintain limits (see "Limit-Setting," later).

Accept the client as a person.

Be nonjudgmental at all times.

Provide structure (ie, structure the client's time and activities).

Have realistic expectations of the client.

Make your expectations clear to the client.

Initially, provide the client with tasks, responsibilities, and activities that can be easily accomplished; advance the client to more difficult tasks as he or she progresses.

Praise the client for his or her accomplishments, however small, giving sincere appropriate feedback for meeting expectations, completing tasks, fulfilling responsibilities, and so on.

Never insincerely flatter the client or be otherwise dishonest.

Minimize negative feedback to the client without giving mixed messages (enforce the limits that have been set, but withdraw attention from the client if possible rather than chastising the client for exceeding limits).

Use confrontation judiciously and in a supportive manner; use it only when the client can tolerate it.

Allow the client to make his or her own decisions whenever possible. If the client is pleased with the outcome of his or her decision, point out that he or she was responsible for the decision and give positive feedback. If the client is not pleased with the outcome, point out that the client, like everyone, can make and survive mistakes, then help the client identify alternative approaches to the problem. Give positive feedback for the client's taking responsibility for problem-solving and for his or her efforts.

Limit-Setting

Setting and maintaining limits are integral to a trust relationship and to a therapeutic milieu. Effective limits can provide a structure and a sense of caring that words alone cannot. Limits also minimize manipulation and secondary gains in therapy.

Before stating the limit and consequence, you may wish to go over briefly with the client the reasons for limit-setting and involve the client in this part of care planning; you may work together to decide on specific limits or consequences. However, if this is impossible, briefly explain the limits to the client, and do not argue or indulge in lengthy discussions or give undue attention to the consequences of an infraction of a limit. Some basic guidelines for effectively using limits are:

1. State the expectation or the limit as clearly, directly, and simply as possible. The consequence that will follow the client's exceeding the limit also must be clearly stated at the outset.
2. Keep in mind that consequences should be direct, simple, have some bearing on the limit, if possible, and be something that the client perceives as a negative outcome, not as a reward or producer of secondary gain. For example, if the consequence is not allowing the client to go to an activity, it will not be effective if (a) the client did not want to go anyway, (b) the client is allowed to watch television instead, which the client may prefer, or (c) the client receives individual attention from the staff at that time, which the client may prefer.
3. The consequence should immediately follow the client's exceeding the limit and must be consistent, both over time (each time the limit is exceeded) and among staff (each staff member must enforce the limit). One staff person may be designated to make decisions regarding the client and limits to ensure consistency; however, when this person is not available, another person must take that responsibility rather than defer the consequences.

Remember, although consequences are essential to setting and maintaining limits, they are not an opportunity to be punitive to a client. The withdrawal of attention is perhaps the best and simplest of consequences to carry out, provided that attention and support are given when the client meets expectations and remains within limits (and that the client's safety is not jeopardized by the withdrawal of staff attention). If the only time the client receives attention and feedback, albeit negative, is when he or she exceeds limits, that client will continue to elicit attention in that way. The client must perceive a positive reason to meet expectations; there must be a reward for staying within limits.

When dealing with limits, don't delude yourself in thinking that a client needs the nurse as a friend or sympathetic person who will be "nice" by making exceptions to limits. If you allow a client to exceed limits, you will be giving the client mixed messages and will undermine the other staff members as well as the client. You will convey to the client that you do not care enough for the client's growth and well-being to enforce a limit, and you will betray a lack of control on your part at a time when the client feels out of control and expressly needs someone else to be in control (see "Nursing Responsibilities and Functions," later).

Sexuality

Human sexuality is an area in which staff members' feelings are often evoked and must be considered. Because it is basic to everyone, sexuality may be a factor with any client in a number of ways. Too often the discomfort of both the nurse and the client interferes with the client's care; you, the nurse, can significantly overcome this discomfort by dealing with your own feelings and approaching this facet of the client's life in a professional way.

A client may be experiencing a problem involving sexual issues or sexuality in various situations. First, the client may be having difficulty adjusting to a change in sexual habits or feelings, such as first sexual activity, marriage, the loss of a sexual partner, or as a result of an injury, an illness, or a disability (see Care Plan 20: Altered Body Image). Second, the client may have been the victim of a traumatic experience that involved a sexual act, such as incest or rape, and may be experiencing subsequent difficulty with sexuality (see Care Plan 46: Post-Traumatic Behavior and Care Plan 53: Sexual, Emotional, and/or Physical Abuse). Third, the client may talk about being charged with or convicted of a crime that is associated with sexual activity, such as incest, exhibitionism, or rape (see "Clients with Legal Problems," later). Finally, certain aspects of sexuality may be posing a problem for the client: The client may be impotent or experiencing menopausal symptoms; the client may be experiencing homosexual feelings that are uncomfortable, confusing, or unacceptable to him or her; or the client may feel guilty about masturbation or sexual activity outside of marriage. These problems may be difficult for a client to reveal initially or to share with more than one staff person or with other clients. In situations like these, it is often helpful to the client for the nurse to initially bring up the topic of sexuality or ask about problems related to sexuality in the initial nursing assessment. Be sensitive to the client's feelings in care planning (the client's participation may be especially helpful in this situation). Remember that both male and female clients have a human need for sexual fulfillment. A matter-of-fact approach to sexuality on your part can help to minimize the client's discomfort.

Sexual activity or sexually explicit conversations may occur on the unit, posing another kind of problem related to sexuality. This may include clients being sexual with one another, a client making sexual advances or displays to a staff member or to other clients, or a client masturbating openly on the unit. Sexual acting out on the unit can be effectively managed by setting and maintaining limits (see "Limit-Setting"), as with other acting out situations. Again, a matter-of-fact approach is often effective.

Some aspects of the client's sexuality or lifestyle may be disturbing to staff members, even though the client may not be experiencing a problem or believe that the issue is a problem. For example, sexual activity in the young or elderly client, sexual practices that differ from those of the staff member, transvestism, or homosexuality may evoke uncomfortable, judgmental, or other kinds of feelings in staff members. Again, it is important to be aware of and deal with these feelings as a part of your responsibility rather than create a problem or undermine the client's perception of himself or herself by defining something as a problem when it is not. Providing nonjudgmental care to a client is especially important in the area of sexuality because the client may have previously encountered or may expect censure from professionals, which reinforces guilt, shame, and low self-esteem.

Homosexuality per se is no longer considered a mental health disorder and, although a client may be gay or lesbian, he or she may not feel that his or her homosexuality is a problem. Indeed, many lesbians and gay men feel positive about their homosexuality and have no desire to change. If a homosexual client seeks treatment for another problem (eg, depression), do not assume that this problem is due to or even related to the client's homosexuality. On the other hand, being a homosexual in our society can present a number of significant stresses to an individual, and these may or may not influence the client's problem. Aside from societal censure in general, the client faces possible loss of familial support and his or her

job, housing, and children by revealing his or her homosexuality. The gay or lesbian client often must deal with these issues on a daily basis, but even these stresses must not be confused with the client's sexuality per se.

Gay and lesbian clients may choose not to reveal their homosexuality to staff members, family members, or others (eg, employers) in their lives. Confidentiality is an important issue in this situation because of the potential losses to the client should his or her homosexuality become known, and it must be respected by the nursing staff. Regardless of whether or not a client's sexual orientation is spoken, his or her primary support persons may be a partner, a lover, a roommate, and friends, rather than family members. It is important to respectfully include this client's significant others in care planning, discharge planning, teaching, and other aspects of care, just as family members are included in the care of heterosexual clients. Remain aware of your own feelings about homosexuality and take responsibility for dealing with those feelings so that you are able to provide effective, nonjudgmental nursing care for all clients.

Sexual concerns also may conflict with the religious beliefs of both clients and staff members. It may be helpful to involve a chaplain or other clergy member in the client's treatment. Having respect for the client, examining your own feelings, maintaining a nonjudgmental attitude toward the client, encouraging expression of the client's feelings, and allowing the client to make his or her own decisions are the standards for working with clients in situations with a moral or religious dimension, whether the issue is abortion, celibacy, sterilization, impotence, transsexualism, or any other aspect of human sexuality.

Stress

Clients come to a mental health facility with a variety of problems; many of these problems may be seen as responses to stress or as occurring when the client's usual coping strategies are inadequate in the face of a certain degree of stress. For example, posttraumatic behavior has been identified as a response to a significant stressor that would evoke distress in most people, and grieving is a process that occurs in response to a loss or change. A stressor is not necessarily only one major event, however, and some problems may be related to the constant presence of long-term or unrelenting stress, such as poverty or minority status and oppression. Stressors are usually perceived as unpleasant or negative events; however, a significant "happy" event, such as marriage or the birth of a child, also can cause a major change in the client's life and overwhelm his or her usual coping strategies.

Stress may be a significant contributing factor to a client's present problem. For example, psychosomatic illnesses, eating disorders, and suicidal behavior have all been linked to stress and to the client's response to stressors. It is important to assess all clients with regard to the stress in their lives (both perceived and observable) and to their response to stress, regardless of the presenting problem.

There is a danger in labeling a severely stressed client as ill when he or she seeks help. Labeling separates the client from other "normal" people and may lead the nurse to expect illness behavior rather than to continue to see the client as a unique and multifaceted person who possesses strengths and who deals with stress in daily life. It is important to realize that stressors are very real and demand responses from all of us: the client, his or her significant others, and staff members. Illness and caregiving are themselves stressors (see Care Plan 5: Supporting the Caregiver and "Staff Considerations"). One of the most important therapeutic aims in nursing care is to help the client deal with the stress of present problems and to build skills and resources to deal with stress in the future. Teaching stress management skills, such as how to identify stress, relaxation techniques, and the problem-solving process, is an important part of client education (see "Client Teaching").

Spirituality

Spirituality is a person's beliefs, values, and/or philosophy of life. The client may consider spirituality to be extremely important or not at all a part of his or her life. The spiritual realm may be a source of strength, support, security, and well-being in a client's life. On the other hand, the client may be experiencing problems that have caused him or her to lose faith, to become disillusioned, or to be in despair. Or, the client's psychiatric symptoms may have a religious focus that may or may not be related to his or her spiritual beliefs, such as religiosity.

Spiritual belief systems differ greatly among people. These systems can range from traditional Western religions (eg, Christianity and Judaism) to Eastern religions (eg, Taoism and Buddhism) to alternative or New Age beliefs (including psychic healing and channeling), or they may reflect individual beliefs and philosophy unrelated to an organized group. As with other aspects of a client, it is important to assess spirituality in the client's life, particularly as it relates to the client's present problem and life situation. It is also important to be respectful of the client's beliefs and feelings in the spiritual realm and to deliver nonjudgmental nursing care regardless of the client's spiritual beliefs. As always, be aware of your own feelings and take responsibility to deal with those feelings in order to avoid giving the client negative messages about his or her spirituality. Remember that the client has a right to hold his or her own beliefs; it is not appropriate for you to try to convince the client to believe as you do or to proselytize your beliefs in the context of nursing care. If the client is experiencing spiritual distress, it may be appropriate to contact your facility's chaplain or to refer the client to a member of the clergy or leader of his or her faith or belief system for guidance. Nursing care can then continue in conjunction with the recommendations of this specialist to meet the client's needs in a respectful, holistic manner.

The Aging Client

People are aging throughout life; developmental growth, challenges, changes, and concomitant losses occur on a continuum from birth to death. As people go through life stages, they experience changes in many aspects of their daily lives. Some of these changes are gradual and barely noticed; others may be sudden or marked by events that result in profound differences in one's life. Aging necessitates adjustment to different roles, relationships, responsibilities, skills and abilities, work, leisure, levels of social and economic status; changes in self-image, independence and dependence; and changes in physical, emotional, mental, and spiritual aspects of life. Adjustment from adolescence into early adulthood entails a major transition in terms of independence, roles, and relationships. Moving from young adulthood into middle age, older age, and becoming elderly results in many changes, some of which affect one's self-esteem and body image, and which may entail significant losses over time. As one becomes increasingly aged, these losses may become major factors in one's life. Loss of physical abilities, altered body image, loss of loved ones, loss of independence, loss of economic security and social status, and the loss of a sense of the future or of recovering from past losses may present significant problems to a client. For example, despair, spiritual disillusionment, depression, or suicidal behavior may occur, in which these life changes are major contributing factors. If the client's presenting problem does not seem to be directly related to aging, factors associated with aging, developmental, or adjustment issues still need to be assessed in order to gain a holistic view of the client.

Because aging is a universal experience that involves multiple losses and grief, it can be a difficult issue for nursing staff members and can result in uncomfortable feelings, denial, and rejection of the client. With aging or aged clients, as with other difficult issues, discomfort on the part of the nurse influences the care given to the older client. Respect for the individual and awareness of both your own feelings and those of the client together contribute to good nursing care that maintains the client's dignity. The elderly client is a whole person with individual strengths and needs. Do not assume that a client over a certain age has organic brain pathology, no longer has sexual feelings, or has no need for independence. It is important to promote independence to the client's optimal level of functioning no matter what the client's age and to provide the necessary physical care and assistance without drawing undue attention to the client's needs. The client may never before have needed someone to care for him or her and may feel humiliated by being in such a dependent position. The client may have previously been proud of his or her independence and may have gained much self-esteem from this. This client may be horrified at the thought of being a burden and may experience both fear and despair. Do not dismiss the client's feelings as inappropriate because of your own discomfort; instead, encourage the client to express these feelings and give the client support while promoting as much independence for the client as possible (see Section 6: Loss).

HIV Disease and AIDS*

Acquired immunodeficiency syndrome (AIDS) and *AIDS-related complex (ARC)* are names for two conditions caused by *human immunodeficiency virus (HIV)*. When a person is diagnosed with AIDS, he or she has been infected with HIV and has one or more diseases that the Centers for Disease Control and Prevention (CDC) has designated as diagnostic for AIDS and that indicate a severe impairment of his or her immune system. When a person is diagnosed with ARC, he or she has been infected with HIV and has one or more conditions that are associated with HIV infection but are not designated as AIDS. Many people, however, are infected with HIV and have no symptoms at all. Many of these people are unaware that they have been infected or are even unaware of their risk for

*Research is ongoing concerning HIV and AIDS-related issues. The recommendations in this Manual are based on information available at the time of this writing. Please consult the resources suggested for current recommendations and new information.

infection. It is not yet known whether every person infected with HIV will develop ARC or AIDS. The incubation period for AIDS after infection with HIV can be 10 years or longer. All persons who have been infected with the virus are presumed to remain infected and to be infectious to others for the remainder of their lives.

HIV infection is usually determined by testing for the presence of *antibodies* to HIV, using a preliminary test (*ELISA*) and a confirmatory test (*Western blot*).

A person who has evidence of antibodies to HIV is said to be *antibody positive* or *HIV seropositive* or *HIV positive*. It is thought that an infected person *usually* has detectable levels of antibodies; however, rarely an infected person may not be seropositive (eg, if he or she has been so recently infected that detectable levels of antibodies are not yet present). Because having an HIV-positive status can lead to discrimination, loss of insurance coverage, and other problems, HIV testing is often governed by strict confidentiality measures and/or state regulations. Be sure to be aware of your state and facility policies regarding all HIV-related issues.

At the time of this writing, there is no cure for HIV infection, ARC, or AIDS. Nursing care is primarily focused on HIV-related illnesses, such as opportunistic infections, symptom management and control, nutrition and other areas of health maintenance, palliative and comfort measures, and psychosocial problems. HIV-related treatments and medications are available through traditional medical care, HIV research protocols, and alternative health resources. Many people who are HIV-positive but free of the symptoms of AIDS take medications and/or treatments to prevent or delay the onset of AIDS or ARC. Also, researchers continue to search for a cure and a vaccine. However, prevention of transmission of HIV is paramount in controlling the AIDS epidemic.

HIV infection occurs when a person is exposed to the virus, primarily through blood or semen. Because the virus has been found in virtually all body fluids, *universal infection precautions* should be *routine* in situations in which one is exposed to body fluids or substances. As nurses, it is important to observe precautions to minimize the risk of transmission from client to nurse, from nurse to client, and from client to client. Clients who are sexually active or who act out sexually may need careful supervision regarding sexual activity as well as transmission-prevention education.

Because it is impossible to identify who may be infected with HIV, precautions *must* be taken with *all* clients and by all health care workers when exposure to blood or body fluids is likely. Remember, routine precautions must be taken in these situations to protect both the health care worker and the client from exposure to HIV. Routine precautions include:

1. Always wash your hands thoroughly before and after performing client care.
2. Avoid needlestick injury. Do not recap needles after use; dispose of needles in proper containers. Place containers near areas where needles are used to avoid transporting used needles.
3. Use an ambu bag or mouthpiece for resuscitation.
4. Wear gloves when exposure to blood or body fluids is likely (eg, when performing wound care or drawing blood). Wash your hands after removing and discarding gloves.
5. Wear a mask or protective eye shields, or both, when aerosolization of body fluids is likely.
6. Wear a gown if splashing of blood or body fluids is likely.
7. If you are pregnant, direct care of clients who have AIDS may present a risk of exposure to cytomegalovirus. This virus is often present in persons with AIDS and may cause birth defects if exposure occurs during pregnancy.

Contact your infection control officer for specific, current recommendations and for your facility's policies regarding accidental exposure (eg, from a needlestick injury). HIV-related information is also available from the CDC (1-800-342-2437; National AIDS Clearinghouse, P.O. Box 6003, Rockville, MD 20850), local and state health departments, and community AIDS organizations.

Remember, no precautions are indicated if exposure to blood or body fluids is not anticipated. Many studies have been done regarding casual contact with HIV-infected persons, and there has been *no* evidence of transmission by casual contact, such as food preparation, talking, or touching skin.

It is important for nurses in any health care setting to educate clients, families or significant others, and the public about HIV infection, transmission, and illness. Clients with psychiatric problems may be particularly in need of education about transmission or of supervision regarding high-risk behaviors. HIV-positive clients in psychiatric settings may present with a complex group of problems and must be carefully assessed regarding symptoms or behaviors related to HIV disease (eg, dementia), psychiatric problems that may be or may not be related to HIV (eg, depression), and other problems that are independent of HIV disease (eg, personality disorder). In addition, clients with AIDS may be more sensitive to the effects of psychotropic medications than other clients and may need dosages lower than those normally given. These clients also may be at risk for serious consequences related to side effects of psychotropic drugs. It is recommended that low-cholinergic agents (eg, haloperidol) be used with AIDS clients rather than high-cholinergic medications (eg, chlorpromazine), because the latter can cause a decrease in oral secretions and result in thrush as well as lead to confusion (Hall, Koehler, and Lewis, 1989).

Education about HIV is aimed at preventing transmission of the virus. Clients who use intravenous drugs are at increased risk of HIV infection through sharing needles with someone who might be infected. Education for these clients includes recommending that they must not share needles with other people and recommending that needles be cleaned with bleach solution (1 part bleach to 10 parts water) and rinsed if they are shared. *All* clients, like all persons, are at risk of HIV infection through sexual activity that involves the exchange of body fluids with someone who is infected. Recommendations for sexual practices that may reduce the risk of infection, or "safer sex" activities, include the use of condoms and nonoxynol-9 (a spermicide that kills the virus) for penile sexual activity and the use of latex barriers (eg, dental dams) for oral–vaginal or oral–rectal sexual activities. Contact your health department or community AIDS organization for specific recommendations and educational materials. *Remember*, it is impossible to know who might be infected with HIV. In the beginning of the AIDS epidemic in the United States, certain groups of people were identified as high-risk groups because HIV infection initially occurred and was transmitted among people in these groups in greater numbers than in the general population. However, HIV-related disease can occur in *anyone* who is exposed to the virus.

HIV-related disease impairs the body's immune system, making the body vulnerable to many opportunistic infections, which result in many types of symptoms, including neurologic problems. HIV can also directly damage the nervous system, causing various neurologic problems, including *AIDS dementia complex*, or *HIV encephalopathy* (see Care Plan 17: Neurological Illnesses) and peripheral neuropathies. In addition, because there is no cure for HIV disease, and because AIDS is considered to be fatal, clients who are HIV-positive or who have been diagnosed with AIDS must deal with having a terminal illness (see Care Plan 21: Living with a Chronic or Terminal Illness and Care Plan 20: Altered Body Image). Clients with HIV infection may be at increased risk for depression and suicide (see Care Plan 23: Depressive Behavior and Care Plan 24: Suicidal Behavior).

Clients with HIV infection face possible discrimination in employment, housing, insurance, medical care, and social services. In addition, because many people infected with HIV early in the epidemic were gay men or intravenous drug users, social stigma related to homosexuals and drug use can occur, whether or not the client is homosexual or has used intravenous drugs. *Remember*, no one deserves to be infected with HIV, and all clients are entitled to non-judgmental nursing care.

The Nursing Process

The nursing process is a dynamic and continuing activity that includes the nurse–client interaction and the problem-solving process. Because the client is an integral part of this process, client input in terms of information, decision-making, and evaluation is important; ideally, the client should participate as a team member as much as possible. In addition, the client's family or significant others may be included in the nursing process because the client affects and is affected by the people in his or her life and may be seen as part of a interactive system of people. Contracting with the client and his or her significant others can be a useful, direct way of facilitating this participation and may help the client and his or her family to see themselves as actively involved in this process of change.

The nursing process includes the following steps:

1. Assessment of data, including identification of personal strengths and resources
2. Formulation of nursing diagnoses with defining characteristics and related factors
3. Identification of expected outcomes, including establishing timing and specific client-centered goals
4. Identification of therapeutic aims, or nursing objectives
5. Identification and implementation of nursing interventions and solutions to possible problems
6. Evaluation and revision of all steps of the process (ongoing)

Because every client is in a unique situation, each care plan must be individualized. The care plans in this *Manual* consist of background information related to a behavior or problem and one or more nursing diagnoses that are likely to be appropriate to clients experiencing the problem. Other related diagnoses also are suggested, but the care plans in the *Manual* are written using the primary diagnoses given as the basis for the nursing process. Within each of these diagnoses, there are lists of possible defining characteristics and related factors that may be assessed, suggestions of general expected outcome statements appropriate to the diagnosis, and therapeutic aims and interventions (with rationale)

that may be effective for clients with that nursing diagnosis. All of this is meant to be used to construct individualized care plans that are based on nursing diagnoses, using specific data, outcomes, and interventions for each client.

Assessment

The first step in the nursing process, the assessment of the client, is crucial. In assessing a client to formulate nursing diagnoses, and to plan and implement care in the area of mental health nursing, the following factors are important:

1. *Client participation.* The client's perceptions should be elicited as well as the client's expectations of hospitalization and the staff. What would the client like to change? How can this happen? What is the client most concerned about right now?
2. *Client's strengths.* What are the client's strengths as perceived by the client and by the nurse?
3. *Client's coping strategies.* How does the client usually deal with problems? How is he or she attempting to deal with the present situation?
4. *Participation by the client's family or significant others.* How are other people's behaviors or problems affecting the client, and how is the client affecting others? Note family patterns and history of behaviors.
5. *Primary language.* What is the client's primary language? Does the client read in his or her primary language? Is the client able to speak and read English? Is there a need for an interpreter for interactions and teaching with the client and his or her significant others?
6. *Transcultural considerations.* What is the client's cultural background? In what kind of cultural environment is the client living (or was the client raised)? What is his or her group identification? If possible, educate yourself and other staff members about the client's culture if it is different from your own. Remember that cultural differences are not only related to ethnic background (eg, Asian, Hispanic, or African American), but are also related to other factors, such as socioeconomic status (eg, poverty or affluence), sexual orientation (eg, gay or heterosexual), or religion (eg, Christian or Buddhist), and so forth. Because there are so many cultures in the United States, you may not realistically be able to learn about all facets of each client's culture that may be pertinent to his or her care. It is important, therefore, to be *aware* that there are significant differences among cultures, to ask the client and his or her significant others about important cultural fea-

tures. Be careful *not* to make assumptions based solely on your own culture or on what you *think* you know about the client's culture when dealing with clients.

7. *Appearance.* Describe the client's general appearance, clothing, and hygiene.

8. *Substance use or chemical dependence.* Consider the client's use of caffeine (symptoms of anxiety and high caffeine intake can be very similar); tobacco; alcohol; and illicit, prescription, and over-the-counter drugs (eg, bromide poisoning can occur with abuse of some over-the-counter medications).

9. *Orientation and memory.* Check for both recent and remote memory as well as the client's orientation to person, place, and time.

10. *Allergies to both food and medication.* It may be necessary to ask the client's significant others for reliable information or to check the client's past records if possible.

11. *Complete physical systems review.* The client may minimize, maximize, or be unaware of physical problems.

12. *Dentures and dentition.* These may be a factor in nutritional problems.

13. *Physical disabilities, prostheses.* Does the client need assistance in ambulation or other activities of daily living?

14. *Present medications.* Include questions about the client's knowledge of medication regimen, effects, and adverse effects as well as when the last dose of medication was taken.

15. *Suicidal ideation.* Does the client have suicidal ideas, or does he or she have a history of suicidal behavior, including plans, gestures, or attempts?

16. *Perceptions, presence of hallucinations or delusions.* Describe the nature and frequency of delusions or hallucinations; how does the client feel about them?

17. *Aggression.* Does the client have a history or a present problem of aggression toward others, homicidal thoughts or plans, or possession of weapons?

18. *Family history.* Have there been mental health problems in the client's family?

19. *Present living situation.* How does the client feel about it?

20. *Relationships with others.* How does the client see others? Are present relationships helpful to the client? Stressful? Does the client have anyone to talk with? To trust? Are relationships dependent? Abusive?

21. *Sexuality.* Are any aspects of sexuality causing problems for the client?

22. *Behavior and activity level.* Describe the client's general behavior during the assessment. What is the client's psychomotor activity level? What can the client do for himself or herself?

23. *Eye contact.* Does the client make eye contact with staff members or significant others? What is the frequency and duration of eye contact?

24. *Affect and mood.* Describe the client's general mood, facial expressions, and demeanor.

25. *Ability to communicate.* Include the nature and extent of both verbal and nonverbal communication. Does the client's significant other speak for him or her?

26. *Tremors or fidgeting.* Describe the nature, extent, and frequency of repetitive movements.

27. *Daily living habits.* What does the client do all day? How do the client's habits differ now from before the client's present problems began?

28. *Health practices.* Does the client get adequate nutrition? Adequate sleep? Regular exercise? General medical care?

29. *Cognition and intellectual functioning.* Include present level of functioning, judgment, and insight as well as educational level and prior abilities and achievements.

30. *Employment.* Include the client's present job and history of employment and the client's perception of his or her work.

31. *Level of income.* Is the client's income level adequate for his or her needs? Is it a stressful factor in the client's life?

32. *Spirituality.* Is spirituality important to the client?

33. *Value system and personal standards.* Does the client have very high standards for himself or herself or others? Does the client manifest a sense of personal responsibility?

34. *Interests and hobbies.* Include the client's hobbies, both before the present problems began and of continuing interest to the client.

35. *Previous hospitalizations.* Include both medical and psychiatric hospitalizations; note length of stay and reason for hospitalization.

Assess the client in a holistic way, integrating any relevant information about the client's life, behavior, and feelings as the initial steps of implementing the nursing process. Remember that the focus of care, beginning with the initial assessment, is toward the client's optimum level of health and independence from the hospital.

Nursing Diagnosis

The second step of the nursing process is to formulate nursing diagnoses. The nursing diagnosis is a statement of an actual or potential problem or situation amenable to nursing intervention. It is based on the nurse's judgment of the client's situation following a nursing assessment. It serves to provide information and a focus for the planning, implementation, and evaluation of nursing care and to communicate that information to the nursing staff.

The nursing diagnosis is not a medical diagnosis. Medical psychiatric diagnoses are used by physicians or psychiatrists to categorize and describe mental disorders. The *Diagnostic and Statistical Manual of Mental Disorders* was first published by the American Psychiatric Association in 1952. The current edition, known as DSM-III-R, or *Diagnostic and Statistical Manual of Mental Disorders, Revised* (1987), is intended to be used primarily by persons trained to provide medical diagnoses. However, it can be useful to nurses and other professionals as a reference. The DSM-III-R classifies mental disorders into similar groups, known as categories. The disorders are described, and diagnostic criteria are provided to distinguish one from another. Descriptors are intended to be as objective as possible and allow for individual differences among clients. The DSM-III-R can be used for medical diagnosis, teaching, and research purposes as well as to provide a foundation for understanding medical treatment of psychiatric disorders.

Nursing diagnoses differ from medical psychiatric diagnoses in that it is the client's *response* to that medical problem, or how that problem affects the client's daily functioning, that is the concern of the nursing diagnosis. Only those problems that lend themselves to nursing's focus and intervention can be addressed by nursing diagnoses. And like other parts of the nursing process, the nursing diagnosis is client-centered; that is, the focus of the nursing diagnosis is the client's problem or situation rather than, for example, a problem the staff may have with a client.

A nursing diagnosis statement consists of the *problem* or client *response* and one or more *related factors*. Related factors influence or contribute to the client's problem or response. Signs and symptoms, or *defining characteristics*, are subjective and objective data that support the nursing diagnosis. The defining characteristics are not usually written as part of the diagnostic statement. The problem may be stated as actual (the problem has been confirmed) or high risk (the problem may develop in the absence of nursing intervention to decrease or minimize risk factors). The second part of the diagnostic statement is written to communicate the nurse' perception of the factors related to the problem or contributing to its etiology. The phrase *related to* reflects the relationship of problem to factor rather than stating cause and effect per se. If the relationship of these contributing factors is unknown at the time the nursing diagnosis is formulated, the problem statement may be written without

them. In the *Manual*, the problem statement or diagnostic category is addressed, leaving the "related to" phrase to be written by the nurse working with the individual client.

The North American Nursing Diagnosis Association (NANDA) is developing a taxonomy of officially recognized nursing diagnoses. The association reviews proposed nursing diagnoses according to certain criteria to assure clear, consistent, and complete statements. The list of official diagnoses is organized into categories based on human response, including "exchanging, communicating, relating, valuing, choosing, moving, perceiving, knowing, and feeling" (NANDA, 1990). Nurses are encouraged by NANDA to develop, use, and submit other nursing diagnoses to NANDA for approval.

Each care plan in this *Manual* is written using the nursing diagnoses most frequently identified with that behavior or problem. In addition, related nursing diagnoses are identified that are often associated with the problems addressed in that care plan. The specific diagnoses in the individualized nursing care plan for a given client will be based on the actual data collected in the nursing assessment of that client.

Expected Outcomes

The next step, the identification of expected outcomes, gives direction and focus to the nursing process and provides the basis for evaluating the effectiveness of the nursing interventions employed. Expected outcomes are client-centered; they are statements that reflect the client's progress toward resolving the problem or nursing diagnosis or preventing problems identified as potential or high risk. Expected outcomes also are called *outcome criteria* or *goals*, and they contain specific information (*modifiers*) and time factors (*deadlines*) so that they are measurable and can be evaluated and revised as the client progresses. The expected outcomes in this *Manual* have been written as general statements to be used in writing specific expected outcomes for an individual client; specific modifiers and timing must be added for outcome criteria for an individualized care plan. The general outcome statements in the *Manual* are identified as initial or discharge outcomes to suggest time frames, but specific timing must be written in the individual nursing care plan. For example, an expected outcome may be written as "The client will talk with a staff member (modifier) about loss (modifier) for 10 minutes (modifier) each day by 11/18 (time factor)." The specific criterion may be an amount of food, fluid, or time, an activity or behavior, a topic of conversation, a certain person or group, and so forth. Expected outcomes should be stated in behavioral or measurable terms and should be reasonable and attainable within the deadlines stated. The suggested outcomes in the *Manual* are not written in any particular order to denote priority; in a specific plan of care, the nurse will designate priorities.

Therapeutic Aims

Therapeutic aims, also known as nursing objectives, are included in this *Manual* to help guide the nurse's thinking about the therapeutic process of working with the client. As the nurse chooses specific interventions designed to resolve the problem stated in the nursing diagnosis or to improve the client's health, an awareness of the therapeutic framework of the nurse's role in working with the client can be helpful, especially to nursing students learning this process.

Implementation

The identification of nursing interventions and their implementation are the next steps in the nursing process. Here, the nurse can choose and implement specific measures to achieve the expected outcomes identified. Nursing interventions may be called *actions*, *approaches*, *nursing orders*, or *nursing prescriptions*. They must be individualized to include modifiers that specify parameters. Interventions address specific problems and suggest possible solutions or alternatives that nurses employ to meet client needs or to assist the client toward expected outcomes. Writing specific nursing interventions in the client's care plan will help ensure consistency among staff members in their approaches to the client and will aid in the evaluation of the client's care. In addition to specific problem-solving measures, nursing interventions include additional data gathering or assessment, health promotion and disease prevention activities, nursing treatments, referrals, and client education.

Evaluation and Revision

The final steps in the nursing process are not actually termination steps at all but ongoing activities incorporated into the entire process—the evaluation and revision of all other steps. New data will be discovered throughout the client's care and must be added to the original assessment; the client may reveal additional (or different) information; and his or her behavior may certainly change over time. Nursing diagnoses must be evaluated: Are the diagnoses accurate? Are there different, or additional, related factors that will change the diagnostic statements? Expected outcomes and therapeutic aims also need evaluation, and their modifiers and time factors will change as the client progresses. The effectiveness of nursing interventions must be ascertained—Should a different approach be used? Specific modifiers within the interventions will be revised over time, and new problems may need to be addressed as well. Other areas to evaluate and revise include the extent of the client's participation and assumption of self responsibility (as the client progresses, he or she may be able to participate and take more responsibility in both treatment and care planning), and staff consistency (Is the staff implementing the specified interventions consistently?).

Ideally, evaluation and revision should be integrated into the client's daily care; each observation or nurse–client interaction provides an opportunity to evaluate and revise the components of the client's care plan. Nursing report (change of shift) meetings are an ideal time to evaluate the effectiveness of and revise interventions and expected outcome criteria. Client care conferences, as regular or impromptu meetings, or nurse–client sessions also may be used to discuss revisions. The nursing staff may want to schedule time to evaluate and discuss care planning each shift, several times per week, or on whatever timetable is appropriate for the unit. Regardless of how it is scheduled, however, it is essential to incorporate evaluation and revision into the planning of care for each client, and to view nursing care as the flexible, dynamic, change-oriented, thoughtful process that it can (and should) be.

Documentation

Another aspect of nursing care for the hospitalized client is documentation. Written records of client care are important in several ways. First, written care plans serve to coordinate and communicate the plan of nursing care for each client to all staff members. Using a written plan of care maximizes the opportunity for all nursing staff to be consistent and comprehensive in the care of a particular client. Ongoing evaluation and revision of the care plan reflect changes in the client's needs and in nursing's response to those needs. Second, a written care plan is an effective, efficient means of communication among different staff members who cannot all meet as a group (that is, on different shifts, float staff, supervisors, and so forth). Third, documentation or charting in the client's medical record serves to communicate nursing observations and nursing care to other members of the health care team (eg, other nurses, physicians, social workers, discharge planners, consultants, and so forth). Information in the chart is also available as a record in the event of transfer to another facility, follow-up care, or future admissions. Fourth, the chart is a legal document, and the written record of nursing care may be instrumental in legal proceedings involving the client. Finally, the documentation of care is important for accreditation and reimbursement purposes. Quality assurance and utilization review departments, accreditation bodies, and third party payors depend on adequate documentation to review quality of care and to determine appropriate reimbursement.

Nurse–Client Interactions

Communication Skills

Effective therapeutic communication between a nurse and a client is a conscious, goal-directed process that differs greatly from a casual or social interaction. Therapeutic communication is grounded in the purposeful, caring nature of nursing care. It is undertaken as a tool with which to develop trust, effect change, promote health, provide limits, reinforce, orient, convey caring, identify and work toward goals, teach, and provide other types of nursing care. The nurse must be aware of the client and his or her needs when communicating with the client, and as with all nursing care, it is the client's needs that must be met, not the nurse's needs. Therapeutic conversations are goal-oriented: they are employed deliberately as nursing interventions to meet nursing objectives or to help a client reach a goal. However, therapeutic communication with a client is not a stiff, rote recitation of predetermined phrases used to manipulate clients. Rather, it is a part of the art and science of nursing, a blend of conversation and caring, of limits and reinforcement, of communication techniques and one's own words. Communicating with a client can range from sitting with a client in silence to speaking in a very structured, carefully chosen way (eg, in behavior modification techniques). An interaction with a client may be in the context of a social or recreational activity, in which the nurse is actively teaching social skills or modeling such skills through her own conscious "social" conversations. Regardless of the situation, it is always important to remember that an interaction with a client is part of your professional role and therefore must be respectful of the client and his or her needs.

A number of communication skills, or techniques, have been found to be effective in therapeutic interactions with clients (see Appendix C). These techniques are tools of communication. They are meant to be consciously chosen to meet the needs of particular clients and may be modified to best meet those needs

and to be best used by the nurse. It is important for you to be comfortable as well as effective in therapeutic communication: Use your own words; integrate purposeful communication techniques into conversations; following an interaction, evaluate its effectiveness and your own feelings, then modify your techniques in subsequent interactions. Like other aspects of nursing care, communication is dynamic: It can, and should, be evaluated and revised. The following are suggestions, or guidelines, to improve therapeutic communication:

Offer yourself to the client for a specific period for the purpose of communication. Tell the client that you would like to talk with him or her.

Call the client by name and identify yourself by name. The use of given (first) names may be decided by the facility or the individual unit philosophies or may depend on the comfort of the client and the nurse or the nature of the client's problem.

Make eye contact with the client as he or she tolerates. However, do not stare at the client.

Listen to the client. Pay attention to what the client is communicating, both verbally and nonverbally.

Be comfortable using silence as a communication tool.

Talk with the client about the client's feelings, not about yourself, other staff members, or other clients.

Ask open-ended questions. Avoid questions that can have one-word answers.

Allow the client enough time to talk.

Be honest with the client.

Be nonjudgmental. If necessary, directly reassure the client of your nonjudgmental attitude.

Know your own feelings and do not let them prejudice your interaction with the client.

Encourage the client to ventilate his or her feelings.

Reflect what the client is saying back to him or her. In simple reflection, repeat the client's statement with an upward inflection in your voice to indicate questioning. In more complex reflection, rephrase the client's statement to reflect the feeling the client seems to be expressing. This will allow the client to validate your perception of what he or she is trying to say, or to correct it. You also can point out seemingly contradictory statements and ask for clarification (this may or may not be confrontational). Do not simply describe what you think the client is feeling in your own terms; instead, use such phrases as "I hear you saying. . . . Is that what you are feeling? Is that what you mean?"

Tell the client if you do not understand what he or she means; take the responsibility yourself for not understanding and ask the client to clarify. This gives the client the responsibility for explaining his or her meaning.

Do not use pat phrases or platitudes in response to the client's expression of feelings. This devalues the client's feelings, undermines trust, and may discourage further communication.

Do not give your personal opinions, beliefs, or experiences in relation to the client's problems.

Do not give advice or make decisions for the client. If you advise a client and your advice is "good" (ie, the proposed solution is successful), the client has not had the opportunity to problem-solve, to take responsibility or credit for a good decision, and to enjoy the increased self-esteem that comes from a successful action. If your advice is "bad," the client has missed a chance to learn from making a mistake and realizing that he or she can survive making a mistake. In effect, the client has evaded responsibility for making a decision and instead may blame the staff member or the hospital for whatever consequences ensue from that decision.

Help the client to use the problem-solving process (see "Client Teaching"). Help the client to identify and explore alternatives.

Give the client honest, nonpunitive feedback based on your observations.

Do not try to fool or manipulate the client.

Do not argue with the client or get involved in a power struggle.

Do not take the client's anger or negative expressions personally.

Use humor judiciously. Never tease a client or use humor pejoratively. Remember that clients with certain problems will not understand abstractions such as humor. Remember to evaluate the use of humor with each individual client.

Expression of Feelings

A significant part of therapy is the client's expression of feelings. It is important for the nurse to encourage the client to ventilate feelings in ways that are nondestructive and acceptable to the client, such as writing, talking, drawing, or physical activity. It also may be desirable to encourage expressions, such as crying, with which the client (or the nurse) may not feel entirely comfortable. You can facilitate the expression of emotions by giving the client direct verbal support, by using silence, by handing the client tissues, and by allowing the client time to ventilate (without probing for information or interrupting the client with pat remarks).

The goal in working with a client is not to avoid painful feelings but to have the client express, work through, and come to accept even "negative" emotions such as hatred, despair, and rage. In accepting the client's emotions, you need not agree with or give approval to everything the client says—you can support the client by acknowledging that he or she is ex-periencing the emotion expressed without agreeing with or sharing those feelings. If you are uncomfortable with the client's ventilation of feelings, it is important that you examine your own emotions and talk with another staff member about them or that you provide the client with a staff member who is more comfortable with expression of those feelings.

Client Teaching

Client teaching, like client advocacy, is an essential component of good nursing care. In mental health nursing, client teaching can take many forms and address many content areas. It is important to consider the learning needs of the client and his or her significant others when performing an initial assessment, planning for discharge, and throughout the client's hospitalization. The assessment of a client (or significant others) with regard to teaching includes consideration of the following:

Level of present knowledge or understanding
Present primary concern (you may need to address the client's major emotional concerns before he or she can attend to learning information)
Client's perceived educational needs
Level of consciousness, orientation, attention span, and concentration span
Hallucinations or other psychotic or neurologic symptoms
Effects of medications
Short- and long-term memory
Primary language
Literacy level
Visual, hearing, or other sensory impairment
Client's preferred learning methods
Cultural factors
Learning disabilities
Motivation for learning
Barriers to learning (eg, denial or shame related to mental illness)

Optimal conditions for client teaching and learning may not exist during an inpatient stay; many factors may be present that diminish the effectiveness of teaching. However, the client's hospital stay may be the only opportunity for teaching, and certain information (especially regarding medications and self-care activities) must be conveyed prior to discharge. In addition, follow-up appointments may be scheduled for continued teaching after discharge, if indicated; significant others can assist in reinforcing teaching; and home care with continued instruction may be possible.

Choosing the mode of education best suited to the client and the situation is also important. Many teaching techniques and tools are available and can be integrated into the teaching plan according to the client's needs, the clinical setting, available resources, and the nurse's expertise. Effective teaching tools include:

Presentation of information to a group or an individual: lecture, discussion, question and answer sessions; verbal, written, or audiovisual materials (eg, slides, overhead transparencies, cassette tapes, or videotapes)

Simple written instructions, drawings or photographs, or both (especially for clients with low literacy or language differences)

Repetition, reinforcement, and restatement of the same material in different ways

Group discussions (to teach common topics, such as safe use of medications and to promote compliance with medication regimens using both teaching and encouraging peer support)

Social or recreational activities (eg, to teach social skills)

Role-playing (to provide practice of skills and constructive feedback in a nonthreatening, supportive milieu)

Role-modeling or demonstration of skills, appropriate behaviors, effective communication

Interpreters or translated materials (for clients whose primary language is different from your own)

Return demonstrations or explanations: Asking for the client's perception of the information presented is crucial. Clients may indicate understanding because they want to please, they are embarrassed about low literacy levels, or because they think they "should" understand. Remember, learning does not necessarily occur because teaching is done.

Topics or content areas appropriate for nurse–client teaching include:

General health and wellness: the relationship between physical and emotional health, nutrition, exercise, rest, and hygiene

Emotional health: ways to increase emotional outlets, expression of feelings, increasing self-esteem

Stress management: identification of stressors, recognizing one's own response to stress, making choices about stress, relaxation techniques, relationships between stress and illness

Problem-solving: the use of the problem-solving process, including assessment of the situation, identification of the problems, identification of goals, identification of possible solutions, choice of a possible solution, evaluation, and revision

Communication skills: effective communication techniques, expressing one's needs, listening skills, assertiveness training

Social skills: development of trust, fundamentals of social interactions, appropriate behavior in public and in social situations, eating with others, eating in restaurants

Leisure activities: identification of leisure interests, how to access community recreation resources, use of libraries

Community resources: identification and use of social services, support groups, and so forth

Vocational skills: basic responsibilities of employment, interviewing skills, appropriate behavior in a work setting

Daily living skills: basic money management (eg, bank accounts, rent, utility bills), use of the telephone, grocery shopping

Specific psychodynamic processes, for example, grieving and developmental stages

Specific mental health problems, for example, eating disorders, schizophrenia, hypochondriacal behavior, and suicidal behavior

Specific physical illness pathophysiology, for example, HIV/AIDS and diabetes mellitus

Prevention of illness, for example, prevention of transmission of HIV

Relationship dynamics: healthy relationships, secondary gains, abusive relationships

Self-care or caregiver responsibilities, for example, how to change dressings, range of motion exercises, safety and supervision concerns for neurologic illness

Medications: purpose, action, side effects (what to expect, how to minimize them, if possible, when to call a health professional), dosage, strategies for compliance, special information (eg, monitoring blood levels), signs and symptoms of overdose or toxicity.

Role of the Psychiatric Nurse

Nursing Responsibilities and Functions

As a nurse, within a healthcare facility and within a therapeutic relationship with a client, you have certain responsibilities. These include:

Recognizing and accepting the client as an individual
Client advocacy (see "Client Advocacy")
Assessing the client and planning nursing care
Involving the client and the client's significant others in the nursing process
Accepting the client's perceptions and expression of discomfort (ie, do not require the client to prove distress or illness to you)
Providing a safe environment, including the protection of the client and others from injury
Providing external controls for the client until such time as the client can maintain self-control

Providing a therapeutic environment

Recognizing and examining your own feelings and being willing to work through those feelings

Respecting the client's stated needs, desires, and goals (within the limits of safety, ethics, and good nursing care) in planning his or her care

Identifying the client's optimum level of health and functioning and making that level the goal of the nursing process

Cooperating with other professionals in various aspects of the client's care; coordination of a multidisciplinary approach to care

Accurately observing and documenting the client's behavior

Maintaining awareness of and respect for the client's culture, cultural values and practices, especially if they differ from your own

Providing safe nursing care, including medication administration and therapy, individual interactions (verbal and nonverbal), formal and informal group situations, activities, role playing, and so forth

Client teaching

Providing feedback to the client based on observations of the client's behavior

Maintaining honesty and a nonjudgmental attitude at all times

Maintaining a professional role with regard to the client (see "Professional Role")

Providing opportunities for the client to make his or her own decisions or mistakes and to assume responsibility for his or her emotions and life

Forming expectations of the client that are realistic and clearly stated

Continuing nursing education and the exploration of new ideas, theories, and research.

Professional Role

Maintaining a professional role is essential in working with clients. A client comes to a health care facility for help, not to engage in social relationships. Remember, the client needs a nurse, not a friend: It is neither necessary nor desirable for the client to like you personally (nor for you to like him or her) in the therapeutic situation.

Because the therapeutic milieu is not a social environment, all social interactions with clients should be directed only toward teaching the skills of social interaction and facilitating the client's abilities to engage in relationships. The nurse must not offer personal information or beliefs to the client nor should the nurse attempt to meet his or her own needs in the relationship. Although this may seem severe, its importance extends beyond the establishment and maintenance of a therapeutic milieu. For example, a client who is considering an abortion but who has not yet revealed this may ask the nurse if he or she is Catholic. If the response is, "Yes," the client may assume that the nurse is therefore opposed to abortion, and the client may then be even more reluctant to discuss the problem. The point is that the client must feel that the nurse, regardless of personal beliefs, will be accepting of him or her as a person and of the client's behaviors and problems. If the nurse reveals personal information about himself or herself, the client may make assumptions about the nurse that preclude such acceptance or that confuse the nature and purpose of the therapeutic relationship.

Because a therapeutic relationship is not social, there is no reason for the nurse to discuss his or her marital status or to give his or her home address or telephone number to the client. If information of a personal nature like this is requested by the client, it is appropriate for the nurse to respond by stating that such information is not necessary to the client and is inappropriate to the therapeutic relationship. The nurse can reinforce the principle and importance of the therapeutic relationship (as opposed to a social relationship) at this time—the client may need to be educated about the nature of a therapeutic relationship because he or she may not have experienced this prior to this health care episode. Giving the client information of a personal nature may encourage a social relationship outside the hospital or health care setting, foster dependence on a staff member after discharge, or endanger the nurse if the client is aggressive or hostile.

Staff Considerations

This *Manual* often refers to the identification, awareness, and expression of feelings staff members have when working with clients. It is essential that you (or any staff member) recognize that you have an emotional response to a client and to his or her problems. Many situations arise that may evoke an emotional response in you (eg, issues of sexuality or religion) or that prompt recollections of experiences similar to your own (present or past). Your response may be painful or uncomfortable; may involve fear, revulsion, or judgment; or may be something vague, something of which you are hardly aware. The importance of recognizing and working through these emotions lies in the fact that if you do not do this, you will respond nevertheless, but in a way that may adversely affect both you and the client. For example, you may unconsciously convey disapproval to the client, or you may avoid interacting with the client on certain topics or problems. You may deny your feelings and project them onto the client, or your frustration tolerance with the client may be very low. If the client's problems remind you of an experience that was painful in your own life, which you may or may not remember (such as abuse or incest), you may minimize the client's feelings or distance yourself from the client. Finally, working with clients may become so stressful to you that you may suffer from burnout and may even leave nursing. Not only do attempts to ignore such emotions often lead to a decreased awareness of the client's feelings and interference with the therapeutic relationship, they also take an emotional toll on the nurse and increase the stress involved in interpersonal work.

It is important to note that emotional responses to clients are to be expected and are not unprofessional. It is indeed not professional behavior to act these out with the client, but it is part of the nurse's professional role to acknowledge and accept responsibility for these issues. A good way to increase awareness of staff feelings is to hold regular (though not necessarily rigidly scheduled or formal) client care conferences and staff meetings. At least a part of these meetings can be devoted to the ventilation of the staff's feelings regarding the client. For example, staff members may be frustrated with a client who is not responding to treatment. At a client care conference, these feelings can be explored and the nursing care plan evaluated and revised, thus improving the client's care as well as dealing with the staff's feelings of hopelessness or averting apathy regarding the client. Staff meetings can provide support for the feelings of staff members and provide the sense that a staff member is not alone in his or her reactions toward a client. Another form of client care conference that can be used in this way is a meeting with the nursing supervisor or psychiatric nurse consultant or specialist on a regular or as-needed basis to discuss emotions and plan nursing care.

In another situation, staff members may find themselves becoming angry with a client who is manipulative, hostile, or aggressive. It is important in an acute situation to identify your own emotions and deliberately withdraw from the client (if safety considerations allow) if those feelings are interfering with your care of the client. If you find yourself reacting in an angry or punitive way, for example, it would be best to ask another staff member to deal with the client. Perhaps a client's behavior is simply difficult to tolerate or work with for extended periods (as with manic behavior). In such a case, the client care conference can be used to structure nursing care assignments to limit individual staff contacts with this client to brief periods (maybe 1 or 2 hours at a time). If a client has become aggressive, requiring interventions such as restraint or seclusion, staff members may meet for a brief conference to discuss the interventions as well as emotions generated by the client's behavior and the measures taken to provide safety.

Remember, however, that expression of emotions by the nursing staff should not involve passing judgment on the client or the client's behavior; it is done, rather, to avoid being judgmental or passive–aggressive in the client's care. Other ways to deal with staff considerations include scheduling and encouraging breaks from the unit, making nursing assignments that vary the staff members' experiences and client interactions, supporting educational activities and other professional growth opportunities for staff members, and using support groups for nursing staff that include peers from other units.

Client Advocacy

The nurse in the mental health care setting has a unique and vital role as a client advocate. Clients who are experiencing emotional problems are often unaware of their rights or unable to act in their own interest. Some clients (those hospitalized or restrained against their will) are almost completely dependent on the staff to safeguard their legal rights. Also, the trauma and confusion of entering a mental health facility may be so overwhelming to the client and his or her significant others that they may become extremely passive in this regard. In addition to planning and implementing individualized nursing care in the best interest of the client, the nurse should be familiar with the rights of hospitalized clients in general as well as specific situations (eg, commitment) and should monitor other aspects of client care with these in mind. As a client advocate, the nurse can offer to help the client and his or her family or significant others.

Clients' Rights

In any nursing practice in which mental health problems are encountered the nurse must be aware of the state and federal laws regarding the client's rights and certain aspects of client care. Anything that is deemed part of treatment but is against the client's will must be examined by the nurse with respect to the law as well as to the client's well-being and the nurse's conscience. Do not assume that someone else on the treatment team or in the facility has taken or will take responsibility for treating the client within legal or ethical limits. Your role as client advocate is especially important here. Commitment of a client to a treatment facility, the use of physical restraints, and the use of medication and electroconvulsive or other invasive therapies against the client's will must be scrutinized and handled carefully by the nurse.

In any situation that might have legal ramifications, the nurse must know the law, must acutely observe the client, and must document those observations accurately. Good documentation is essential and should be specific in all respects. For example, if a client is physically restrained, the nurse must chart the precipitating factors, situation, behaviors, and reason for restraints; the time and way in which the client was restrained; actions taken to meet the client's basic needs and rights while he or she was restrained (for example, removing one limb restraint at a time and performing range of motion exercises and offering liquids, food, and commode); frequent individual observations of the client for the duration of the restraint; the time the client was released from restraints; the client's behavior on release; and any other pertinent information (see "Documentation").

Difficult situations may arise when the nurse and another member of the treatment team (such as a physician) disagree regarding the treatment of a client when legal considerations may be a factor. For example, the nurse may believe that a client is actively suicidal, while the other members of the treatment team feel that the client is ready for a weekend at home. In this kind of situation, the nurse must document all observations that led to this judgment and should seek help from the nurse manager, nursing supervisor, director of nursing, or other administrators at the facility.

Clients with Legal Problems

Another potentially difficult situation is the treatment of a client who has been charged with or convicted of a violent crime, such as rape, domestic abuse, child abuse or molestation, incest, murder, or arson, or who talks about these behaviors while in the hospital. Again, it is essential to be aware of legal factors pertinent to the client's treatment. For example, why is the client at the treatment facility? Has a court ordered observation to establish competence or insanity? Is treatment at this facility ordered by the court instead of or as part of a sentence for a crime? Was the client being treated at the facility for another problem and during treatment confessed a crime to the staff?

If a client is at the facility for observation, it must be determined if there will be any treatment given (beyond safety considerations) or if the staff will only observe the client and document those observations. This observation, in any case, must be accurate and well-documented in the client's chart (a client's chart is a legal document and may be presented as evidence in court).

Examination of your own feelings about the client is crucial in situations in which criminal activity is involved. You must become and remain aware of your feelings in order to work effectively with the client and remain nonjudgmental. For instance, whether you feel that the client "could not possibly be guilty" or "is absolutely despicable.... How could anyone do something like that?" you will not be treating the client objectively. And yet it is simply realistic to expect that anyone working with the client will indeed have feelings about a crime. Use staff conferences and interactions to ventilate, explore, and deal with emotions and try to remain objective in your nursing care of the client.

Role of the Client

In a therapeutic relationship, the client also plays an active role. It is important to engage the client in as much of his or her care planning and treatment as possible. Encouraging the client to identify his or her own goals for treatment will help the client see his or her role as an active one and to be more invested in the outcome of the strategies employed. Asking the client to help evaluate the effectiveness of nursing interventions can promote the client's sense of control and responsibility as well as maintain a focus on expected results from treatment, progress, and eventual discharge from the facility.

Client's Responsibilities

A client has certain responsibilities within the therapeutic relationship. The client's ability to accept or fulfill some of these responsibilities may vary according to his or her mental state or problems. As the client progresses, the degree of self-responsibility he or she assumes should increase. Client responsibilities include:

Recognizing and accepting hospitalization or treatment as a positive step toward the goal of optimum health

Recognizing and accepting the nurse as a therapist

Recognizing and accepting his or her emotional problems

Accepting responsibility for his or her own feelings, even though that may be difficult or distasteful or conflict with the client's desired self-image

Accepting an active role in his or her own treatment and being motivated toward pursuing the goal of optimum health

Actively participating in care planning and implementation as soon and as much as possible

Recognizing and accepting that there is a relationship between physical and mental health

Reporting honest information, even if it is perceived as undesirable, to form an accurate data base on which to plan and evaluate care.

Part 3

Care Plans

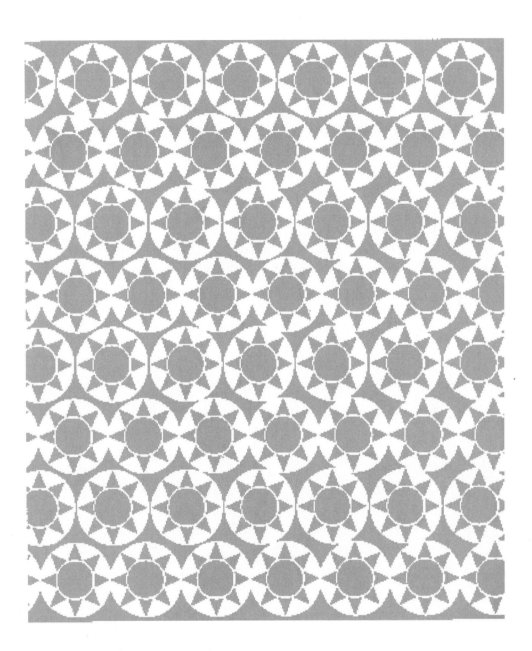

Schultz JM, Videbeck SD: MANUAL OF
PSYCHIATRIC NURSING CARE PLANS, 4th ed.
© 1994 J. B. Lippincott Company.

The *Manual of Psychiatric Nursing Care Plans* is intended as a resource in planning for each client's care. Because each client is a person with a unique background, home environment, and support system, and a particular set of behaviors, problems, strengths, needs, and goals, each client needs an individual plan of nursing care. The following care plans present general information concerning clients' behaviors and the nursing diagnoses most likely to be used in the client's care plan (and other possible nursing diagnoses); for each diagnosis addressed in the care plan, suggestions are given for defining characteristics and related factors that may be assessed with a client, expected outcomes for two time frames (initial and prior to discharge), therapeutic aims or nursing objectives, and nursing interventions and rationale. Because of individual differences and because the care plans in this manual are based primarily on behaviors (as opposed to medical and psychiatric diagnoses or symptom complexes), a plan from this *Manual* should not be copied verbatim for an individual client's plan of care. Some care plans, in fact, contain seemingly contradictory problems that call for different approaches or suggest different possible approaches for the same problem. Therefore, each plan in the *Manual* may be viewed as a resource from which to glean appropriate information and suggestions for use in each client's case.

This *Manual* focuses primarily on the client's behavior. This is essential because not only is each client unique, but in general, clients do not always present a textbook picture of a medical diagnosis or problem. The *Manual's* behavioral approach also enables the nurse to use the *Manual* to plan care in the absence of a specified psychiatric diagnosis. Thus, nursing care can be planned using nursing diagnoses formulated on the basis of nursing assessment, rather than depending on a medical and psychiatric diagnosis. This is important for several reasons: not all clients with emotional or psychiatric problems are found in psychiatric settings or carry a psychiatric diagnosis, psychiatric diagnoses are not always immediately determined, and most important, good nursing care must involve seeing the client holistically, using a nursing framework, rather than solely in terms of a psychiatric diagnosis.

The nursing process includes assessment, formulation of nursing diagnoses, determination of expected outcomes, identification of nursing interventions that may lead to expected outcomes, establishment of deadlines or a timetable for evaluation of all parts of the process, and revision of each step when appropriate. Each part of this dynamic and continuing process is specific to the person and must be determined for each client. The sections included in each plan in this

Manual are ones the authors have found could be used as resources and references. In planning nursing care for a client, the nurse must select appropriate items from these care plans or use them as ideas or a framework from which to write others more appropriate for the individual client and then supply timing, evaluation, and revision specific to the situation. The following is a brief explanation of each section found in each of the care plans in the *Manual*.

The section that begins each care plan contains information about the behaviors or problems addressed in the care plan. This information may include a basic description of the problem(s), key definitions, and background or explanatory information, pertinent reminders, suggestions about related problems, and specific symptom complexes or medical diagnoses in which the problem(s) may occur.

Nursing Diagnoses

The nursing diagnoses most likely to be formulated from the assessment of clients exhibiting these behaviors or problems and to be addressed in the care plan are presented, followed by a list of other nursing diagnoses (not addressed specifically in the care plan) that may be useful in planning care for some clients with these behaviors or problems. Neither list is intended as a complete list of all nursing diagnoses that may be generated; rather, those diagnoses presented address problems that commonly occur; they are guides for the nurse to use in formulating diagnoses appropriate for individual clients.

For each nursing diagnosis addressed in the care plan, the following elements of care planning are given:

Assessment Data. This section includes *Defining Characteristics* and *Related Factors*, likely to be present in the client's appearance, behavior, and situation.

Expected Outcomes. This section presents expected outcomes, or outcome criteria, that the nurse and the client may identify to include in the care plan as a focus for nursing care, for the client's progress, and for evaluating the effectiveness of the care plan. The outcome criteria, or goals, are written in terms of the client's behavior. The nurse should write these outcomes in terms that are as specific as possible, so that they can be used as a basis for evaluation and revision. Deadlines or other timing criteria need to be included in the individual client's care plan for each outcome. Other specifications (or modifiers), such as the amount of interaction, specific people or types of people involved (eg, staff members, other clients), amounts of food or fluids, and so forth, also should be included. An example of an expected outcome written for a client's care plan is: "The client will talk with a staff member about loss for 10 minutes each day by 3/6" (see Basic Concepts: The Nursing Process).

Therapeutic Aims. Therapeutic aims are included in the *Manual's* care plans as an indication of nursing objectives in the planning of care for the client. They can be used by the nurse or the student to guide thinking about nursing goals and the use of their therapeutic relationship with the client, but they do not need to be included in the client's written plan of care.

Implementation, including *Nursing Interventions* and *Rationale*. This section presents choices and alternatives that the nurse can select (with the client, if possible) as a means of achieving the expected outcomes. Interventions, also called nursing orders or nursing prescriptions, are given as specific practical suggestions, and often details are given for more than one approach so that care can be tailored to individual differences within a general behavior or problem. When writing an individual's care plan, the nurse should add modifiers to the interventions presented in the *Manual*, similar to those written for expected outcomes. Rationale for nursing interventions is an important part of the nursing process, although it is seldom written out in an individual client's care plan. It has been included in this *Manual* as a means of communicating the principles on which the suggested interventions are based and to show that nursing interventions are to be written based on rationale. That is, rationale exists whether it be explicitly written or only implicit in the construction of each care plan. As nursing research expands the body of nursing knowledge, rationale for nursing interventions will become more distinct and specific.

Section One

General Care Plans

The first two care plans in this section should be used with every client's care plan because they address two of the most important facets of treatment: establishing the therapeutic relationship and planning for the client's independence from treatment. In order for work with any client to be most effective, that work must be soundly based in a trusting relationship. The client and the nurse must see each other and their work as valuable, must strive toward mutually agreed on goals, and must enter into the problem-solving process together as described in Care Plan 1: Building a Trust Relationship.

Equally important is the client's discharge from treatment or from the therapeutic relationship. Discharge planning should begin immediately when therapy begins, providing a focus for goals and an orientation toward as much independence as possible for the client. Discussing discharge plans with the client from the outset will help minimize the client's fears of discharge and will facilitate goal identification and an active role for the client in therapy. By using Care Plan 2: Discharge Planning, the nurse may anticipate the client's optimum level of functioning, the quality of the client's home situation and relationships with significant others, and the need for client teaching throughout nursing care planning and implementation.

Care Plan 3: Knowledge Deficit speaks to the situation in which clients and their significant others may lack knowledge or understanding of their condition, treatment, safe use of medications, and other self-care needs. Clients who are unable or unwilling to adhere to their treatment plans, regardless of their primary problems or behaviors, are addressed in Care Plan 4: Noncompliance. The nursing diagnoses and care planning found in these plans may be appropriate for use in clients with any of the behaviors addressed elsewhere in the *Manual*.

Many times clients are cared for at home by a family member, partner, or friend. Caregivers often undertake the care of a client with little preparation or knowledge and with little attention to their own needs. Care Plan 5: Supporting the Caregiver examines some of the considerations related to caregiving and the needs of caregivers. Using it will help the nurse in planning care for the client after discharge and in addressing the needs of caregivers to ensure continued success.

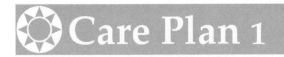
Building a Trust Relationship

The nurse–client relationship is an interpersonal process that is intended to support the client's growth as he or she evaluates needs, solves problems, shares feelings and thoughts, and acquires new coping skills (Stuart and Sundeen, 1991). The therapeutic relationship is client focused and built on trust between the nurse and the client. In contrast to personal or social relationships, the therapeutic relationship has specific goals and expectations; is time-limited; and is focused on the client in terms of learning, meeting needs, and growing. The client has a right to expect participation in the relationship to be a meaningful part of his or her treatment. The nurse has the responsibility to facilitate and guide the relationship to achieve that end.

The trust relationship between client and nurse can be viewed in four phases or stages. Each phase has primary tasks and characteristics, but transition from one phase to the next is gradual and is not always clearly delineated. These stages follow:

1. *Introductory or orientation phase.* This phase is the foundation of the relationship. The nurse becomes acquainted with the client, begins to establish rapport, and gains mutual trust. The purpose, goals, limits, and expectations of the relationship are established.
2. *Testing phase.* The nurse's truthfulness, sincerity, and reliability are in question at this time. The client may say or do things to shock the nurse to see if he or she will reject the client. During this time the client may become manipulative in an attempt to discover the limits of the relationship or test the nurse's sincerity and dependability. The client's attitude and behavior may vary a great deal, for example, from pleasant and eager to please to uncooperative and angry. This phase can be extremely trying and frustrating for the nurse.
3. *Working phase.* Transition to this phase is accompanied by the client's willingness to assume a more active role in the relationship. This usually is the longest phase of a trust relationship and the most overtly productive. The client begins to trust the nurse and starts to focus on problems or behaviors that need to be changed. During times of frustration the client may revert to testing behaviors. The nurse should anticipate this and avoid becoming discouraged or giving up on the relationship.

4. *Termination Phase.* This phase provides closure of the relationship. Ideally, planning for termination of the relationship begins during the orientation phase or as soon as the client is able to comprehend it. As the client begins to rely more on himself or herself, plans to return home, to the community, or to a more permanent placement can be made. (See Care Plan 2: Discharge Planning.) When the client leaves the relationship (or facility) for unanticipated reasons, termination is less organized and usually more difficult. In that situation it is important to try to talk with the client, even very briefly, to put some closure in the relationship.

Nursing Diagnosis Addressed in this Care Plan

Impaired Social Interaction

Related Nursing Diagnoses

Impaired Verbal Communication
Ineffective Individual Coping
Altered Role Performance
Anxiety

Nursing Diagnosis

Assessment Data

Impaired Social Interaction (3.1.1)
The state in which an individual participates in an insufficient or excessive quantity or ineffective quality of social exchange.

Defining Characteristics	• Discomfort in social or interactive situations
	• Poor social skills
	• Difficulty trusting others
	• Difficulties in relationships with significant others
	• Difficulties with others in school or work environment
	• Feelings of anxiety, fear, hostility, sadness, guilt, or inadequacy

Related Factors	• History of unsatisfactory relationships
	• Negative feelings regarding past hospitalizations or contacts with health care providers
	• Psychiatric problems (The client's behavior may range from slightly withdrawn and quiet to openly hostile and aggressive, depending on the nature of the client's problems.)

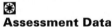
Expected Outcomes

Initial	*The client will:*
	• Participate in the trust relationship
	• Demonstrate ability to interact with staff and other clients within the therapeutic milieu

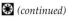 *(continued)*
Expected Outcomes

Discharge	*The client will:*
	• Assume increasing responsibility within the context of the therapeutic relationship
	• Identify relationships outside the hospital environment to be used as a support system
	• Terminate the nurse–client relationship successfully

Therapeutic Aims

- Define the purpose of the relationship.
- Establish the roles and responsibilities of the client and the nurse.
- Begin planning for termination of the relationship.
- Set and maintain acceptable limits for the therapeutic relationship.
- Assist the client in establishing a support system outside the hospital environment.
- Terminate the relationship.

Implementation

Nursing Interventions	Rationale
Introduce yourself to the client. Explain your role on the unit or within the treatment team.	An introduction and explanation will help the client know what to expect from you, other staff, and the hospitalization.
Assess the client's behavior, attitudes, problems, and needs.	Baseline data are essential for developing a plan of nursing care.
Obtain the client's perception of his or her problems and what the client expects to gain from the relationship or hospitalization.	The client's actions are based on his or her perceptions, which may or may not be the same as other people's perceptions or objective reality.
Make your expectations for the relationship clear to the client.	Defining your expectations helps the client identify his or her role and understand what is expected of him or her.
Be honest in all interactions with the client. Avoid glossing over any unpleasant topics or circumstances. Take a matter-of-fact approach to such problems as commitment, legal difficulties, and so forth.	Honesty is essential if a trusting relationship is to develop. You are not doing the client a favor by avoiding unpleasant areas; he or she will need to deal with these problems. You show that you are trustworthy by discussing these issues without judging or rejecting the client.
Let the client know that you will work with him or her for a specified period of time, and when the client is no longer in treatment, the relationship will end.	Explaining the time limitations helps to set the limits of the professional relationship. It also conveys your positive expectation that the client will improve and leave the hospital.
Be consistent with the client at all times.	Your consistency demonstrates that you are trustworthy, and it reinforces limits.

✸ *(continued)*
Implementation

Nursing Interventions	Rationale
Show the client that you accept him or her as a person.	Conveying acceptance can help the client feel worthwhile. It is possible to accept the client yet not accept "negative" or undesirable behaviors.
Avoid becoming the only one the client can talk to about his or her feelings and problems.	Becoming the sole confidant of the client may seem flattering, but it may be manipulative on the part of the client, and it inhibits the client's ability to form relationships with others.
Let the client know that pertinent information will be communicated to other staff members. Do not promise to keep secrets (that is, from other staff) as a way of obtaining information from the client.	A promise of keeping secrets is not one you can keep. The client has a right to know how information is communicated and used in his or her treatment.
Set and maintain limits on the client's "negative" or unacceptable behavior; withdraw your attention from the client if necessary.	Lack of attention can help extinguish unacceptable behavior.
Do not allow the client to bargain to obtain special favors, to avoid responsibilities, or to gain privileges.	Allowing bargaining permits the client to be manipulative and undermines limits and trust.
Give attention and positive feedback for acceptable or positive behavior.	Desirable behaviors increase when they are positively reinforced.
When limiting the client's behaviors, offer acceptable alternatives (for example, "Don't try to hit someone when you're angry—try punching your pillow instead"). See Basic Concepts: Limit-Setting.	By offering alternative ways to express feelings, you teach acceptable as well as unacceptable behavior. The client is more likely to abandon old behaviors if new ones are available to him or her.
Establish a regular schedule for meeting with the client (such as 1 hour each day or 10 minutes every hour), whatever fits your schedule and the client is able to tolerate.	Regular schedules provide consistency, which enhances trust. The client also can see that your interest in him or her continues.
At the beginning of your interaction with the client, inform him or her of how much time you have to spend. If you must interrupt the interaction, tell the client when you expect to return.	Discussing your schedule conveys your respect for the client and lets the client know what to expect from you.
Do whatever you say you will do, and conversely, do not make promises you cannot keep. If extenuating circumstances prevent your following through, apologize and honestly explain this to the client. Expect the client to be disappointed or angry; help him or her to express these feelings appropriately, and give support for doing so.	The client must know what to expect and will trust you more when you follow through. Extenuating circumstances that necessitate a change of plans happen in everyday life; the client has the opportunity to deal with the frustration or disappointment that may ensue in an acceptable manner.
Assist the client in identifying personal behaviors or problem areas in his or her life situation that interfere with relationships or interactions with others.	The client must identify what behaviors or problems need modification before change can occur.

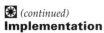 *(continued)*
Implementation

Nursing Interventions	Rationale
Teach the client a step-by-step approach to solving problems: identifying the problem, exploring alternatives, evaluating the possible consequences of the alternative solutions, making a decision, and implementing the solution.	The client may be unaware of a logical process for examining and resolving problems.
Help the client identify and implement ways of expressing emotions and communicating with others.	The client's ability to identify and express feelings and to communicate with others is impaired.
Teach the client social skills. Describe and demonstrate specific skills, such as eye contact, attentive listening, nodding, and so forth. Discuss the types of topics that are appropriate for social conversation, such as the weather, news, local events, and so forth.	The client may never have learned basic social skills and how to use them appropriately.
Assist the client in identifying more effective methods of dealing with stress.	The client may be dealing with stress in the most effective way he or she can and may need to learn new skills and behaviors.
Anticipate the client's anxiety or insecurity about being discharged from the hospital and terminating the therapeutic relationship, including the possibility that the client may revert to manipulative behavior or his or her presenting problem behavior as termination approaches. Remember: The termination phase of the therapeutic relationship actually should begin in the introductory or orientation phase and should be reinforced as a goal and as a positive outcome throughout the entire therapeutic relationship.	Once the client is comfortable in the relationship, you may expect that he or she will perceive the end of the relationship as threatening and the beginning of other relationships as entailing risk. In addition, the termination of the relationship is a loss for the client (and for the staff).
Assist the client in identifying sources of support outside the hospital, including agencies or individuals in the community, as well as significant others in his or her personal life.	Community support may help the client deal with future stress and avoid hospitalization.
Assist the client in making plans for discharge (returning home, employment, and so on). See Care Plan 2: Discharge Planning.	Making specific discharge plans enhances the client's chances for success in the community.

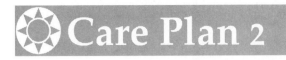

Discharge Planning

Discharge planning is a process that should begin on the client's admission to the hospital and should first be addressed in his or her initial care plan. Planning for eventual discharge should underlie the client's plan of care throughout the hospital stay in recognition of the temporary nature of hospitalization. The basic discharge goal is that the client will reach his or her optimal level of wellness and independence. Such an approach will encourage goal-oriented planning and discourage the client and the staff from seeing hospitalization as an end in itself or a panacea. Ideally, the client should work with the staff as soon as possible to develop an ongoing plan of care that is oriented to his or her discharge. In the assessment of the client with regard to discharge plans, it is important to obtain the following information:

The client's ability to function independently before hospitalization
The client's home environment
The type of situation to which the client will be discharged
The client's optimal level of functioning outside the hospital
The client's own support system outside the hospital
The client's need for follow-up care, including frequency, type, location, or specific
    therapist

It also is important to assess the client's feelings about hospitalization and discharge and the client's motivations to remain hospitalized or to be discharged and to change his or her out-of-hospital behavior or situation to prevent readmission. The nurse should remain aware of any secondary gains the client obtains from being hospitalized.

Discharge planning, like other nursing care planning, is a dynamic process and must undergo evaluation and change throughout the client's care. If the client needs continued care or will not be returning to his or her former environment, it may be necessary to consider the following:

Transfer to another hospital or institution
Discharge to a sheltered or transitional setting
Discharge to other supportive services in the community
Relocation to a community other than the client's prehospitalization community

Nursing Diagnoses Addressed in this Care Plan

Impaired Home Maintenance Management
Anxiety

Related Nursing Diagnoses

Ineffective Individual Coping
Altered Health Maintenance

Nursing Diagnosis

Assessment Data

Impaired Home Maintenance Management (6.4.1.1)
The state in which an individual or family is unable or potentially unable to maintain a safe, hygienic growth-promoting environment independently.

Defining Characteristics	• Lack of skills with which to function independently outside the hospital • Lack of confidence • Dependence on hospital • Perceived helplessness • Nonexistent or unrealistic goals and plans • Lack of knowledge
Related Factors	• Inadequate support system • Inadequate financial resources • Cognitive deficits • Disorganized or dysfunctional living environment

Expected Outcomes

Initial	*The client will:*
	
	• Verbalize concrete realistic plans regarding:
	  Meeting essential physical needs (housing, employment, financial resources, necessary transportation, and physical care, if needed)
	  Meeting emotional needs through significant relationships, social activities, a general support system, and so forth
	  Dealing with stress or problems
	  Dealing with other facets of living specific to the client (legal problems, physical or health limitations, and so forth)

Discharge	*The client will:* • Demonstrate the ability to meet essential needs (self-reliance when possible) • Verbally identify and contact resource people in the community for various needs

❀
Therapeutic Aims

- Promote compliance with treatment regimen.
- Maximize independence.
- Prepare the client for discharge—home, community, or another setting—as appropriate.

❀
Implementation

Nursing Interventions	Rationale
On admission, ask the client about his or her expectations for hospitalization and plans for discharge. Attempt to keep the discharge plans as a focus for discussion throughout the client's hospitalization.	Discussing discharge plans will reinforce the idea that the client's hospitalization is temporary and that discharge is the eventual goal.
Encourage the client to identify his or her goals and expectations after discharge.	Focusing on the client's life outside the hospital may help to diminish fears of discharge.
Help the client assess personal needs for specificity and structure. If it is indicated, assist the client in making a time schedule or other structure for activities (work, study, recreation, solitude, social activities, and significant relationships).	The client may be overwhelmed by the lack of structure in the home environment after a stay in an institution, which often is very structured and in which the client's choices and need for decision making are limited.
Encourage the client to continue working toward goals that have been identified but not yet realized during hospitalization (for example, obtaining a high school diploma, vocational plans, divorce). Give positive support for goal identification and work that has begun.	The client is leaving a supportive environment and may need encouragement to continue working toward goals outside the hospital.
Talk with the client regarding medication or other treatment schedules and reasons for continuing therapy. Attempt to involve the client in treatment decisions, especially regarding postdischarge therapies.	The client's participation in decisions may increase his or her motivation to continue therapies.
Talk with the client about ways to meet personal needs after discharge (for example, obtaining food, money, shelter, clothing, transportation, and a job).	The client may need direction or assistance in making these plans.
Assess the client's skills related to meeting the above needs (for example, using a telephone and directory, managing a checkbook and bank accounts, contacting other community resources, and arranging job interviews). Work with the client and obtain help from other disciplines if indicated, such as vocational rehabilitation, therapeutic education, and so forth.	The client may lack daily living skills and may need to develop and practice them before discharge.
Before discharge, encourage the client to make arrangements as independently as possible (for example, find housing, open bank accounts, obtain a job). Give support for these activities. Refer the client to social services if he or she needs additional assistance in obtaining housing.	The client will be leaving the support of the hospital and staff and needs to be as independent as possible.

(continued)
Implementation

Nursing Interventions	Rationale
Use role playing and setting up hypothetical situations with the client when discussing discharge plans.	Anticipatory guidance can be effective in preparing the client for future situations. Role playing and hypothetical situations allow the client to practice new behaviors in a nonthreatening environment and to receive feedback on new skills.
Teach the client about his or her illness, medications (action, toxic symptoms, and side effects), nutrition, exercise, and medical conditions requiring physical care, if needed.	The client needs health information to participate effectively in his or her own care and to achieve independence and optimal health outside the hospital.
If the client is transferring to another facility: Give the client factual feedback regarding his or her progress, and discuss the need for further treatment. Point out the reasons for the transfer, if possible, such as the need for long-term care, another type of care, different treatment structure, or another location. Involve the client in the decision-making process and offer the client choices as much as possible.	It is important that the client understand the reasons for continued treatment, transfer decisions, and so forth, as much as possible. Giving the client choices or input will help diminish feelings of helplessness and frustration.
Stress that the transfer is not a punishment.	The client may see the need for continued care as a failure on his or her part.
Attempt to give the client information about his or her new environment; arrange a visit prior to the transfer, if possible, or provide the name of a contact person at the new facility.	Information about the new environment will help diminish the client's anxiety.

Nursing Diagnosis	*Anxiety (9.3.1)* *A vague uneasy feeling of which the source often is nonspecific or unknown to the individual.*

Assessment Data

Defining Characteristics	• Verbalized nervousness, apprehension • Fear of failure • Withdrawn behavior • Reappearance of symptoms as discharge is near • Refusal to discuss future plans
Related Factors	• Perception of discharge as rejection • History of unsuccessful attempts at independent living • Dependency on hospital staff

(continued)
Assessment Data

| Related Factors | • Excessive comfort within hospital environment
• Secondary gains from hospitalization
• Plans for discharge to an unfamiliar or changed environment |

Expected Outcomes

| Initial | *The client will:*

• Discuss termination of staff–client relationships
• Verbally acknowledge eventual discharge
• Verbalize feelings about discharge and hospitalization |
| Discharge | *The client will:*

• Participate actively in discharge planning
• Demonstrate alternative ways to deal with stress or problems
• Evaluate own skills related to proposed discharge realistically
• Terminate staff–client relationships |

Therapeutic Aims

• Provide anticipatory guidance.
• Promote self-confidence and independence.
• Terminate staff–client relationships without the perception of rejection.

Implementation

Nursing Interventions	Rationale
Help the client identify factors in his or her life that have contributed to hospitalization (for example, living situation, relationships, drug or alcohol use, work problems, inadequate coping mechanisms). Discuss each contributing factor, how the client sees these now, what can be changed, what the client is motivated to change, and how the client will deal differently with these things to prevent rehospitalization.	The client's therapy and work inside the hospital must be integrated with his or her life outside the hospital to remain effective. Outside influences or situations may need to be changed to promote the client's well-being. Anticipatory guidance can be effective in helping the client prepare for future situations.
Always orient discussions with the client toward his or her eventual discharge.	Providing a focus on discharge will minimize the client's focusing only on the hospitalization and will promote the client's acceptance of discharge plans.
Support the client and give positive feedback when the client plans for discharge or talks positively about discharge.	Positive support may reinforce the client's positive anticipation of discharge.
Encourage the client to view discharge as a positive step or sign of growth, not as being "kicked out" of the hospital. Try to convey this in your attitude toward the client.	The client may see discharge as punishment or rejection.

✳ (*continued*)
Implementation

Nursing Interventions	Rationale
Encourage the client to express feelings about leaving the hospital, including a discussion of anticipated problems, fears, and ways to deal with the outside world.	The client may be fearful of being outside a structured, supportive environment; may fear a return of symptoms; or may be anxious about dealing with significant others, his or her job, and so forth.
Use formal and informal group settings for discussions. A discharge group that includes all clients who are near discharge may be helpful.	Groups can offer support for feelings by others in similar situations, and they provide a nonthreatening environment in which to explore new behaviors.
Talk with the client about the feelings he or she may experience after discharge (such as loneliness) and how the client will deal with those feelings.	Identifying feelings and exploring ways to deal with them can help diminish the client's fears.
Give the client a telephone number and name (if possible) to call in case of a crisis or situation in which the client feels overwhelmed.	Tangible information can help decrease the client's fears and prepare for dealing with crises in ways other than returning to the hospital.
Deliberately terminate your relationship with the client, and talk with him or her about this. First, try to acknowledge and deal with your own feelings about the client and the client's discharge; try not to merely withdraw attention from or avoid the client because he or she will be leaving.	Your relationship with the client is a professional one and must be terminated at the time hospitalization ends. The client needs to develop and maintain optimal independence. Your own feelings of discomfort must not prevent you from helping the client acknowledge and work through termination of the relationship.
Encourage the client to express his or her feelings regarding termination of therapeutic relationships and loss of the hospitalization.	Discharge from the safety, security, and structure of the hospital environment represents a real loss to the client for which grief is an expected and appropriate response. Encouraging the client to work through his or her feelings regarding this loss will foster acceptance and growth.
Do not encourage the client's dependence on the staff members or hospital by suggesting the client pay casual visits to the unit or by giving the client home addresses or telephone numbers of staff members. It may be necessary to establish a policy that clients may not visit the unit socially after being discharged.	It is not desirable or therapeutic for clients to become friends with staff members or to engage in social relationships with them after discharge.

Knowledge Deficit

Knowledge deficit, or the "state in which specific information is lacking" (Kim, McFarland, and McLane, 1991) in the client or his or her significant others or caregiver(s), is a common finding when assessing clients with psychiatric problems. Although there is controversy in the nursing literature regarding the validity of Knowledge Deficit as a nursing diagnosis per se (Dennison and Keeling, 1989; Fleming, 1990; Jenny, 1987; Tennant, 1990), a client or his or her significant others who lack information necessary to regain, maintain, or improve health is suited to nursing intervention and is therefore addressed in this care plan. (The nursing process described here can be integrated into other diagnoses if the knowledge deficit is determined to be a defining characteristic, related factor, or etiology in another diagnosis rather than a separate diagnosis.)

A knowledge deficit can occur in a client or his or her significant others or caregiver(s) in concert with virtually any of the behaviors or problems addressed in this *Manual*. The specific deficit may be knowledge of the client's specific behavior, problem, medical diagnosis, or health state; basic knowledge of self-care needs, social skills, problem solving, or other general daily living activities; prevention of future problems; resources related to any of the above; treatment plan or regimen; or safe use of medications. The client's or caregiver's knowledge deficit may be related to a wide range of factors, including cognitive deficits, skill deficits, or physical or psychiatric problems. (See "Related Factors," later)

Client teaching is the basic nursing intervention related to a knowledge deficit. Many nursing and other health care organizations have mandated client teaching as a basic part of all clients' right to health care (Goldblum, 1992). Specific techniques regarding assessment, content areas, and methods of client teaching are found in the sections "Basic Concepts: Client Teaching" in this *Manual*.

Nursing Diagnosis Addressed in this Care Plan

Knowledge Deficit (Specify)

Related Nursing Diagnoses

Altered Thought Processes
Sensory/Perceptual Alterations
Self-Care Deficit
Impaired Verbal Communication
Altered Role Performance
Ineffective Individual Coping
Impaired Adjustment
Ineffective Denial
Noncompliance (Specify)
Altered Health Maintenance
Anxiety

Nursing Diagnosis

Knowledge Deficit (Specify) (8.1.1)

The state in which specific information is lacking in the client, his or her significant others, or caregiver(s) regarding the client's self-care, treatment plan, safe use of medications, or other health care needs.

Assessment Data

Note: The following steps of the nursing process are written in terms of the client but may be equally or more appropriate for the client's significant others and caregivers.

Defining Characteristics

- Verbalization of knowledge deficit or need for learning
- Incorrect or inadequate demonstration of self-care skills
- Incorrect verbal feedback regarding self-care information
- Inappropriate behavior related to self-care

Related Factors

- Lack of exposure to information
- Inability to recall prior learning
- Cognitive limitations
- Misinterpretation of information
- Previously held misconceptions
- Resistance to learning
- Denial of problem or need for learning
- Feelings of being overwhelmed
- Feelings of being discouraged or despondent
- Passivity or apathy and lack of motivation for learning
- Low self-esteem
- Lack of motivation for self-care

✸ *(continued)*
Assessment Data

Related Factors	• Psychiatric problems that interfere with cognition or retention of information, such as altered thought processes, withdrawn behavior, and so forth • Physical problems (such as impaired hearing) or lack of learning skills (such as low literacy) that may interfere with learning (especially if the nurse is unaware of these problems)

✸
Expected Outcomes

Initial	*The client will:*
	• Demonstrate decreased denial • Demonstrate decreased problems that impair learning ability (such as altered thought processes, sensory-perceptual alterations, and so forth) • Demonstrate interest in learning • Participate in learning about self-care needs; behaviors, problems, or illness; treatment program; or safe use of medications
Discharge	*The client will:*
	• Verbalize accurate information related to self-care needs • Demonstrate adequate skills related to self-care needs • Verbalize knowledge of resources and their use for anticipated needs

✸
Therapeutic Aims

• Accurately assess knowledge deficit.
• Accurately assess ability to learn information and skills.
• Promote learning and return verbalization or demonstration of information and skills.

✸
Implementation

Nursing Interventions	Rationale
Assess the client in terms of current level of knowledge, misconceptions, ability to learn, readiness to learn, and knowledge needs for optimal self-care. Assess the client's level of anxiety and his or her perceptions of greatest needs and priorities.	To be effective in meeting the client's needs, your teaching plan must be based on an accurate assessment of the client's knowledge deficit and ability to learn. In addition, if the client is anxious, his or her ability to learn will be impaired until the level of anxiety decreases. In the same way your interventions will be most effective if you focus first on meeting the client's perceived needs and priorities, then progress to other necessary teaching.
Provide information and teach skills as appropriate to the specific knowledge deficit. In a specific individual's care plan, write a formal teaching plan with specific information, techniques, timing, and outcome criteria appropriate to that individual client. (See Basic Concepts: Client Teaching.)	Different clients may have very different learning needs, abilities, and situations. It is just as important to individualize a client's teaching plan as it is to write an individual nursing care plan for each client. A written, formal teaching plan will help ensure consistency among nursing staff, a focus, and a method of evaluating progress.

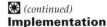 *(continued)*

Implementation

Nursing Interventions	Rationale
Provide written information or other supporting materials as appropriate.	Informational materials or sample products can support and reinforce learning and recall especially after the client is discharged.
Provide information in a matter-of-fact, nonjudgmental, reassuring manner.	Information concerning psychiatric problems or illnesses can be threatening or have negative connotations to a client; he or she may have misconceptions or internalized judgment, humiliation, shame, and so forth, related to his or her behaviors, experiences, or psychiatric diagnoses. Conveying information in a nonjudgmental manner can reassure the client and help with his or her acceptance of his or her condition or situation.
Provide information at a pace at which the client can learn effectively. Do not try to teach all necessary information at one time: Use as many teaching sessions as the client needs to learn, if at all possible.	The client's ability to learn may be impaired.
Ask the client to verbalize or demonstrate his or her understanding of the information given or skill taught. Ask the client directly if he or she has any questions; assure the client that asking questions or asking for clarification is an important part of the learning process. Allow the client sufficient time to formulate and ask questions.	The client may feel inadequate or intimidated in a learning situation and may therefore indicate understanding (for example, by nodding his or her head or answering "yes" to the question, "Do you understand?") when he or she actually does not understand or has not learned the information or skill. Adequate assessment of learning requires verbalization or active demonstration of learning.
Give the client positive feedback for asking questions, verbalizing information, demonstrating skills, and otherwise participating in the teaching–learning process.	Recognition and positive support will reinforce the client's efforts and encourage further participation.
Document teaching, the client's response to teaching, and indications of understanding verbalized or demonstrated by the client.	It is important to document teaching and learning for the successful communication within and implementation of the teaching plan and to protect the nurse from later claims that such teaching and learning did not occur.
Repeat your assessment of the client's learning and understanding at another time (that is, after the instructional episode) prior to the client's discharge.	Repeated assessment of learning is essential to ensure that the client has retained the information.
If possible, allow and encourage the client to assume increasing responsibility in performing his or her own self-care prior to discharge.	Learning is most effective when the client actually practices and integrates new information and skills. Encouraging the client to integrate and demonstrate new information and skills in a protected environment allows the client to ask questions, clarify understanding, and build confidence in his or her self-care abilities.

Noncompliance

Noncompliance, or failure to adhere to a therapeutic regimen, is a common phenomenon in health care. Research indicates that one third of the clients studied failed to follow the prescribed regimen (Young, 1986). These clients often can verbalize their understanding of the therapeutic regimen, but their behavior (noncompliance) indicates a problem. In mental health clients noncompliance regarding prescribed medications is a primary problem that often leads to rehospitalization. Noncompliance with medication can take many forms, including complete refusal to take any medications, taking a larger or smaller dose than prescribed, erratic or sporadic ingestion of the medication, or taking the medication of others.

Working with the noncompliant client can be frustrating. The nurse may feel angry or impatient when the client fails to follow the prescribed regimen, which can damage the therapeutic relationship. It is important for the nurse to recognize and deal with his or her own feelings regarding the client's noncompliant behavior if the nurse expects to remain effective in the nurse–client relationship.

Initially, neither the nurse nor the client may be aware of the reasons for noncompliance. It is essential to explore the factors underlying noncompliant behavior to assist the client to make positive changes in this area. Wilson and Kneisl (1992) summarize the following factors related to noncompliance:

Psychologic factors, including lack of knowledge; clients' attitudes, values, and beliefs; denial of the illness or other defense mechanisms; personality type; and anxiety levels.

Environmental and social factors, including lack of support system, finances, transportation, housing, and other problems that may distract from health needs.

Characteristics of the regimen, such as not enough benefit perceived by the client, demands too much change from the client, too difficult or complicated, distressing side effects, leads to social isolation or stigma.

Characteristics of the provider–client relationship, such as faulty communication in which the client perceives the provider as cold, uncaring, or authoritative; the client feels discouraged or treated as an object; or the client and the provider are engaged in a struggle for control.

Through exploration of these factors and with patience and understanding, the client and the nurse can come to an agreement about the therapeutic regimen through the use of the nursing process. The nurse's and the client's goal is to maximize the effectiveness of the therapeutic regimen for the client.

In this care plan two approaches to noncompliant behavior are presented. The first approach, using the nursing diagnosis Noncompliance, is designed for use with clients who refuse to comply or make a specific decision to be noncompliant. The second approach uses the nursing diagnosis Ineffective Management of Therapeutic Regimen for the client who is unable to follow the therapeutic regimen.

Nursing Diagnoses Addressed in this Care Plan

Noncompliance
Ineffective Management of Therapeutic Regimen

Nursing Diagnosis

Noncompliance (Specify) (5.2.1.1)

A person's informed decision not to adhere to a therapeutic recommendation.

Assessment Data

Defining Characteristics	• Objective tests indicating noncompliance, such as low neuroleptic blood levels • Statements from the client or significant others describing noncompliant behavior • Exacerbation of symptoms • Appearance of side effects or complications • Failure to keep appointments • Failure to follow through with referrals
Related Factors	• Inaccurate or incomplete knowledge • Unsupportive home or community environment • Conflict between therapeutic regimen and personal beliefs • Denial of illness • Experiencing unpleasant side effects of therapy • Unsatisfactory relationship(s) with health care professional(s) • Inadequate resources, for example, financial and transportation

Expected Outcomes

Initial	*The client will:* • Identify barriers to compliance • Recognize the relationship between noncompliance and undesirable consequences (ie, increased symptoms, hospitalization) • Express feelings about therapeutic regimen
Discharge	*The client will:* • Verbalize acceptance of illness • Identify risks of noncompliance • Negotiate acceptable changes in the therapeutic regimen that the client is willing to follow

Therapeutic Aims

- Facilitate acceptance of the illness.
- Promote participation in the therapeutic process.
- Promote adherence to an acceptable therapeutic regimen.

Implementation

Nursing Interventions	Rationale
Teach the client and his or her family or significant others about the client's illness, treatment plan, medications, and so forth.	The client and his or her significant others may have incomplete or inaccurate information that is contributing to the client's noncompliance.
Observe the client closely to ensure that medications are ingested. Remain with the client long enough to see that the medication was swallowed.	The client must ingest medications because he or she is being evaluated for the drug's effectiveness, side effects, or any problems associated with the prescribed medication.
Explain the need for medications honestly and directly. Give the client full explanations (for example, "This is an antidepressant to improve your mood so you'll feel less suicidal").	Honest and complete explanations foster trust. The client may be more likely to comply if he or she feels fully informed.
Help the client to draw a connection between noncompliance and the exacerbation of symptoms.	The client may not have made this connection previously. The client is more likely to comply if he or she can see the benefits of compliance.
Explore the client's feelings about his or her illness, need for ongoing treatment (such as medications), and so forth.	The client may be hesitant to express feelings, especially negative ones, without explicit permission from the nurse.
If the client expresses feelings of being stigmatized (that is, being observed taking medications by friends or coworkers), assist the client to arrange dosage schedules when he or she can take medications unobserved.	Taking medications regularly in the presence of others may have elicited unwanted questions about the client's illness, need for medications, and so forth.
If the client stops taking medications when he or she "feels better," discuss the role of the medication in keeping the client free of symptoms.	Many people believe that people take medications when they are sick and should not have to take them when they are not sick or feel better. The client on long-term or maintenance therapy needs a different perspective to remain compliant.
If the client is noncompliant because he or she feels "dependent" on the medication, assist the client to gain a sense of control over his or her medication regimen. This would include supervised self-administration of medication, selecting convenient and acceptable times to take the medication, and setting limits on essentials and allowing control of nonessentials (for example, "You may take the medication before or after breakfast, but you must take it before 10:00 a.m.").	Allowing the client to make choices or decisions about some aspects of the therapeutic regimen enhances his or her sense of personal control, thus decreasing feelings of helplessness and dependency.

❊ *(continued)*
Implementation

Nursing Interventions	Rationale
Encourage the client to express his or her feelings about having a chronic illness and the continued need for medication.	Discussing feelings about chronic illness and the continued need for medication can be an initial step toward the client's acceptance of his or her health status. The client may begin to see long-term medication as a positive way to remain more healthy rather than a negative indication that the client is sick.
If the client is experiencing distressing side effects, encourage him or her to report them rather than stopping medication entirely.	A negotiated change of dosage or medication may alleviate side effects and eliminate noncompliance.
If the client still refuses to be compliant, encourage him or her to report this decision accurately. Remain matter-of-fact and nonjudgmental in your approach to the client when he or she is discussing this decision. Give positive feedback for honest reporting.	If the client perceives a greater reward for honesty than for strict compliance, he or she is more likely to report accurately. It is essential to have accurate information before decisions regarding changes in medication or dosages are made; therefore, it is preferable to know whether the client is taking the medication. If the client refuses to comply and subsequently experiences the return of symptoms or rehospitalization, you can use these data for future discussions about compliance.

Nursing Diagnosis

Ineffective Management of Therapeutic Regimen (5.2.1)
A pattern of regulating and integrating into daily living a program for treatment of illness and the sequelae of illness that is unsatisfactory for meeting specific health goals.

Assessment Data

Defining Characteristics	• Verbalized desire to comply with therapeutic regimen • Objective tests indicating noncompliance, for example, neuroleptic blood levels outside therapeutic range • Exacerbation of symptoms • Appearance of side effects, toxic effects, or complications • Difficulty integrating therapeutic regimen into daily life
Related Factors	• Knowledge or skill deficits • Cognitive deficits • Sensory-perceptual alterations • Inadequate home or community support • Lack of resources (ie, financial, transportation, and so forth) • Complex treatment regimen • Decisional conflicts

Expected Outcomes

Initial

The client will:

- Learn skills needed for compliance
- Verbalize knowledge of illness and therapeutic regimen
- Identify barriers to compliance
- Identify resources needed to ensure compliance

Discharge

The client will:

- Demonstrate skills or knowledge needed for compliance
- Arrange needed services or resources in the community
- Follow through with discharge plans, including evaluation of adherence to and effectiveness of therapeutic regimen

Therapeutic Aims

- Remove barriers to compliance.
- Provide education and skill training needed for adequate management of therapeutic regimen.

Implementation

Nursing Interventions	Rationale
Teach the client and his or her family or significant others about the client's illness and therapeutic regimen.	The client and his or her significant others may have incomplete or inaccurate information about the client's illness or therapeutic regimen.
Explore reasons for noncompliance with the client: for example, Can the client perform needed skills for compliance? Can the client afford the medication? Does he or she forget to take medicines? Does he or she forget that medicine was taken and repeat doses? Can the client find transportation to appointments to get refills or new prescriptions?	Identifying reasons for noncompliance or barriers to compliance will determine the interventions needed to gain compliance.
If the client does not have appropriate skills, teach him or her the skills required for compliance. Break skills into small steps, and proceed at a pace with which the client is comfortable. Give positive feedback for the client's efforts and progress.	The client must know the needed skills before he or she can become independent in performing them and remain compliant. Positive feedback will enhance the client's confidence and thus will enhance his or her chances for success.
Do not limit skill teaching and evaluation of the client's mastery of skills to one session. Evaluate the client on several occasions if necessary to determine confidence and mastery of the skill. (See Care Plan 3: Knowledge Deficit.)	The client may be able to perform the skill once adequately if it has just been demonstrated to him or her. That does not mean the client knows all he or she needs to know to comply at home.
If the client cannot afford medicines, refer him or her to social services.	The client may need financial assistance if that is the only barrier to compliance.

✳ *(continued)*
Implementation

Nursing Interventions	Rationale
If the client cannot remember to take medicines or forgets he or she has already taken medicines and repeats doses, set up a concrete system to eliminate this type of problem. For example, make a chart the client can use to cross off doses as they are taken, or use a pill box with separate compartments for each daily dose that the client can have filled at the pharmacy.	A concrete system for taking medicines eliminates the client's problems with trying to remember dosages and schedules.
If the client has difficulty finding transportation to appointments or to the pharmacy for new prescriptions or refills, help the client identify what he or she needs in this area. If public transportation is available, teach the client the specific routes he or she will need to take and procedures necessary to access public transportation (for example, if exact change is required). If the client forgets appointments, arrange to have someone at the client's clinic call to remind him or her of the appointment.	Once a specific barrier has been identified, plans can be made to eliminate that barrier, resulting in the client's compliance.
If the client is taking a medication that is available as a long-acting intramuscular preparation, such as fluphenazine (Prolixin) or haloperidol (Haldol), investigate the possibility of its use with the client and his or her physician.	Many clients prefer receiving injections once every 2 to 4 weeks to taking oral medications on a daily or more frequent basis.
If the client has areas of noncompliance other than medication, such as a prescribed or restricted diet, use the interventions described previously to solve that area of noncompliance.	Exploring reasons for noncompliance, teaching and validating needed skills, and arranging needed resources are effective methods of dealing with this type of noncompliant behavior.

Supporting the Caregiver

In the past, clients with debilitating or terminal illnesses were placed in institutional facilities, particularly in the later stages of the illness. Today an increasing number of these individuals receive home care. This trend is occurring because of the high costs of institutional care, dissatisfaction with the lack of personalized care in long-term settings, and the institution's rejection of some clients as "unsuitable" due to the nature of their illness or the behaviors that result from the illnesses. In addition, many clients and their families have a desire to draw closer together, viewing death as a natural part of life, rather than experience the isolation that may occur when the client is in an institutional setting.

The effect on the family unit of caring for a client is profound, and it has given rise to a new phrase, *caregiver's syndrome.* Jed (1989) identified four aspects of support that are crucial for the caregiving family: emotional support, tangible support, advice, and social interaction. Jed found that adequate support in these areas not only promoted the well-being of caregivers, but also reduced the need for re-hospitalization of the clients.

The caregiver must be involved in the client's hospital treatment if home care is being considered. The caregiver is in a dual role of being part of the team caring for the client and needing to be a recipient of nursing care. Too often the caregiver is overlooked as a consumer of services. In a long-term home care situation, a frustrated caregiver may say, "No one asks how *I* am. He or she (the client) is the center of attention—what about me and my needs?" The caregiver may show signs of emotional wear and tear, such as frustration, resentment, apathy, and inattention to personal needs.

The rise in the number of reported incidents of *elderly abuse* or *dependent adult abuse* (emotional or physical abuse of an adult who is dependent on others for his or her care for financial, physical, or mental health reasons) is a major cause for concern. Inadequate knowledge, meager financial resources, and inadequate training or support from professionals are some of the factors thought to influence this alarming trend. This care plan is designed to include the caregiver as a team member yet identify the special needs of the caregiver in this dual role.

Nursing Diagnoses Addressed in this Care Plan

Caregiver Role Strain
Social Isolation

Related Nursing Diagnoses

Altered Role Performance
Altered Family Processes
Sleep Pattern Disturbance
Diversional Activity Deficit
Ineffective Family Coping: Disabling
High Risk for Violence: Self-Directed or Directed at Others
Knowledge Deficit

Nursing Diagnosis

Caregiver Role Strain (3.2.2.1)
A caregiver's difficulty in performing the family caregiver role.

Assessment Data

Defining Characteristics

- Change in role or responsibility
- Lack of knowledge or needed skills in providing the client's care
- Intermittent apathy toward the client
- Ambivalence (feelings of resentment and guilt, as well as concern and care) toward the client
- Inattention to own needs
- Fatigue
- Conflict between caregiver role and other roles, for example, spouse and parent

Related Factors

- Lack of confidence in new role skills or abilities
- Changes in others' perceptions of caregiver's role
- Disruption of established routines and habits
- Inadequate emotional or financial support for caregiver

Expected Outcomes

Initial

The caregiver will:

- Participate in the care of the client
- Verbalize knowledge of the client's treatment plan
- Learn psychomotor skills needed for client's care

Discharge

The caregiver will:

- Identify community and agency resources for assistance, if indicated
- Follow through with discharge plans
- Verbalize knowledge of client's illness, care requirements, safe use of medications, and so forth
- Demonstrate needed psychomotor skills independently

Therapeutic Aims

- Teach needed physical care skills.
- Provide necessary information and support.
- Promote a safe environment.
- Facilitate establishment of new routines.

Implementation

Nursing Interventions	Rationale
Help the caregiver identify potential hazards in the home.	The home situation must be physically safe for the client.
If the client requires constant supervision at home, help the caregiver plan to do daily chores, errands, and recreational activities when someone else is available to stay with the client.	The caregiver must be able to manage the home and do necessary chores. Also, the caregiver needs periods of relief from constant involvement with the client.
Discourage the caregiver from making unnecessary changes in the client's immediate environment. Encourage the development of a routine for the client's activities at home. (This routine does not have to be strictly rigid but should have some structure.)	Familiar activities help the client to maintain reality orientation, which also helps the caregiver. The caregiver needs to feel that some flexibility is acceptable so that he or she does not feel like a slave to the client and his or her routine.
Help the caregiver plan how to manage visitors at home (not too many in one day, preferably one or two people at a time, and so forth).	The client will be less confused and be able to enjoy visitors more if he or she is not too fatigued by too many people at once. Too much stimulation can increase confusion or acting-out behavior.
Remind the caregiver that the client's memory may be very poor and that this is out of the client's control.	Recognition of the client's memory impairment can help the caregiver avoid the frustration of repeated explanations and avoid expecting the client to work harder to remember.
Allow the caregiver to observe you working with the client during meals and other activities of daily living.	The caregiver can learn techniques by watching you and practicing them with supervision.
Gradually increase the caregiver's responsibility for mealtimes and other activities of daily living until he or she is ready for the primary role in each area.	Gradual assumption of responsibility will enable the caregiver to feel less overwhelmed and move at his or her own pace, which will enhance the chances for success.
Encourage the caregiver to discuss any feelings he or she may have about meeting the client's personal needs.	The caregiver may be repulsed or upset by the idea of an adult parent or family member needing help with bathing, dressing, and so forth.
Encourage the caregiver to discuss feelings associated with role reversal. ("My mother used to help me dress when I was a child, and now I'm helping her get dressed.")	It may be difficult for the caregiver to see a parent, spouse, or partner (on whom the caregiver used to depend) become dependent on the caregiver.
Remind the caregiver that the client is not a child. In fact a child can be expected to learn to provide self-care independently—the client may not be able to do so.	When seeing childlike behaviors (such as the inability to dress oneself), it is easy to begin treating the client like a child. This must be avoided to preserve the client's dignity.

❋ *(continued)*
Implementation

Nursing Interventions	Rationale
Encourage structure in daily routines. Caution the caregiver to avoid letting the client sleep whenever he or she desires, such as all day.	An established regular routine also allows the caregiver to sleep at night, which is a more normal pattern. This also enables the caregiver to meet his or her own needs for sleep.
Ask the caregiver about the client's previous bedtime routines, and encourage adherence to prior routines.	The client may be unable to provide this information. Replicating prior habits will enhance successful adherence in the future.

Nursing Diagnosis

Social Isolation (3.1.2)

Aloneness experienced by the individual and perceived as imposed by others and as a negative or threatened state.

❋
Assessment Data

Defining Characteristics

- Disinterest in previous hobbies or other pleasurable activities
- Refusal to leave the client in the care of someone else
- Feelings of helplessness
- Feelings of frustration
- Absence of other support people
- Failure to use available resources

Related Factors

- Reluctance to engage in social activities related to the client's inappropriate social behavior
- Embarrassment of caregiver
- Use of alcohol, tranquilizers, or other mood-altering drugs

❋
Expected Outcomes

Initial

The caregiver will:

- Verbalize plans to meet his or her own needs independent of the caregiving situation
- Express feelings related to his or her unmet needs

Discharge

The caregiver will:

- Implement plans for using resources to help care for the client
- Manage his or her own feelings regarding the client's behavior
- Implement plans to meet his or her own needs independent of the caregiving situation
- Use coping strategies to deal with stress without abusing alcohol or drugs

❀ Therapeutic Aims

- Decrease feelings of hopelessness.
- Minimize social isolation.

❀ Implementation

Nursing Interventions	Rationale
Encourage the caregiver to discuss his or her feelings of embarrassment related to the client's inappropriate social behavior.	The caregiver can use you as a sounding board—he or she may not be able to share these feelings with the client or other family members.
Remind the caregiver that indiscriminate undressing, profanity, and other inappropriate behaviors are not within the client's conscious control; they are part of the illness.	Out of frustration, the caregiver may become angry with the client about his or her behavior. It is important that the caregiver make a distinction between the client and his or her behavior and deal with behaviors without punishing the client. The caregiver can then express anger to others and not become angry at the client.
Role play with the caregiver to help him or her have a short explanation to give visitors or others regarding the client's behavior.	If the caregiver practices what to say and how to prepare others for the client's behavior, he or she can alleviate some of the shock or discomfort experienced when the client displays such behavior. The caregiver is less likely to become isolated if feelings of guilt or embarrassment are minimized.
Encourage the caregiver to continue any activities in which the client can engage and feel successful and that the client and caregiver enjoy.	Fun activities between the client and caregiver can enhance their relationship. Not all of the interactions between the client and the caregiver have to be centered on care and physical or emotional dependence.
Encourage the caregiver to plan time away from home regularly to meet his or her own needs. The caregiver should not wait until the client is better or until the caregiver "can't take anymore."	The caregiver needs to spend personal time away from the client regularly. Burnout can occur quickly if the caregiver has no relief.
Refer the caregiver or family members to local or national support groups as indicated by the client's problem.	These groups can offer support, education, and resources to the client's significant others.

Section Two

Chronic Mental Illness

Clients who are chronically mentally ill have a broad range of problems. Many clients have spent years in a long-term hospital setting and were then discharged through the process of deinstitutionalization. Some of these clients may have been hospitalized as adults, with problems such as schizophrenia or bipolar affective disorder. Others may have been institutionalized in facilities for the mentally retarded when they were children and have been discharged into the community as adults. In addition to the difficulties encountered because of retardation or a major psychiatric illness, these clients have special needs as a result of having lived in a long-term facility. Their basic needs may have been cared for by the staff of the institution, sometimes for many years; consequently, they have become very dependent. Often, they have minimal skills in meeting their own needs independently. These are skills that the community assumes that any adult can do, such as using the telephone or public transportation, buying groceries, preparing meals, doing laundry, and so forth. The inability of such clients to care for themselves in these ways may have nothing to do with their psychiatric illness or retardation but may be the result of long-term institutional living.

Another segment of the chronically ill population, one that is rapidly expanding, are clients who have not been in long-term care facilities for extended time periods. Instead, these clients have lived in the community, either on their own or in an environment that is structured or supervised to some degree. Such clients often are intermittently admitted to acute care facilities and discharged to a community setting. They may or may not receive care on an outpatient basis between hospital admissions.

The care plans in this section are designed to assist nurses in providing care for chronically mentally ill clients in the hospital during an acute episode of the illness and in the community setting between episodes of acute care or addressing problems following long-term institutionalization.

Acute Episode Care

Chronically ill clients living in the community often need short-term hospitalizations periodically or extended supervision in a sheltered setting. This may result from an exacerbation of psychiatric symptoms or from a lack of success in community living, often related to failure to take medication as prescribed or to disordered water balance (DWB). DWB, also called psychogenic polydipsia, can lead to water intoxication and has become a major management problem for many clients with chronic mental illness. Financial difficulties, whether from lack of successful employment or limited governmental support, usually complicate the client's problems. Often, the type of services the client may need for success does not exist in his or her community or may have waiting lists.

Psychiatric treatment and nursing care of chronically ill clients usually center around minimizing inpatient hospitalization, maximizing client independence and self-reliance, decreasing dependence on institutions and services, and placing the client in the community in an environment that has the least restriction. Nurses must work closely with community agencies and personnel to achieve these objectives.

The nurse also must be aware of his or her attitudes toward the chronically ill client. It can be quite frustrating to see the client return to the hospital setting repeatedly or not to succeed after careful planning for follow-up or placement. Another pitfall in working with the chronically ill is failing to view these clients as adults. This may be particularly true if the client exhibits immature or attention-seeking behavior. Though it is difficult for the professional, it is necessary to take a "fresh look" at the client's behavior, problems, and situation with each admission to provide effective care and promote the client's chances for future success. It also is important not to take the client's readmissions personally or to see them as failures of the staff or of the client.

Nursing Diagnoses Addressed in this Care Plan

Impaired Adjustment
Ineffective Management of Therapeutic Regimen (individuals)
Altered Health Maintenance

Related Nursing Diagnoses

Altered Thought Processes
Sensory/Perceptual Alterations
High Risk for Injury

Nursing Diagnosis

Impaired Adjustment (5.1.1.1.1)

The state in which the individual is unable to modify his or her life-style or behavior in a manner consistent with a change in health status.

Assessment Data

Defining Characteristics	• Poor impulse control
	• Difficulty making decisions and choices
	• Limited ability to deal with stress or changes
	• Feelings of fear, hopelessness, and inadequacy
	• Low self-esteem
	• Anxiety
Related Factors	• Self-destructive behavior
	• Acting-out behavior
	• Disrupted sleep patterns
	• History of repeated hospitalizations
	• Mental retardation
	• Major mental illness
	• Personality disorder
	• Limited financial resources

Expected Outcomes

Initial	*The client will:*
	• Be free of injury
	• Decrease acting-out behavior
	• Verbally express feelings of fear, hopelessness, inadequacy, if present
Discharge	*The client will:*
	• Return to the community to the least restrictive environment that is safe
	• Establish interpersonal relationships in the community setting that are unrelated to the hospital

⬛
Therapeutic Aims

- Provide a safe environment.
- Assist the client to express feelings.

⬛
Implementation

Nursing Interventions	Rationale
Ask the client about any ideas or plans for suicide.	The client's safety is a priority.
Remove any potentially harmful objects from the client's possession (razor, nail file, and so forth).	These items may be used for self-destructive actions or acting out toward others.
Remove the client to a quiet area or seclusion if he or she is acting out.	Acting-out behavior usually decreases when the client is alone or has no one to pay attention to the behavior.
Withdraw your attention when the client is acting out. Tell the client you will return when he or she is more in control.	Your inattention to the client's behavior will facilitate the extinction of the behavior. Your stated intent to return conveys your acceptance of the client.
Encourage the client to talk about his or her feelings when the client is not upset or acting out.	The client will be better able to verbalize feelings when he or she is not overwhelmed by them, or is not in control of his or her behavior.
As the client gains skill in discussing feelings, encourage the client to talk with someone when he or she begins to become upset rather than acting out.	After the client is able to verbalize feelings, he or she can begin to use expression of feelings to replace acting out.
Teach the client a step-by-step problem-solving process. For example, identify the problem, examine alternatives, weigh the pros and cons of each alternative, and select an approach.	The client may not know the steps of a logical, orderly process to solve problems.

Nursing Diagnosis

Ineffective Management of Therapeutic Regimen (5.2.1.)

A pattern of regulating and integrating into daily living a program for treatment of illness and the sequelae of illness that is unsatisfactory for meeting specific health goals.

⬛
Assessment Data

Defining Characteristics

- Noncompliance with prescribed medications
- Psychogenic polydipsia (excessive intake of water or other fluids)
- Increase or worsening of psychiatric symptoms

Related Factors

- Episodic, excessive intake of alcohol or other substances
- Inadequate financial resources
- Lack of knowledge or understanding of therapeutic regimen
- Mistrust of health care professionals or system

❋
Expected Outcomes

Initial	*The client will:*

- Ingest all medications as prescribed
- Establish fluid intake–output balance

Discharge	*The client will:*

- Verbalize intent to comply or demonstrate ingestion of prescribed medication
- Demonstrate ability to monitor own fluid intake without staff intervention

❋
Therapeutic Aims

- Promote compliance with therapeutic regimen.
- Facilitate development of self-care skills.

❋
Implementation

Nursing Interventions	Rationale
Observe the client closely to ensure ingestion of medications.	The client must ingest medications as prescribed before their effectiveness can be determined.
Explore the client's reasons for noncompliance with medications: Can the client afford the medication? Does he or she forget to take it? Is the client resistant to taking medications?	Identifying the reason for noncompliance will determine your interventions to gain the client's compliance.
If the client cannot afford to purchase the medication, refer him or her to social services for help to obtain financial assistance.	The client may need financial assistance if that is the only barrier to compliance.
If the client cannot remember to take medications, set up a system with him or her to check off the medication times or use a pill box with separate compartments for each dose.	A concrete system for taking medications minimizes problems the client has with trying to remember without being reminded.
If the client is resistant, you may wish to discuss with the physician use of long-acting intramuscular medications or attempting to manage without medications.	Noncompliance due to resistance is the most difficult to change. The client does have the right to refuse medications. It is preferable to know that the client is not taking medication rather than to assume compliance.
Teach the client about polydipsia or disordered water balance (DWB).	The client may lack knowledge about the severe medical consequences of DWB or may fail to understand how drinking water (or other "harmless" fluids) could be a problem.
If the client is severely water "intoxicated," medical treatment may be required. The client may require seclusion and be allowed only supervised access to water.	Severe water intoxication causes confusion, increased psychosis, hyponatremia, lethargy, and seizures. The client must be "dried out" to a normal baseline of fluid balance before he or she can benefit from any teaching to learn self-control of water intake.

✪ *(continued)*
Implementation

Nursing Interventions	Rationale
If the client is able to monitor his or her own weight, a target weight protocol can be used in the management of DWB. The client is taught to regulate fluid intake to keep his or her weight under a preset "target" of no more than a 7% weight increase.	Clients with the internal control to regulate water consumption based on the frequent monitoring of body weight have been reported to have success in preventing further episodes of water intoxication (Snider and Boyd, 1991).
Another behavioral approach to management of DWB involves setting a designated amount of fluid to be consumed every 30 to 60 minutes throughout the day. Assist the client to form a checklist to monitor compliance with this type of approach.	This structured approach can be useful with clients experiencing difficulty delaying gratification (drinking fluids) or making decisions about whether or not to drink fluids, how much to drink, and so forth.
If the client experiences anxiety in concert with the desire for increased fluids, teach the client a relaxation technique, such as progressive muscle relaxation.	Relieving the client's anxiety will enhance his or her ability to resist drinking increased amounts of fluid.
Offer the client gum or hard candy if he or she complains of excessive thirst.	Gum or hard candy can help the client limit fluid intake.
Assess the client's use of alcohol or other chemicals. If chemical use is a major problem for the client, you may consider a referral to a treatment program.	Alcohol and other mood-altering drugs can interfere with the effectiveness of the client's prescribed medication, fluid and electrolyte balance, and general health status.

Nursing Diagnosis

Altered Health Maintenance (6.4.2)

Inability to identify, manage, and/or seek help to maintain health.

Assessment Data

Defining Characteristics	• Lack of independent living skills • Lack of social skills • Difficulty handling unstructured time • Poor nutritional intake • Ineffective interpersonal relationships
Related Factors	• Lack of supportive relationships with family or significant others • History of repeated hospitalizations • Social isolation

❊
Expected Outcomes

Initial	*The client will:*

- Establish nutritious eating habits
- Participate in activities or hobbies
- Demonstrate adequate personal hygiene skills

Discharge	*The client will:*

- Verbalize plans for use of unstructured time
- Demonstrate basic independent living skills
- Accept referral to planned programs, such as vocational or sheltered workshops, recreational or outpatient groups, or community support services

❊
Therapeutic Aims

- Promote knowledge about nutrition.
- Maximize independent living skills.
- Minimize reliance on hospital.
- Promote return to the community.

❊
Implementation

Nursing Interventions	Rationale
Encourage the client to eat nutritious meals. Assess the client's selection of food at mealtimes.	You will be able to evaluate the client's knowledge about basic foods needed for a nutritious diet.
Help the client plan meals in advance, perhaps for 1 week. Consider the client's food preparation skills and income; does he or she receive financial assistance for food?	Making a plan and following through each week will help the client budget enough money for nutritious food and will avoid the necessity for daily decisions about what to eat.
Assess the client's ability to perform essential daily skills, such as using the phone book, using the transportation system, knowing how to get emergency assistance, and so forth. Have the client demonstrate these skills when possible.	A baseline of the client's skill level is necessary for you to determine how well he or she performs certain skills. You can then determine the interventions needed to assist the client to learn the skills. Demonstrations are helpful, because the client may be unable to explain what he or she can do, or the client may say "I know that" because he or she is too embarrassed to admit a knowledge deficit.
For any skill the client needs to learn, give simple step-by-step directions.	Small parts of a task are easier to learn than tackling the whole task at once.
Perform the skill with the client initially, and gradually progress to the client's independent performance of the skill.	It may be easier for the client to learn the skill by observing how it is done before he or she can progress to independence.
Encourage the client to develop routines for personal hygiene and grooming activities.	The client is more likely to follow through if he or she is following a routine rather than having to decide each time whether or not to bathe, change clothes, wash hair, and so forth.

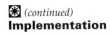 *(continued)*
Implementation

Nursing Interventions	Rationale
Give the client honest praise for accomplishments.	Positive feedback for independent skills will increase the frequency of the behavior and enhance the client's self-esteem.
Assess the client's level of interest and participation in leisure or recreational activities.	If you can build on previous interests, it may be easier to obtain the client's involvement.
Explore possible alternatives for "fun" activities. Help the client try new activities. Keep in mind the cost of the activity and whether it requires the participation of other people.	The client may not have had many successful leisure activities. It would be frustrating to the client to begin a new hobby that he or she could not afford or to learn card games or board games if most of the client's leisure time is solitary.
Involve the client in social interactions with others to practice social skills. The client may need to learn what topics generally are acceptable for social conversation.	You can be a role model for the client in social interchanges. The client may need to learn to avoid certain topics when in social situations, for example, not discussing hospitalizations when he or she first meets someone.
Ask the client to describe what he or she does during a usual day, week, and weekend. Writing down the activities may be helpful.	You can obtain data regarding the amount of unstructured time the client has available.
Help the client make a specific plan for unstructured time. It can include activities alone or with others, leisure activities, or whatever the client desires.	The client is more likely to follow a plan for dealing with unstructured time. This will decrease the chance of the client ruminating and becoming more isolated.
Indicate your expectation at the beginning of the hospitalization that the client will return to the community setting.	Your positive approach may help decrease the client's dependence on an institution.
Do not allow the client to become too comfortable or settled while hospitalized. Always focus your behavior and interaction on the client's achievement of expected outcomes and discharge. The client who returns frequently to the hospital should not be greeted as a friend but as a person who is hospitalized on a short-term basis for specific reasons.	The client's hospitalization must be focused on therapeutic work toward expected outcomes and discharge. If the client views hospitalization as a comfortable rest from the challenges of life, he or she is more likely to become dependent on the institution and the staff and less likely to participate in treatment and work toward discharge as a goal.
Help the client make plans to deal with changes or problems that may occur while he or she is living in the community. Role playing might be helpful.	If the client has an idea of what he or she can anticipate and alternative ways to deal with stress or change, he or she is less likely to return to the hospital as soon as he or she encounters any crisis.

Community Based Care

In the United States more clients with chronic mental illness (CMI) are receiving care in the community than at any other time. This is due, in part, to the continued goals of deinstitutionalization and short-term hospitalizations for younger clients to avoid the problems of institutionalization. Many people are now in the 25- to 45-year-old age group as a result of the "baby boom." This also is the age group in which the majority of people with CMI are found. In addition, symptoms are now controlled better with medications currently used in mental illness care, thus enabling clients to remain in the community for longer periods of time.

Nurses work with chronically mentally ill clients in many settings other than the acute psychiatric units of hospitals. These clients are seen in emergency rooms with increasing frequency and are being referred to public health and community health nurses for ongoing care. Nurses also are providing a wide variety of services as nurse–case managers. Community support programs are spreading across the country in an effort to serve the needs of this population.

One of the reasons that traditional methods of treatment are unsuccessful with clients who are functionally impaired is that these methods do not address the primary problems of this group. Clients with CMI typically are readmitted to hospitals due to frustration, stress, and the poor quality of their lives, not just due to the reemergence of psychiatric symptoms. Drew (1991) writes that the "diminished mental and emotional resources suffered by those with CMI often lead to impoverished relationships that fail to produce satisfying connections with others. As a result, people with CMI frequently are chronically lonely" (p. 17).

Clients with chronic mental illness experience "positive" signs of illness, such as delusions and hallucinations, which usually respond in some degree to chemotherapy. Frequently, the presence or absence of these signs is the criterion for admission and discharge in the acute setting. Gomez and Gomez (1991) identify the need to reduce the "negative" signs of schizophrenia to avoid outcomes of nonproductivity and emptiness for the client. The negative signs are social withdrawal, anhedonia (inability to experience pleasure), anergy (lack of energy), and apathy. Unfortunately, these do not necessarily respond to medications and are some of the major barriers to a successful adjustment in the community for the client.

Skills needed for community living fall into five categories:

1. *Activities of daily living.* This includes personal hygiene, grooming, room care, laundry upkeep, restaurant utilization, cooking, shopping, budgeting, public transportation, telephone use, and procurement of needed services and financial support. Many clients have difficulty in more than one of these major areas. These difficulties may be due to lack of knowledge, skill, experience, or support.
2. *Vocational skills.* This area may include paid employment in a competitive or sheltered work setting, volunteer work, or any productive, useful service that the client perceives as making a contribution. Clients may lack specific work skills or good work habits, job-seeking or job-keeping skills, or interest or motivation.
3. *Leisure skills.* This area involves the ability to choose, plan, and follow through with pleasurable activities during unstructured time. Clients may lack the interest or skills to fill their free time or may lack leisure habit patterns, such as watching television, reading the newspaper, and so forth.
4. *Health maintenance.* Managing medications, keeping appointments, preventing or treating physical illnesses, and crisis management are included in this area. Clients with chronic mental illness frequently use medications inappropriately, use chemicals, drink alcohol, or trade medications with friends. These clients often do not recognize or seek treatment for physical illness, and they are reluctant to return for appointments for a variety of reasons: denial of illness, lack of control over their lives, fear of hospitals and physicians, and so forth.
5. *Social skills.* This is a broad category ranging from social conversation to dealing with landlords and service providers to talking about feelings and problems. When clients have severe social skill deficits, it results in increased difficulties in the other four areas, as well as the inability to maintain a state of well-being.

Outreach programs, in which practitioners go to the clients in their own environments, have been most successful in working with clients to develop needed skills. Neutral settings, such as community support services and drop-in centers, also have been more successful than traditional outpatient or hospital-based day programs. This can be partially attributed to a "less clinical" approach and the lack of association with inpatient treatment. The ability to generalize knowledge frequently is impaired with chronic clients; learning skills in their own homes or community eliminates that very difficult step.

Nursing Diagnoses Addressed in this Care Plan

Altered Health Maintenance
Impaired Social Interaction
Diversional Activity Deficit

Related Nursing Diagnoses

Social Isolation
Self-Esteem Disturbance
Impaired Home Maintenance Management
Altered Thought Processes
Ineffective Individual Coping

Nursing Diagnosis	*Altered Health Maintenance (6.4.2)*
	Inability to identify, manage, or seek help to maintain health.

Assessment Data

Defining Characteristics	• Lack of daily living skills
	• Difficulty making choices
	• Deficient problem-solving skills
	• Apathy
	• Anergy
	• Low frustration tolerance

Related Factors	• Inadequate financial support
	• Mistrust of agencies or professionals
	• Information processing deficits
	• History of sporadic compliance with treatment
	• Self-medication
	• Recurrent psychiatric symptoms

Expected Outcomes

Initial

The client will:

- Maintain contact with community professionals
- Communicate accurate information regarding symptoms, medication compliance, eating habits, and so forth
- Participate in planning self-care

Discharge

The client will:

- Verbalize knowledge of illness, treatment, safe use of medications, and independent living skills
- Seek medical treatment for health-related needs
- Demonstrate maintenance of safe home environment
- Demonstrate adherence to established daily routine
- Demonstrate adequate independence in activities of daily living

Therapeutic Aims

- Increase client participation in treatment.
- Promote independent living skills.
- Promote health maintenance behavior.

Implementation

Nursing Interventions	Rationale
Engage the client in mutual goal setting, such as avoiding hospitalization, becoming more satisfied with his or her life, meeting needs, and so forth.	The client's willingness to participate is increased if he or she values the reasons for doing so.
Use an assertive approach when attempting to engage the client in a particular activity.	A positive attitude is conveyed with this approach. The client may respond to a tentative approach with a negative answer, and there will be no opportunity to proceed.
Be directive with the client, and do not ask "yes/no" questions or questions that require a choice. For example, say "It is time for group," rather than "Do you want to go to group?"	The client is likely to respond "no" to "yes/no" questions because of the negativism he or she feels, or it may simply seem easier not to do something.
Use a behavioral approach when teaching skills.	A behavioral approach decreases reliance on the client's verbal skills and ability to think abstractly.
Model the skill or behavior for the client.	Modeling provides a clear, concrete example of what is expected.
Coach the client to replicate the skill or behavior.	Coaching allows *shaping*—a behavioral procedure in which successive approximations of a desired behavior are positively reinforced—toward successful completion of the target behavior.
Prompt the client to continue practicing the skill or behavior. Reinforce success with verbal praise and tangible rewards, such as a soda, a snack, and so forth.	The client may need reminders because of a lack of interest or initiative. Coupling verbal praise with tangible rewards is the most successful means of reinforcement. It helps the client perpetuate the behavior or skill until it becomes part of his or her daily routine.
Teach the client a basic problem-solving sequence. It may help to write the steps.	Problem solving in a methodic fashion may be a skill the client has never had, or it may have been impaired by his or her illness.
Help the client establish a daily schedule. Writing on a daily or weekly calendar is usually helpful. Once the client agrees to a particular appointment or activity, instruct the client to write it on the calendar.	A written schedule provides a visual aid to which the client can refer. Once the client has written it on the calendar, it is more likely that he or she will follow through, much as with a written contract.
Assess the client for living skills that are absent or need improvement. Include hygiene, grooming, shopping, obtaining housing, budgeting, using telephones and transportation, cooking, and ability to call a doctor or other agencies for service.	A variety of skills is needed for independent living. It is imperative to identify deficient areas as the initial step of the learning process.
Teach the client about cooking and requirements for adequate nutrition. Referral to a dietitian may be indicated.	The client may have little or no knowledge of nutritional needs or food preparation skills.

⚛ *(continued)*
Implementation

Nursing Interventions	Rationale
Have the client demonstrate skills if possible. If skills are assessed verbally, avoid asking "Do you know how to . . .?" Rather, say "Tell me how you . . . ."	Areas such as hygiene or grooming are easily assessed by the client's appearance. Skill demonstration may be necessary in less evident areas, such as use of telephone or transportation. If you ask the client if he or she has a particular skill, the response may be "yes" because the client is embarrassed at not having the skill or because the client mistakenly believes that he or she has the skill.
Teach skills in the client's own environment when possible. For example if teaching how to do laundry, use the laundromat the client will use regularly.	Transferring or generalizing knowledge from one situation to another may be difficult for the client.
Review with the client the events that have led to increases in psychiatric symptoms or hospitalizations.	The client's awareness can be increased regarding the relatedness of particular health behaviors and recurrence of his or her illness.
Instruct the client about signs of physical illness that require medical attention. Give specific parameters, such as a "fever of 102°F."	Specific indicators are easier for the client to recognize, because the client's judgment often is ineffective.
Assist the client to identify the clinic or physician services that he or she will contact if physical illness occurs.	It is easier to choose health care providers when the client is well, before an urgent situation develops. Knowing who to call when a need arises will help the client follow through.
Encourage the client to discuss with his or her physician any difficulties with medications or needs for changes before the client initiates changes on his or her own.	This strategy preserves the client's sense of participation in managing his or her health, while providing a way for the client to meet perceived needs regarding medication changes.
Tell the client that if he or she does alter the pattern of medications without professional help, you would like him or her to report this honestly.	It is more important to have accurate information on which to base decisions than to create the illusion of a "good" patient.
Give the client positive feedback for attempts in the self-care area and for honesty in reporting.	Even if attempts at self-care are unsuccessful initially, it is important to reinforce the client's sense of personal control over his or her life and honesty in relationships with health care providers.
Teach the client and his or her family and significant others, if any, about the client's illness, treatment, and safe use of medications.	The client and his or her significant others may have little or no knowledge of the client's illness, treatment, or medications.

Nursing Diagnosis

Impaired Social Interaction (3.1.1)

The state in which an individual participates in an insufficient or excessive quantity or in-effective quality of social exchange.

Assessment Data

Defining Characteristics	• Feelings of worthlessness • Difficulty initiating interaction • Lack of social skills • Social withdrawal
Related Factors	• Low self-esteem • Overstimulation from environmental stress • Mental illness • Absence of available significant others

Expected Outcomes

Initial	*The client will:* • Engage in social interactions • Demonstrate acceptance of feedback from others
Discharge	*The client will:* • Verbalize increased feelings of self-worth • Continue to participate in social activities • Verbalize decreased anxiety during social interactions • Communicate with others in sufficient quantity to meet basic needs

Therapeutic Aims

• Facilitate development of social skills.
• Promote self-esteem.

Implementation

Nursing Interventions	Rationale
Teach the client social skills. Describe and demonstrate specific skills, such as eye contact, attentive listening, nodding, and so forth. Discuss the type of topics that is appropriate for casual social conversation, such as the weather, local events, news, and so forth.	The client may have little or no knowledge of social interaction skills. Modeling provides a concrete example of the desired skills.
Assist the client to approach someone and ask a question. Use real-life situations, such as seeking assistance in a store, asking directions, or renting an apartment.	Asking questions is an essential skill in daily life. Using real situations makes the exercise more meaningful for the client.

✳ *(continued)*
Implementation

Nursing Interventions	Rationale
Practice giving and receiving compliments with the client. Make sure compliments are sincere.	Chronically mentally ill clients rarely notice things about other people without practicing that skill. Likewise, receiving compliments can be an awkward situation due to low self-esteem.
Role play situations in which the client must accept "no" to a request and in which the client must appropriately refuse a request from someone else.	Low frustration tolerance makes hearing a negative answer difficult for the client. Clients frequently comply with requests from others, then regret doing so because they are unable to refuse in a socially appropriate manner.

Nursing Diagnosis

Diversional Activity Deficit (6.3.1.1)

The state in which an individual experiences decreased stimulation from or interest or engagement in recreational or leisure activities.

✳
Assessment Data

Defining Characteristics

- Anhedonia
- Inattentiveness
- Feelings of boredom
- Expressed desire for purposeful activity
- Lack of leisure skills
- Inability to manage unstructured time

Related Factors

- Inadequate financial resources or transportation
- Impaired functional abilities

✳
Expected Outcomes

Initial

The client will:

- Participate in leisure activities
- Express feelings of satisfaction with a leisure activity

Discharge

The client will:

- Engage in leisure activities independently
- Participate in productive activities

✳
Therapeutic Aims

- Promote development of leisure skills and productive activities.
- Promote self-esteem.
- Relieve boredom.

Implementation

Nursing Interventions	Rationale
Encourage the client to develop some leisure habits, such as reading the newspaper or watching television at a certain time each day. It may be beneficial to have the client write these activities on a daily schedule.	Lack of interest or past pleasure experiences in activities causes clients to be reluctant to try them. Establishing routine habits eliminates the need to make a decision about whether or not to pursue an activity each day.
Engage the client with others. If a drop-in center or other service is available, accompany the client to acquaint him or her with others. Plan a group activity that three or four clients attend.	It is important for the client to establish a social network, because professionals cannot meet all of his or her needs. The client is not likely to form relationships independently.
Assist the client in identifying and trying activities that are free or low cost, such as taking walks, attending free concerts, and so forth.	Chronically mentally ill clients usually have limited financial resources. The cost of movies, bowling, or independent transportation prohibits frequent participation in these types of activities.
Assist the client in finding a suitable volunteer activity or an activity involving helping other people, animals, or the environment. Refer to vocational services as appropriate.	Many clients resist doing things just for fun, because these activities don't provide a sense of productivity or of making a useful contribution. Feeling useful or needed enhances self-esteem.

Section Three

Adolescent Clients

Adolescence is often described as a phase of development characterized by turmoil, crises, and acting-out behavior. Anna Freud (1961) wrote that adolescent turmoil is "... by its nature an interruption in peaceful growth ... the upholding of a steady equilibrium during the adolescent process is in itself abnormal. It is normal for an adolescent to behave for a considerable length of time in an inconsistent and unpredictable manner." Others postulate that the intense turmoil some adolescents experience is due to lack of success in completing developmental tasks. The adolescent who is unable to cope with the stress and challenge of developing a sense of identity and sexuality, separation from family, and attainment of social and vocational competence may exhibit clinical symptoms that require mental health intervention and are addressed in this section: attention deficit disorders, conduct disorders, and adjustment reactions.

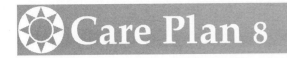

Attention Deficit Disorders

Attention deficit disorders (ADD) involve developmentally inappropriate degrees of inattention, impulsivity, and hyperactivity (DSM-III-R, 1987). ADD usually is identified when a child enters the educational system. It is common to observe hyperactivity as a major component of the disorder in younger children, though this is less likely to be a primary feature in adolescents. It also is possible to have ADD without hyperactivity; however, this occurs less frequently. Many of the interventions for treatment of childhood ADD are similar to those for the adolescent. The participation of school personnel is a crucial element in the successful treatment of both.

It is important to distinguish ADD from other childhood disorders, as well as from behavior in a child who is simply difficult to manage. Diagnosis of ADD by trained professionals is required, because children from chaotic environments often are mislabeled as hyperactive, when problem behaviors are occurring due to other factors (for example, abuse, head injuries, or learning disabilities). Manifestations of ADD are prevalent in all of the child's environments (home, school, social situations), whereas other types of problems often occur only in particular situations.

In the educational setting the client frequently experiences poor performance or failure. Problems include incomplete assignments, difficulty with organization, and incorrect and messy work. Verbally, the client disrupts others, fails to heed directions, interrupts, and is unable to take turns in conversations. At home the client is accident prone, knocks things over, and is intrusive with family members. With peers the client is unable to follow the rules of games, fails to take turns, and appears oblivious to the desires or requests of others. By adolescence hyperactive behavior usually is reduced to fidgeting and an inability to sit for sustained periods of time.

Many individuals experience problems with ADD into adulthood. This is particularly true if no effective treatment was received earlier. The client may have a long history of unsuccessful experiences, both socially and academically. It is estimated that one third of the children with ADD have some type of major difficulty as an adult, such as adjustment disorders or underachievement.

Children with ADD frequently are given medication to decrease hyperactive and distracting behavior. Stimulant medication, such as methylphenidate hydrochloride (Ritalin) or pemoline (Cylert), is given for the paradoxic effects of calming the child's behavior. This medication is discontinued when the child reaches puberty, because it is no longer effective.

Nursing Diagnoses Addressed in this Care Plan

High Risk for Injury
Impaired Social Interaction

Related Nursing Diagnoses

Ineffective Management of Therapeutic Regimen (individuals)
Self-Esteem Disturbance
Ineffective Family Coping: Disabling

Nursing Diagnosis	***High Risk for Injury (1.6.1)*** *A state in which the individual is at risk of injury as a result of environmental conditions interacting with the individual's adaptive and defensive resources.*

Risk Factors

- Motor-perceptual dysfunction, for example, poor hand–eye coordination
- Inability to perceive potentially harmful situations
- Intrusive behavior with others

Expected Outcomes

Initial	*The client will:*

- Be free of injury or unnecessary risks
- Respond to limits regarding intrusion on others

Discharge	*The client will:*

- Engage in activities without taking unnecessary risks
- Demonstrate decreased intrusive behavior

Therapeutic Aims

- Provide a safe environment.
- Decrease intrusive behavior.

Implementation

Nursing Interventions	Rationale
Talk with the client about safe and unsafe behavior. Explain to the client that accidents will result in increased supervision and that purposeful unsafe behavior will have consequences.	This provides the client with clear expectations.
Assess the frequency and severity of accidents.	It is necessary to establish a baseline prior to planning interventions.

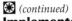 *(continued)*
Implementation

Nursing Interventions	Rationale
Provide supervision for potentially dangerous situations. Limit the client's participation in activities when safety cannot be assured.	The client's ability to perceive harmful consequences of a behavior is impaired.
Attempt to distinguish between accidents and behaviors that are deliberate.	Physical safety is a priority. Accidents will require increased supervision, but deliberate actions can be altered with behavioral techniques.
Assist the client's parents or caregivers to make the distinction between accidental and purposeful incidents.	This will enable them to deal with behaviors at home more effectively.
If the situation is determined to be accidental, institute safeguards or limitations as appropriate.	Different interventions are instituted for accidents than for deliberate actions.
If the situation is determined to be deliberate, institute consequences in a nonpunitive manner.	Logical consequences for an undesirable behavior can diminish the occurrence of the behavior.
Do not assume that the client knows proper or expected behavior. State expectations for behavior in clear terms.	Developmentally, the client may be unable to process social cues to guide reasonable behavior choices.
Make corrective feedback as specific as possible.	Specific feedback will help the client understand expectations.
Provide consequences that are directly related to the undesirable behavior. Institute consequences as soon as possible after the occurrence of the behavior.	The client will be better able to draw the correlation between undesirable behavior and consequences if the two are related to each other.

Nursing Diagnosis

Impaired Social Interaction (3.1.1)
The state in which an individual participates in an insufficient or excessive quantity or ineffective quality of social exchange.

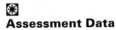
Assessment Data

__Defining Characteristics__

- Short attention span
- High level of distractibility
- Labile moods
- Low frustration tolerance
- Inability to complete tasks
- Inability to sit still or fidgeting
- Excessive talking
- Inability to follow directions

❋ *(continued)*
Assessment Data

Related Factors	• Academic underachievement • Low self-esteem • Frequent loss of possessions and necessary items

❋
Expected Outcomes

Initial	*The client will:* • Successfully complete tasks or assignments with assistance • Demonstrate acceptable social skills while interacting with staff or family member
Discharge	*The client will:* • Participate successfully in the educational setting • Demonstrate the ability to complete single tasks independently • Demonstrate the ability to complete tasks with reminders • Verbalize positive statements about himself or herself • Demonstrate successful interactions with family members

❋
Therapeutic Aims

• Promote self-esteem.
• Decrease distractibility.
• Maximize attention span.
• Promote successful interactions.

❋
Implementation

Nursing Interventions	Rationale
Identify the factors that aggrevate and alleviate the client's performance.	The external stimuli that exacerbate the client's problems can be identified and minimized. Likewise, any that positively influence the client can be effectively used.
Provide an environment as free of distractions as possible. Institute interventions on a one-to-one basis. Gradually increase the amount of environmental stimuli.	The client's ability to deal with external stimulation is impaired.
Engage the client's attention before giving instructions (that is, call the client's name and establish eye contact).	The client must hear instructions as a first step toward compliance.
Give instructions slowly, using simple language and concrete directions.	The client's ability to comprehend instructions (especially if they are complex or abstract) is impaired.
Ask the client to repeat instructions before beginning tasks.	Repetition demonstrates that the client has accurately received the information.
Separate complex tasks into small steps.	The likelihood of success is enhanced with less complicated components of a task.

✸ *(continued)*
Implementation

Nursing Interventions	Rationale
Provide positive feedback for completion of each step.	The client's opportunity for successful experiences is increased by treating each step as an opportunity for success.
Allow breaks, during which the client can move around.	The client's restless energy can be given an acceptable outlet, so he or she can attend to future tasks more effectively.
State expectations for task completion clearly.	The client must understand the request before he or she can attempt task completion.
Initially, assist the client to complete tasks.	If the client is unable to complete a task independently, having assistance will allow success and will demonstrate how to complete the task.
Progress to prompting or reminding the client to perform tasks or assignments.	The amount of intervention gradually is decreased to increase client independence as the client's abilities increase.
Give the client positive feedback for performing behaviors that come close to task achievement.	This approach, called *shaping,* is a behavioral procedure in which successive approximations of a desired behavior are positively reinforced. It allows rewards to occur as the client gradually masters the actual expectation.
Gradually decrease reminders.	Client independence is promoted as staff participation is decreased.
Assist the client to verbalize by asking sequencing questions to keep on the topic ("Then what happens?" and "What happens next?").	Sequencing questions provide a structure for discussions to increase logical thought and decrease tangentiality.
Teach the client's family or caregivers to use the same procedures for the client's tasks and interactions at home.	Successful interventions can be instituted by the client's family or caregivers by using this process. This will promote consistency and enhance the client's chances for success.

Conduct Disorders

Clients with *conduct disorders* exhibit persistent patterns of behavior in which the "basic rights of others and major age-appropriate societal rules and norms are violated" (DSM-III-R, 1987). The client's difficulties exist in all major life areas: at home, at school, with peers, and in the community.

Typically, the onset of the client's behavior patterns is in the prepubertal years. Conduct disorders are four times more prevalent in males than females. Eleven percent of the U.S. population is diagnosed with a conduct disorder (DSM-III-R, 1987). Conduct disorders are more common in children whose parents are chemically dependent or have an antisocial personality disorder. However, isolated acts of antisocial behavior do not warrant a diagnosis of conduct disorder.

The degree of impairment related to conduct disorders can range from mild to severe. In cases with mild impairment, improvement is demonstrated as the adolescent matures and may require only special education classes and supportive therapy for the family. *TOUGHLOVE* is a national parent support group that assists parents in setting basic rules the adolescent must follow or leave home. These limits are established in an atmosphere of love and caring, hence the name of the organization. In severe cases problems related to conduct disorders tend to be chronic and often require placing the client in an institutional setting. As the adolescent grows older, additional complications often develop, including school suspension, legal difficulties, substance use, sexually transmitted diseases, pregnancy, high rates of injury from accidents and fights, and suicidal behavior. Persistent illegal activity and diagnoses of adult antisocial behavior, antisocial personality disorder, and chemical dependence are common for these individuals when they reach adulthood.

Nursing Diagnoses Addressed in this Care Plan

Noncompliance
High Risk for Violence: Self-Directed or Directed at Others
Ineffective Individual Coping

Related Nursing Diagnoses

Ineffective Family Coping: Disabling
Impaired Social Interaction
Self-Esteem Disturbance

Nursing Diagnosis	*Noncompliance (5.2.1.1)*
	A person's informed decision not to adhere to a therapeutic recommendation.

Assessment Data

Defining Characteristics	• Egocentrism • Disobedience • Feelings of frustration • Lack of remorse for unacceptable behavior
Related Factors	• Truancy or dropping out of school • Manipulative behavior • Theft • Cheating (school work, games, sports)

Expected Outcomes

Initial	*The client will:*
	• Be truthful • Adhere to rules • Participate in treatment program
Discharge	*The client will:*
	• Demonstrate compliance with negotiated rules and expectations with parents and teachers

Therapeutic Aims

• Decrease manipulative behavior.
• Facilitate compliance.

Implementation

Nursing Interventions	Rationale
Inform the client of expectations and limits in a matter-of-fact manner.	This allows the client to be aware of expectations without being "challenged" by them.
Do not make exceptions to stated expectations or rules. Avoid making promises; instead, say, "If at all possible, I will."	Consistency will discourage manipulative behavior.
Validate the client's feelings of frustration when expressed, but remain firm with denials of requests for exceptions to limits.	Validation of feelings conveys empathy yet allows consistency in setting and maintaining limits.
Avoid power struggles with the client. Do not engage in lengthy explanations or debating once expectations have been stated.	Debating promotes opportunity for manipulation. If engaged in a power struggle, the adolescent may escalate his or her behavior to "save face" or "win" the struggle.

(continued)
Implementation

Nursing Interventions	Rationale
Demonstrate consistency with your response to the client, and ensure consistency among all the staff members.	Consistent staff response is a primary way to avoid manipulation.
Designate one staff member each shift to be the primary contact person for the client. Other staff should refer requests to the designated staff person. See Basic Concepts: Limit Setting.	Designation of one staff person for decisions regarding client behavior decreases the opportunity for lying and manipulating.
Protect other clients from being drawn into the client's influence, especially those who might be nonassertive or vulnerable.	Clients with conduct disorders have well-established patterns of using others for their own gain.
Institute a daily schedule for getting up, going to bed, doing homework, studying, performing activities of daily living, enjoying free time, and so forth.	Increased structure will increase chances for compliance with expectations.
Give positive feedback for completion of each component of the schedule.	Positive reinforcement of a desired behavior increases the frequency of its occurrence.
Contract with the client (ahead of time) for any special requests or privileges. It may be beneficial to write and sign the agreement.	Using a contract with the client allows him or her to be rewarded for setting a goal and attaining it. A written agreement leaves no room for "forgetting" and minimizes the opportunity for manipulation.

Nursing Diagnosis

High Risk for Violence: Self-Directed or Directed at Others (9.2.2)
A state in which the individual experiences behaviors that can be physically harmful either to the self or others.

Risk Factors

- Temper outbursts
- Reckless, thrill-seeking behavior
- Inability to express feelings in a socially acceptable, safe manner
- Lack of remorse for destructive behavior
- Destruction of property
- Cruelty to animals
- Physical aggression
- Running away from home
- Use of tobacco, alcohol, and drugs
- Involvement in violent situations or crimes

❋
Expected Outcomes

Initial	*The client will:*
	• Be free of injury • Not harm others or destroy property • Eliminate physically aggressive behavior
Discharge	*The client will:*
	• Verbalize feelings in a socially acceptable, safe manner • Reside in the least restrictive environment necessary for safety of self and others • Participate in chemical dependence treatment, if indicated

❋
Therapeutic Aims

• Decrease acting-out or suicidal behavior.
• Facilitate internal control of behavior.

❋
Implementation

Nursing Interventions	Rationale
If the client is losing behavioral control, remove him or her from the situation.	The reinforcement for acting-out is diminished when there is no audience.
Institute *time out* procedure (retreat to a neutral environment to provide the opportunity to regain internal control). Tell the client that the time out period is a positive opportunity for "cooling off," not a punishment for behavior. Remain matter-of-fact when instituting this procedure.	The purpose of time out periods is to allow the client to regain control in a neutral setting.
Encourage the client to work toward instituting time out for himself or herself when unable to handle a situation in any other way.	Time out is a skill the client can use in other situations. This promotes development of the client's internal self-control.
Following the time out period, when the client is more calm, discuss the situation with him or her.	Any discussion will be more productive when feelings and behavior are not excessive or out of control. Remember, time out is not a punishment or a "solution," rather a means to facilitate more effective methods of coping.
Investigate any threats or talk of suicide seriously, and institute interventions as indicated. See Care Plan 24: Suicidal Behavior.	Client safety is a priority.
Encourage the client to keep a diary of his or her feelings, the situation in which the feelings were experienced, what he or she did to handle the situation or feelings, and so forth.	Adolescents often have difficulty identifying and discussing feelings. A written journal provides more concrete information about the connection between the client's feelings and his or her behavior.
Assist the client in examining alternatives to acting-out behavior.	This allows the client to develop a repertoire of choices for future situations.

Nursing Diagnosis

Ineffective Individual Coping (5.1.1.1)

A person's impairment of adaptive behaviors and problem-solving abilities in meeting life's demands and roles.

Assessment Data

Defining Characteristics	• Few or no meaningful peer relationships • Inability to empathize with others • Inability to give and receive affection • Low self-esteem, masked by "tough" act
Related Factors	• Academic underachievement or failure • Use of alcohol or drugs • Unsafe sexual behavior

Expected Outcomes

Initial	*The client will:* • Engage in social interaction • Verbalize feelings • Learn problem-solving skills
Discharge	*The client will:* • Demonstrate development of relationships with peers • Verbalize real feelings of self-worth • Perform at a satisfactory academic level

Therapeutic Aims

• Facilitate successful, appropriate peer relationships.
• Promote ability to make acceptable choices.
• Promote development of positive self-esteem.

Implementation

Nursing Interventions	Rationale
Encourage the client to openly discuss his or her thoughts and feelings.	Verbalizing feelings is an initial step toward dealing with them in an appropriate manner.
Give positive feedback for appropriate discussions.	Positive feedback increases the likelihood of continued performance.
Tell the client that he or she is accepted as a person, though his or her particular behavior may not be acceptable.	Clients with conduct disorders frequently experience rejection. The client needs support to increase self-esteem, while understanding that behavioral changes are necessary.

⊛ *(continued)*
Implementation

Nursing Interventions	Rationale
Give the client positive attention when his or her behavior is not problematic.	The client may have been receiving the majority of attention from others when he or she was engaged in problematic behavior, a pattern that needs to change.
Teach the client about limit setting and the need for these limits. Include time for discussion.	The client may have no knowledge of the concept of limits and how limits can benefit him or her. The client has an opportunity to ask questions when manipulation is not needed. This allows the client to hear about the relationship between aberrant behavior and consequences.
Teach the client a simple problem-solving process as an alternative to acting out (identify the problem, consider alternatives, select and implement an alternative, evaluate the effectiveness of the solution).	The client may not know how to solve problems constructively or may not have seen this behavior modeled in the home.
Help the client practice the problem-solving process with situations on the unit, then situations the client may face at home, school, and so forth.	The client's ability and skill will increase with practice. He or she will experience success with practice.
Role model appropriate conversation and social skills for the client.	This allows the client to see what is expected in a nonthreatening situation.
Specify and describe the skills you are demonstrating.	Clarification of expectations decreases the chance that the client will misinterpret expectations.
Practice social skills with the client on a one-to-one basis.	As the client gains comfort with the skills through practice, he or she will increase their use.
Gradually introduce other clients into the interactions and discussions.	Success with others is more likely to occur once the client has been successful with the staff.
Assist the client to focus on age- and situation-appropriate topics.	Peer relationships are enhanced when the client is able to interact as other adolescents do.
Encourage the client to give and receive feedback with others in his or her age group.	Peer feedback can be influential in shaping the behavior of an adolescent.
Facilitate expression of feelings among clients in supervised group situations.	Adolescents are reluctant to be vulnerable to peers, and they may need encouragement to be open and honest with their feelings.
Teach the client about transmission of human immunodeficiency virus (HIV) infection and other sexually transmitted diseases (STDs).	All clients need to know how to prevent transmission of HIV and STDs. Because these clients may act out sexually or use intravenous drugs, it is especially important that they be educated about HIV infections.

Adjustment Disorders of Adolescents

An *adjustment disorder* involves a maladaptive reaction to an identified psychosocial stressor. The problem occurs within 3 months after the onset of the stressor but does not persist longer than 6 months. Adjustment disorders are expected to remit when the stressor is no longer present or when the client reaches a new level of adaptation (DSM-III-R, 1987). Stressors for adolescents may be easily identifiable, such as separation or divorce of parents, moving to a new community or school, pubertal changes, and so forth. Less evident stressors, such as emerging sexual feelings, desire for increased autonomy, and the growing significance of a peer group, can be a primary source of conflict or add stress to the other more tangible difficulties.

Rubin (1986) identified three common behavioral manifestations of adolescent adaptive difficulties: 1) juvenile delinquency, 2) maladaptive sexual behavior, and 3) substance use. Adolescents with these problems are at highest risk for pregnancy and sexually transmitted diseases, including human immunodeficiency virus (HIV) infection. The ultimate problem area for adolescents is suicidal behavior; suicide is the second leading cause of death in the 15- to 24-year-old age group, according to the National Center for Health Statistics. Lamb and Pusker (1991) cite the promotion of coping ability in teens as a major objective in the prevention of teen suicide. Killeen (1990) indicates that the "combination of vulnerable children and risky environments poses the greatest challenge" for today's health care system.

Nursing care for the adolescent experiencing an adjustment disorder centers around providing a protective environment in which the adolescent can have corrective emotional experiences. These experiences include limits for behavior, opportunities for interpersonal relationships, peer group support and feedback (Rubin 1986), development of coping skills (Puskar, Lamb, and Martsolf, 1989), and successful progression in achievement of developmental tasks.

Nursing Diagnoses Addressed in this Care Plan

Ineffective Individual Coping
Altered Family Processes
Self-esteem Disturbance

Related Nursing Diagnoses

High Risk for Violence: Self-Directed or Directed at Others
Impaired Social Interaction

Nursing Diagnosis

Ineffective Individual Coping (5.1.1.1)

Impairment of adaptive behaviors and problem-solving abilities of a person in meeting life's demands and roles.

Assessment Data

Defining Characteristics

- Impulsive behavior
- Acting-out behavior
- Discomfort with sexual feelings
- Poor social skills
- Anxiety
- Lack of leisure skills
- Suicidal behavior
- Difficulty expressing feelings

Related Factors

- Unmet needs for affection, closeness, and peer group acceptance
- Inaccurate or incomplete knowledge about sexual issues
- Alcohol and drug use
- Ineffective relationships

Expected Outcomes

Initial

The client will:

- Not harm self or others
- Abstain from using alcohol and drugs
- Identify consequences of maladaptive behavior patterns
- Comply with structured daily routine, including educational, social, and recreational activities

Discharge

The client will:

- Eliminate maladaptive coping patterns (alcohol and drug use, acting out, suicidal behavior)
- Demonstrate use of the problem-solving process in decision making
- Complete daily expectations independently
- Verbalize accurate information regarding substance use, sexual activity, and prevention of HIV transmission

❂ Therapeutic Aims

- Decrease anxiety, acting out, and suicidal behavior.
- Promote expression of feelings.
- Decrease impulsive behavior.
- Promote decision-making skills.

❂ Implementation

Nursing Interventions	Rationale
State rules, expectations, and responsibilities clearly to the client, including consequences for exceeding limits.	Clear expectations give the client limits to which his or her behavior must conform and what to expect if he or she exceeds those limits.
Use time out (removal to a neutral area) when the client begins to lose behavioral control.	Time out periods are not punishment but an opportunity for the client to regain control. Instituting time out as soon as the client's behavior begins to escalate may prevent acting out and give the client a successful experience in self-control.
Encourage the client to verbalize feelings.	Identifying and verbalizing feelings is difficult for an adolescent but is a necessary initial step toward resolving difficulties.
Allow the client to express all feelings in an appropriate, nondestructive manner.	The client may have many negative feelings that he or she has not been allowed or encouraged to verbalize.
Ask the client to clarify feelings if he or she is vague or is using jargon.	Clarification avoids any misunderstanding of what the client means and helps the client develop skill in verbally expressing himself or herself.
Encourage a physical activity if the client is better able to discuss difficult issues while doing something physical (for example, take a walk with the client while talking).	Physical activity such as walking provides an outlet for anxious energy, which is common in stressful situations. Also, eye contact, which may be difficult for the client who feels uncomfortable, can be diminished while walking with someone.
Provide a safe environment for the client.	The client's safety is a priority.
Provide factual information about sexual issues, substance use, and consequences of high-risk behavior. Teach the client about transmission of HIV infection and how to prevent it.	Adolescents frequently have inadequate or incorrect information. Any client who may be sexually active or who may use intravenous drugs is at increased risk for HIV infection.
Written information, such as pamphlets, often is helpful.	Written information allows the client to be exposed initially to the material privately, which may be less embarrassing for him or her.
Assess the client's understanding of information through discussion and feedback (for example, return explanation by the client in his or her own words). Do not rely on asking "Did you understand?" or "Do you have any questions?"	Adolescents frequently will deny questions or say they understand when they do not to decrease discomfort, avoid admitting they do not understand, or avoid further discussion.

✷ *(continued)*

Implementation

Nursing Interventions	Rationale
Use a matter-of-fact approach when discussing these emotionally charged issues with the client.	A matter-of-fact approach will decrease the client's anxiety and demonstrate that these issues are a part of daily life, not topics about which one needs to be ashamed.
Avoid looking shocked or disapproving if the client makes crude or outrageous statements.	Testing behavior, to see your reaction, is quite common in adolescents.
Teach the client a simple problem-solving process: Describe the problem, list alternatives, evaluate choices, and select and implement an alternative.	The adolescent client has probably not thought about using a systematic approach to solving problems and may not know where to begin.
Have the client list actual concerns or problems he or she has been having.	Listing concerns helps clarify the client's thinking and provides data about the problems that he or she would like to resolve.
Assist the client in applying the problem-solving process to situations in his or her life.	Personal experience in using the problem-solving process is more useful to the client than using hypothetical examples.
Discuss the pros and cons of possible choices the client has made.	Guiding the client through the process while discussing actual concerns shows him or her how to use the process.
Avoid offering personal opinions. Ask the client, "Knowing what you know now, what might you do next time that happens?"	The client's ability to make more effective decisions is a priority. Your opinions diminish the client's opportunity to develop skills in this arena.

✷

Nursing Diagnosis

Altered Family Processes (3.2.2)
The state in which a family that normally functions effectively experiences a dysfunction.

✷
Assessment Data

Defining Characteristics	• Inadequate parent–child interactions
	• Ineffective communication about family roles, rules, and expectations
	• Rigid family roles
	• Inability to express feelings openly and honestly
Related Factors	• Academic problems
	• Situational, developmental, or maturational transition or crisis

Expected Outcomes

Initial	*The client will:*
	• Express feelings within the family group
	• Listen to feelings of family members

Discharge	*The client will:*
	• Participate in family problem solving
	• Negotiate behavioral rules and expectations with parents
	• Demonstrate compliance with negotiated rules

Therapeutic Aims

• Facilitate family adaptation to current situation.
• Promote family communication.

Implementation

Nursing Interventions	Rationale
Help the client clarify issues he or she would like to discuss with his or her parents. A written list may be helpful.	Anticipatory discussion may decrease the client's discomfort and help the client be specific and avoid generalizations. Writing the ideas ensures that important issues will not be forgotten due to anxiety and provides a focus to keep the client on task.
Encourage the client to use "I" statements to describe what he or she thinks or feels, rather than general statements.	Statements using "I" assume responsibility for the statement of feelings and are less likely to be blaming in nature. The client learns how to share his or her own thoughts and feelings in this way.
Encourage the client's parents to communicate with the client in the same way (see above).	Parents also can benefit from assistance to make "I" statements and focus on feelings rather than blaming.
Arrange and facilitate family sessions for sharing feelings, concerns, and ideas. Establish limits in these meetings that encourage mutual support, self-responsibility, and emotional safety for the participants.	Such meetings can be a semiformalized method for initiating family interaction. Adolescents and their parents may find this difficult to do without assistance.
Help the client and his or her parents take turns talking and listening. Do not get drawn into giving opinions or advice.	Your role is to facilitate communication for all concerned, not to get involved in family dynamics. You must not give the perception of taking sides.
Help clarify statements, and provide a summary for the family group saying "Sounds like . . ."	Your communication skills can be helpful in clarifying ideas; a summary statement can reiterate important discussion points and provide closure on the discussion.

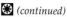 *(continued)*
Implementation

Nursing Interventions	Rationale
Guide the client and his or her parents toward negotiating expectations and responsibilities to be followed at home. A written contract may be helpful.	Negotiating may be unfamiliar to the adolescent and his or her parents. It is a skill that can be the beginning of the adolescent's separation from his or her parents, which is an important developmental task for this age group. Writing the agreement increases the chance that all parties are clear about the expectations, and it decreases the chances for future manipulation or misunderstanding.

Nursing Diagnosis	*Self-Esteem Disturbance (7.1.2)* *Negative self-evaluation or feelings about self or self-capabilities, which may be directly or indirectly expressed.*

Assessment Data

Defining Characteristics	• Negative self-image • Low self-esteem • Feelings of doubt • Minimizing strengths • Underachievement
Related Factors	• Emotional distancing of significant others • Absence of satisfactory peer relationships • Ineffective communication skills

Expected Outcomes

Initial	*The client will:* • Identify feelings of doubt and uncertainty • Give and receive honest feedback with peer group • Make realistic, positive self-statements
Discharge	*The client will:* • Verbalize increased feelings of self-worth • Express feelings in an acceptable manner • Report increased satisfaction with peer relationships

❂ Therapeutic Aims

- Promote development of peer relationships.
- Facilitate communication skills.
- Promote accurate and realistic self-assessment skills.

❂ Implementation

Nursing Interventions	Rationale
Provide direct, honest feedback on the client's communication skills.	The client may not have had feedback about his or her communication skills.
Be specific with feedback. Do not assume the client will know what you mean by general or abstract comments.	General statements are less helpful to the client than specific feedback.
Role model specific communication skills (that is, listening, validating meaning, clarifying, and so forth).	Modeling desired behaviors and skills gives the client a clear picture of what is expected. Practicing skills enhances comfort with their use.
Encourage clients to practice skills and discuss feelings with each other. Suggest to the client that he or she may have concerns similar to others and that perhaps they could share them with each other.	The stage can be set for honest sharing if the client feels he or she is not too different from peers.
Give positive feedback for honest sharing of feelings and concerns.	Positive feedback increases the frequency of desired behavior.
Do not allow the client to dwell on past problems and difficulties, "reliving" mistakes, or making self-blaming, negative statements. Help the client separate his or her behavior from his or her sense of personal worth.	The client may believe that past unacceptable behavior makes him or her a "bad" person.
Help the client make the transition from a focus on the past to a focus in the present. For example, the questions "What might you do differently now?" or "What can be learned from ...?" can be used to help the client with that transition.	Once you have heard the client express feelings about past behavior, it is not useful to allow the client to ruminate—the past cannot be changed.

Section Four

Psychotic Behavior

Psychotic behavior may be encountered in clients who are experiencing a variety of problems and disorders. The care plans in this section address common types of psychotic symptoms (such as delusions and hallucinations) as well as problems or disorders that may produce psychotic behavior (such as chemical, toxic or physical damage, or critical care unit psychosis or schizophrenia).

Psychotic behavior can include many different symptoms resulting from disturbed thought processes, distorted perceptions, brain damage (either trauma-induced or from another physical cause), or chemical toxicity (due to alcohol or drug use, poison, or excessive levels of medications). The role of the nurse in working with a client who is exhibiting psychotic behavior may include providing nursing care in cooperation with other health care team members to treat the client's underlying problem, providing reality orientation, preventing injury to the client or others, helping the client build self-esteem and express feelings, or any number of other nursing interventions.

Delusions

Delusions are false beliefs that have no basis in reality. The client is thought to be attempting to meet some need through the delusion, such as increased self-esteem, security, reassurance, punishment, or freedom from anxiety associated with feelings of guilt, fear, and so forth. The client may have delusional ideas in more than one area. The client may have insight into the delusional state but may be unable to alter it. Sometimes the delusion of the client is the antithesis of what he or she thinks or feels. For example, a client who feels insignificant and unimportant may believe himself or herself to be Jesus Christ, or a client who is poverty stricken or destitute may believe himself or herself to be a powerful, wealthy financier.

Delusions can be one of several symptoms manifested by the client, as in schizophrenia or bipolar affective disorder, or the primary symptom, as in a delusional disorder. Common categories of delusions are grandiose, persecutory, somatic, religious, poverty or wealth, contamination, and infidelity.

Some clients (especially those with paranoia) may have *fixed delusions*—delusions that may persist throughout their lives. Most psychotic clients have *transient delusions*—delusions that are episodic and do not persist with time. Three phases have been identified in the process of delusional thinking. First, the client is totally involved in the delusions. Second, reality testing and trust in others coexist with the delusions. Third, the client no longer experiences the delusions (or is not bothered by them in the case of fixed delusions). Two important factors should be considered when working with the delusional client. First, the delusions are a protection and can be abandoned only when the client feels more safe and secure in the reality of his or her environment. Second, the delusions are not within the client's conscious, voluntary control.

Nursing Diagnoses Addressed in this Care Plan

Altered Thought Processes
Altered Health Maintenance

Related Nursing Diagnoses

Ineffective Management of Therapeutic Regimen (individuals)
Anxiety

Nursing Diagnosis

Altered Thought Processes (8.3)
A state in which the individual experiences a disruption in cognitive operations and activities.

Assessment Data

Defining Characteristics	• Non–reality-based thinking • Disorientation • Labile affect • Short attention span • Impaired judgment • Distractibility
Related Factors	• Major mental illness • Sensory deprivation or overload • Alcohol or drug withdrawal • Renal or metabolic disorders • Medication noncompliance

Expected Outcomes

Initial	*The client will:* • Be free of injury • Demonstrate decreased anxiety level • Interact on reality-based topics
Discharge	*The client will:* • Verbalize recognition of delusional thoughts • Be free of delusions or demonstrate the ability to function without responding to persistent delusional thoughts

Therapeutic Aims

• Provide safety and security.
• Promote reality orientation and contact.
• Relieve fears, anxiety, and mistrust.

Implementation

Nursing Interventions	Rationale
Be sincere and honest when communicating with the client. Avoid vague or evasive remarks.	Delusional clients are very sensitive about others and can recognize insincerity. Evasive comments or hesitation reinforces mistrust or delusions.
Be consistent in setting expectations, enforcing rules, and so forth.	Clear, consistent limits provide a secure structure for the client.
Do not make promises that you cannot keep.	Broken promises reinforce the client's mistrust of others.

🧩 *(continued)*

Implementation

Nursing Interventions	Rationale
Encourage the client to talk with you, but do not pry or cross-examine for information.	Probing increases the client's suspicion and interferes with the therapeutic relationship. When the client has full knowledge of procedures, he or she is less likely to feel tricked by the staff.
Explain procedures, and try to be sure the client understands the procedures before carrying them out.	When the client has full knowledge of procedures, he or she is less likely to feel tricked by the staff.
Recognize the client's delusions as the client's perception of the environment.	It is important to recognize the client's environmental perceptions to understand the feelings he or she is experiencing.
Initially, do not argue with the client or try to convince the client that the delusions are false or unreal.	Logical argument does not dispel delusional ideas and can interfere with the development of trust.
Interact with the client on the basis of real things; do not dwell on the delusional material.	Interacting about reality is healthy for the client.
Show empathy regarding the client's feelings; reassure the client of your presence and acceptance.	The client's delusions can be distressing. Empathy conveys your acceptance of the client and your caring and interest.
Do not be judgmental or belittle or joke about the client's beliefs.	The client's delusions and feelings are not funny to him or her. The client may feel rejected by you or feel unimportant if approached by attempts at humor.
Never convey to the client that you accept the delusions as reality.	You would reinforce the delusion (thus, the client's illness) if you indicate belief in the delusion.
Directly interject doubt regarding delusions as soon as the client seems ready to accept this. Do not argue with the client, but present a factual account of the situation as you see it.	As the client begins to trust you, he or she may become willing to doubt the delusion if you express your doubt.
Attempt to discuss the delusional thoughts as a problem in the client's life; ask the client if he or she can see that the delusions interfere with his or her life.	Discussion of the problems caused by the delusions is a focus on the present and is reality based.
Give positive feedback for the client's successes.	Positive feedback for genuine success enhances the client's sense of well-being and helps make nondelusional reality a more positive situation for the client.
Recognize and support the client's accomplishments (activities or projects completed, responsibilities fulfilled, or interactions initiated).	Recognition of accomplishments can lessen the client's anxiety and the need for delusions as a source of self-esteem.
Engage the client in one-to-one activities at first, then activities in small groups, and gradually activities in larger groups.	The client who is distrustful can best deal with one person initially. Gradual introduction of others when the client can tolerate it is less threatening.

Nursing Diagnosis

Altered Health Maintenance (6.4.2)

Inability to identify, manage, or seek help to maintain health.

Assessment Data

Defining Characteristics	• Poor diet • Insomnia, unrestful sleep • Inadequate food and fluid intake • Inability to follow through with activities of daily living
Related Factors	• Delusions regarding food, poison, persecution, contamination • Low neuroleptic levels • Perceptual and cognitive impairment

Expected Outcomes

Initial	*The client will:* • Establish a balance of rest, sleep, and activity • Ingest adequate amounts of food and fluids • Take medications as administered
Discharge	*The client will:* • Take medications as prescribed • Maintain a balance of rest, sleep, and activity • Maintain adequate nutrition, hydration, and elimination

Therapeutic Aims

• Promote homeostasis.
• Facilitate compliance with medications.

Implementation

Nursing Interventions	Rationale
If the client has delusions that prevent or limit rest, sleep, or food or fluid intake, it may be necessary to institute measures that deal directly with physical health.	The client's safety and physical health are a priority.
If the client thinks that his or her food is poisoned or that he or she is not worthy of food, it may be necessary to alter routines to increase the client's control over issues involving food. As a trust relationship develops, gradually introduce more routine procedures.	Any steps taken to directly increase the client's nutritional intake must be taken without validating the client's delusional system. They must be taken unobtrusively and should be used if the client's nutritional status is severely impaired.
If the client is too suspicious to sleep, try to allow the client to choose a place and time in which he or she will feel most comfortable sleeping. Sedatives as needed may be indicated.	If the client feels he or she can select the most comfortable place to sleep, he or she may feel more trusting and feel secure enough to sleep. Again, care must be taken to avoid validating any of the client's delusions.

Hallucinations

Hallucinations are perceptions of an external stimulus without a source in the external world. They may involve any of the senses—hearing, sight, smell, touch, or taste. Clients often act on these inner perceptions, which may be more compelling to them than external reality. Hallucinations may occur with any of the following conditions:

Withdrawal from alcohol, barbiturates, and other substances
Organic brain diseases
Schizophrenia
Hallucinogenic drugs (mescaline, PCP, LSD)
Drug toxicity or adverse effects (amphetamine psychosis, digitalis toxicity)
Bipolar affective disorder, severe mania
Alcoholic hallucinosis (the client may be oriented to person, place, and time while hallucinating)
Endocrine imbalance (steroid psychosis, thyrotoxicosis)
Sleep or sensory deprivation

Current theories regarding the etiology of hallucinations include a metabolic response to stress, an unconscious attempt to defend the ego, and symbolic expressions of dissociated thoughts. It is most important to remember that hallucinations seem real to the client. The client may perceive the hallucination as reality and reject the reality of the surrounding environment or persons. Occasionally, the client may be aware that he or she is hallucinating.

Nursing Diagnoses Addressed in this Care Plan

Sensory/Perceptual Alterations
High Risk for Violence: Self-Directed or Directed at Others

Related Nursing Diagnoses

Fear
Altered Health Maintenance
Altered Thought Processes

Nursing Diagnosis

Sensory/Perceptual Alterations (Specify) (Visual, Auditory, Kinesthetic, Gustatory, Tactile, Olfactory) (7.2)
A state in which the individual experiences a change in the amount of pattern of oncoming stimuli accompanied by a diminished, exaggerated, distorted, or impaired response to such stimuli.

Assessment Data

Defining Characteristics

- Hallucinations (auditory, visual, tactile, gustatory, kinesthetic, or olfactory)
- Listening intently to no apparent stimuli
- Talking out loud when no one is present
- Rambling, incoherent, or unintelligible speech
- Inability to discriminate between real and unreal perceptions
- Attention deficits
- Inability to make decisions
- Feelings of insecurity
- Confusion

Related Factors

- Attention deficits
- Delusions
- Sleep disturbances
- Refusal to eat
- Feelings of guilt, remorse, or embarrassment when recognizing hallucinatory experiences

Expected Outcomes

Initial

The client will:

- Demonstrate decreased hallucinations
- Interact with others in the external environment
- Participate in the real environment

Discharge

The client will:

- Verbalize plans to deal with hallucinations, if they recur
- Verbalize knowledge of hallucinations or illness and safe use of medications

Therapeutic Aims

- Interrupt pattern of hallucinations.
- Encourage contact with real people, interactions, and activities.
- Assist in dealing with guilt if and when the client remembers psychotic behavior.
- Anticipate ways to deal with possible recurrence of hallucinations.

Implementation

Nursing Interventions	Rationale
Be aware of all surrounding stimuli, including sounds from other rooms (such as television or stereo in adjacent areas).	Many seemingly normal stimuli will trigger or intensify hallucinations. The client can be overwhelmed by stimuli.
Try to decrease stimuli or move the client to another area.	Decreased stimuli provide fewer opportunities for misperception. The client has a diminished ability to deal with stimuli.
Avoid conveying to the client the belief that hallucinations are real. Do not converse with the "voices" or otherwise reinforce the client's belief in the hallucinations as reality.	You must be honest with the client, letting him or her know the hallucinations are not real.
Communicate with the client verbally in direct, concrete, specific terms. Avoid gestures, abstract ideas, and innuendos.	The client's ability to deal in abstractions is diminished. The client may misinterpret your gestures or innuendos.
Avoid placing the client in a situation in which choices need to be made. Don't ask "Would you like to talk or be alone for a while?" Rather, suggest that the client talk with you.	The client's ability to make decisions is impaired. Also, if given a choice, the client may choose to be alone (and hallucinate) rather than deal with reality (talking to you).
Respond verbally to anything real that the client talks about; reinforce the client's conversation when he or she refers to reality.	Positive reinforcement increases the likelihood of desired behaviors.
Encourage the client to make staff members aware of hallucinations when they occur or when they interfere with the client's ability to converse and carry out activities.	The client has the chance to seek others (in reality) and to cope with problems caused by hallucinations.
If the client appears to be hallucinating, attempt to engage the client's attention, and provide conversation or a concrete activity of interest to the client.	When the client is engaged in real activities and interactions, it becomes more difficult for him or her to respond to hallucinations.
Maintain simple, basic topics of conversation to provide a base in reality.	The client is more able to talk about basic things; complexity is more difficult.
Provide simple activities that can be easily or realistically accomplished by the client (such as small, uncomplicated craft projects).	Long or complicated tasks may be frustrating for the client. He or she may be unable to complete them.
If the client tolerates it, use touch in a nonthreatening manner to provide a reality base; allow the client to touch your forearm or hand. Remember: some clients are too threatened by touching; evaluate each client's response carefully.	Your physical touch is reality, and it can help the client to reestablish ego boundaries.
Encourage expression of any feelings of guilt, remorse, or embarrassment the client may have once he or she is aware of psychotic behavior; be supportive.	It may help the client to express such feelings, particularly if you are a supportive, accepting listener.

✺ *(continued)*
Implementation

Nursing Interventions	Rationale
Show acceptance of the client's behavior and of the client as a person; do not joke about or judge the client's behavior.	The client may need help to see that hallucinations were a part of the illness, not under the client's control. Joking or being judgmental about the client's behavior is not appropriate and can be damaging to the client.
Note: Not all clients will remember previous psychotic behavior, and they may ask you what they did. Be honest in your answers, but do not dwell on the psychotic behavior.	Honest answers may relieve the client. Many times the client's fears about his or her behavior are worse than the actual behavior.

❂

Nursing Diagnosis

High Risk for Violence: Self-Directed or Directed at Others (9.2.2)
A state in which the individual experiences behaviors that can be physically harmful to the self or others.

✺
Risk Factors

- Fear
- Mistrust or suspicion
- Agitation
- Rapid, shallow breathing
- Clenched teeth or fists
- Rigid or taut body
- Hostile or threatening verbalizations
- History of aggression toward property or others
- History of violent family patterns
- Low neuroleptic level

✺
Expected Outcomes

Initial	*The client will:*

- Be free of injury
- Not injure others or destroy property
- Verbalize feelings of anger, frustration, or confusion
- Express decreased feelings of agitation, fear, or anxiety

Discharge	*The client will:*

- Demonstrate satisfying relationships with others
- Demonstrate effective coping strategies

❋
Therapeutic Aims

- Provide a safe environment.
- Decrease fear, anxiety, or agitation.
- Facilitate expression of fear, anxiety, and other feelings.

❋
Implementation

Nursing Interventions	Rationale
Provide protective supervision for the client, but avoid hovering over him or her.	The safety of the client and others is a priority. Allowing the client to have some personal distance may diminish agitation.
Remain aware of cues indicating that the client is hallucinating (intent listening for no apparent reason, talking to someone when no one is present, muttering to self, inappropriate facial expression).	The client may act on what he or she "hears." Your early response to cues indicating active hallucinations decreases the chance of acting out or aggressive behavior.
Provide a structured environment with as many routine activities of daily living as possible. Explain unexpected changes. Make your expectations clear to the client in simple, direct terms.	Lack of structure and unexplained changes usually will increase agitation and anxiety. Structure enhances the client's security.
Be alert for signs of increasing fear, anxiety, or agitation so that you may intervene as early as possible and prevent harm to the client, others, or property.	The earlier you can intervene, the easier it is to calm the client and prevent harm.
Avoid backing the client into a corner either verbally or physically.	If the client feels threatened or trapped, he or she is more likely to be aggressive.
Intervene with one-to-one contact, seclusion, and medication as needed (as ordered) as appropriate.	The safety of the client and others is a priority.
Be realistic in your expectations of the client; do not expect more (or less) of the client than he or she is capable of doing.	Expecting too much of the client will be frustrating, and he or she may not even try to comply. Expecting too little may undermine the client's self-esteem, confidence, and growth.
As agitation subsides, encourage the client to express his or her feelings, first in one-to-one contacts, then in small groups, and then in larger groups as tolerated.	The client will be more at ease with just one person and will gradually tolerate more people when he or she feels less threatened.
Help the client identify and practice ways to relieve anxiety when the client is able to verbalize such feelings. See Care Plan 24: Suicidal Behavior.	With decreased anxiety, the client will be able to solve problems, learn new behaviors, and establish relationships with others.

Schizophrenia

Schizophrenia is a disorder that involves characteristic psychotic symptoms (delusions, hallucinations, disturbances in mood and thought) and a decrease in the individual's level of functioning in major life areas. According to DSM-III-R, 1987, the illness lasts at least 6 months and may have residual symptoms that necessitate long-term management.

The characteristic symptoms of schizophrenia (DSM-III-R, 1987) are listed below. Clients typically experience symptoms in several of these areas.

1. *Thought content.* Delusional thoughts are fragmented, sometimes bizarre, and frequently unpleasant for the client. Many clients believe that their thoughts are "broadcast" to the external world, so others are able to hear them (*thought broadcasting*); that the thoughts are not their own but are placed there by others (*thought insertion*); and that thoughts are being removed from their head (*thought withdrawal*). The client believes all this *thought control* takes place against his or her will and feels powerless to stop it.

2. *Form of thought.* This refers to the client's inability to communicate meaningful information to others. Frequently, there are *loose associations,* or jumping from one topic to an unrelated topic. The client may be unaware that others cannot comprehend what he or she is saying. There also may be *poverty of speech* (little verbalization), *poverty of content* (much verbalization but no substance), *neologisms* (invented words), *perseveration* (repetitive speech), *clanging* (rhyming speech), or *blocking* (inability to verbalize thoughts).

3. *Perception.* The major perceptual disturbance is hallucinations, most commonly auditory (voices). The voices may be familiar to the client, or they may command the client to do things (including acts that may be harmful to the client or others). Auditory hallucinations may be multiple, that is, more than one voice "speaking" at once. Other types of hallucinations (visual, tactile, gustatory, kinesthetic, and olfactory) can occur, but they are less common.

4. *Affect.* The client has a disturbance of mood, which is usually a flat or inappropriate affect. With a flat affect, there is a lack of expression, monotonous tone of voice, and immobile facies. The client may feel numb or lack the intensity of normal feelings. (*Note:* Many psychotropic medications produce effects that resemble a flat affect.) An inappropriate affect is when the client's expression or feeling tone is incongruent with the situation or topic being discussed. For example, the client may talk of a sad or frightening event yet be laughing loudly and appear amused.

5. *Sense of self.* This refers to the client's inability to feel like a unique, separate person. It also is called loss of ego boundaries and is expressed as identity confusion, lack of meaning in life, or delusions.

6. *Volition.* This is a disturbance in self-initiated, goal-directed activity. Ambivalence is sometimes so severe that even simple decisions are impossible. This symptom can persist into a residual phase, which causes marked impairment in the client's social, vocational, and personal functioning.

7. *Interpersonal functioning and relationship to the external world.* The client frequently is socially withdrawn, isolative, and emotionally detached from others. He or she may be preoccupied with delusional thoughts, distort the external world, and fail to observe others' personal space.

8. *Psychomotor behavior.* Psychomotor disturbances are most commonly seen during acute psychotic episodes and in severely chronically ill clients. The client may respond excitedly to the environment, resulting in agitated pacing or other movements. At the other extreme, the client may be almost unresponsive to the environment and exhibit motor retardation, posturing, or stereotyped movements.

The symptoms of schizophrenia often are categorized as *hard* or *soft* signs. Hard signs include delusions and hallucinations, which are more amenable to the therapeutic effects of medication. The soft signs, such as lack of volition, impaired socialization, and affective disturbances can persist, causing the client continued distress, even though major symptoms of psychosis have abated.

Schizophrenia has a familial tendency, but studies have not found a totally genetic basis for the disorder. It is equally prevalent in males and females; onset usually occurs in late adolescence or early adulthood.

The major types of schizophrenia follow:

1. *Catatonic–excited.* Characterized by excessive and sometimes violent motor activity and excitement; *catatonic–withdrawn:* characterized by a generalized inhibition manifested by stupor, mutism, negativism, or waxy flexibility

2. *Paranoid.* Characterized by persecutory or grandiose delusions, hallucinations, sometimes by excessive religiosity, or hostile, and aggressive behavior

3. *Disorganized.* Characterized by grossly inappropriate or flat affect, incoherence, loose associations, and extremely disorganized behavior

4. *Undifferentiated.* Characterized by mixed schizophrenic symptoms (of other types) along with disturbances of thought, affect, and behavior

5. *Residual.* Characterized by at least one previous episode, but not currently psychotic; other symptoms: social withdrawal, flat affect, or looseness of associations

Previously, schizoaffective disorder was categorized as a subtype of schizophrenia. The DSM-III-R (1987) now places this into a separate category. The symptoms are not exclusively those of a major mood disorder nor of a schizophrenia, rather they are a combination of both. Nursing care of the client with this disorder is based on the nursing diagnoses most appropriate for the individual client.

The prognosis for a client with schizophrenia is better when the client has a history of good social, occupational, and sexual adjustment; when the onset of the illness is acute; or when a precipitating event is present.

Note: The client with schizophrenia probably will be taking medications, such as major tranquilizers or antipsychotic agents.

Nursing Diagnoses Addressed in this Care Plan

Personal Identity Disturbance
Social Isolation
Self-Care Deficits

Nursing Diagnosis	*Personal Identity Disturbance (7.1.3)*
	Inability to distinguish between self and nonself.

Assessment Data

Defining Characteristics	• Bizarre behavior
	• Regressive behavior
	• Loss of ego boundaries (inability to differentiate self from the external environment)
	• Disorientation
	• Disorganized, illogical thinking
	• Flat or inappropriate affect
	• Feelings of anxiety, fear, or agitation
	• Aggressive behavior toward others or property

Related Factors	• Hallucinations
	• Delusions
	• Psychomotor retardation
	• Sexual conflicts

Expected Outcomes

Initial	*The client will:*
	• Be free of injury
	• Not harm others or destroy property
	• Establish contact with reality
	• Express feelings in an acceptable manner
	• Demonstrate or verbalize decreased psychotic symptoms and feelings of anxiety, agitation, and so forth
	• Participate in the therapeutic milieu

Discharge	*The client will:*
	• Reach or maintain his or her optimal level of functioning
	• Cope effectively with his or her illness
	• Demonstrate compliance with prescribed regimen, such as medications

Therapeutic Aims

• Provide a safe environment for the client and others.

• Orient the client to reality.

• Provide structured, goal-directed activity.

• Decrease bizarre, regressive behavior.

• Decrease anxiety and agitation.

Implementation

Nursing Interventions	Rationale
Reassure the client that the environment is safe by briefly and simply explaining routines, procedures, and so forth.	The client is less likely to feel threatened if the surroundings are known.
Protect the client from harming himself or herself or others. Remove items that could be used in self-destructive behavior. See Care Plan 24: Suicidal Behavior.	Client safety is a priority. Self-destructive ideas may come from hallucinations or delusions.
Remove the client from the group if his or her behavior becomes too bizarre, disturbing, or dangerous to others.	The benefit of involving the client with the group is outweighed by the group's need for safety and protection.
Help the client's group accept the client's "strange" behavior: Give simple explanations to the client's group as needed (for example, "[client] is very sick right now; he [or she] needs our understanding and support").	The client's group benefits from awareness of others' needs and can help the client by demonstrating empathy.
Consider the other clients' needs. Plan for at least one staff member to be available to other clients if several staff members are needed to care for this client.	Remember that other clients have their own needs and problems. Be careful not give attention only to the "sickest" client.
Explain to other clients that they have not done anything to warrant the client's verbal or physical threats; rather, the threats are the result of the client's illness.	Other clients may interpret verbal or physical threats as personal or may feel that they are doing something to warrant or bring about the threats.
Set limits on the client's behavior when he or she is unable to do so (when the behavior interferes with other clients or becomes destructive). Do not set limits to punish the client.	Limits are established by others when the client is unable to use internal controls effectively. Unacceptable behaviors decrease as more effective behaviors increase.
Decrease excessive stimuli in the environment. The client may not respond favorably to gym activities, competitive activities, or activities in large groups if he or she is still actively psychotic.	The client is unable to deal with excess stimuli. The environment should not be threatening to the client.
Be aware of PRN medications and the client's varying need for them.	Medication can help the client gain control over his or her own behavior.
Reorient the client to person, place, and time as indicated (call the client by name, tell the client where he or she is, and so forth).	Repeated presentation of reality is concrete reinforcement for the client.
Spend time with the client even when he or she is unable to respond verbally or in a coherent manner. Convey your interest and caring.	Your physical presence is reality. Nonverbal caring can be conveyed to the client even when verbal caring is not understood.

(continued)
Implementation

Nursing Interventions	Rationale
Make only promises that you can realistically keep.	Breaking your promise can result in increasing the client's mistrust of others.
Limit the client's environment to enhance his or her feelings of security.	Unknown boundaries or a perceived lack of limits can foster insecurity in the client.
Help the client establish what is real and unreal. Validate the client's real perceptions, and correct the client's misperceptions in a matter-of-fact manner. Do not argue with the client, but do not give support for misperceptions.	The unreality of psychosis must not be reinforced; reality must be reinforced. Reinforced ideas and behavior will recur more frequently.
Stay with the client when he or she is frightened. Touching the client can sometimes be therapeutic. Evaluate the effectiveness of the use of touch with the client before using it consistently.	Your presence and touch can provide reassurance from the real world. However, touch may not be effective if the client feels that his or her boundaries are being invaded.
Be simple, direct, and concise when speaking to the client.	The client is unable to process complex ideas effectively.
Talk with the client about simple, concrete things; avoid ideologic or theoretic discussions.	The client's ability to deal with abstractions is impaired.
Direct activities toward helping the client accept and remain in contact with reality.	Increased reality contact decreases the client's retreat into unreality.
Initially, assign the same staff members to work with the client.	Consistency can reassure the client.
Begin with one-to-one interactions, and then progress to small groups as tolerated (introduce slowly).	Initially, the client will better tolerate and deal with limited contact.
Establish and maintain a daily routine; explain any variation in this routine to the client.	The client's ability to adapt to change is impaired.
Set realistic goals. Set daily goals and expectations.	Unrealistic goals will frustrate the client. Daily goals are short term and easier for the client to accomplish.
Make the client aware of your expectations for him or her.	The client must know what is expected before he or she can work toward meeting those expectations.
At first, do not offer choices to the client ("Would you like to go to activities?" "What would you like to eat?"). Instead, approach the client in a directive manner ("It is time to eat. Please pick up your fork.").	The client's ability to make decisions is impaired. Asking the client to make decisions at this time may be very frustrating.
Gradually, as the client can tolerate it, provide opportunities for him or her to accept responsibility and make personal decisions.	The client needs to gain independence as soon as he or she is able. Gradual addition of responsibilities and decisions gives the client a greater opportunity for success.

Nursing Diagnosis	*Social Isolation: (3.1.2)*

Aloneness experienced by the individual and perceived as imposed by others and as a negative or threatened state.

Assessment Data

Defining Characteristics	• Inappropriate or inadequate emotional responses • Poor interpersonal relationships • Feeling threatened in social situations • Difficulty with verbal communication • Exaggerated responses to stimuli
Related Factors	• Alteration in mental status • Unacceptable social behavior • Lack of reality contact • Disordered, illogical thinking • Lack of supportive significant others • Low self-esteem

Expected Outcomes

Initial	*The client will:* • Report increased feelings of self-worth • Identify strengths and assets • Engage in social interaction
Discharge	*The client will:* • Communicate effectively with others • Demonstrate use of strengths and assets

Therapeutic Aims

• Promote self-esteem and feelings of self-worth.
• Promote appropriate social interactions.
• Decrease social interactions.

Implementation

Nursing Interventions	Rationale
Provide attention in a sincere, interested manner.	Flattery can be interpreted as belittling by the client.
Support any successes—responsibilities fulfilled, projects, interactions with staff members and other clients, and so forth.	Sincere and genuine praise that the client has earned can improve self-esteem.
Avoid trying to convince the client verbally of his or her own worth.	The client will recognize unfounded praise or flattery and can feel worse because of it. The client must

✹ *(continued)*
Implementation

Nursing Interventions	Rationale
	demonstrate a positive behavior before you can genuinely recognize it.
Teach the client social skills. Describe and demonstrate specific skills, such as eye contact, attentive listening, nodding, and so forth. Discuss the type of topics that are appropriate for casual social conversation, such as the weather, local events, news, and so forth.	The client may have little or no knowledge of social interaction skills. Modeling provides a concrete example of the desired skills.
Help the client improve his or her grooming; assist when necessary in bathing, doing laundry, and so forth.	Good physical grooming can foster feelings of well-being and self-esteem.
Help the client accept as much responsibility for personal grooming as he or she can do (don't do something for the client that he or she can do alone).	The client must be encouraged to be as independent as possible to foster self-esteem and continued self-care practices.

✹

Nursing Diagnosis

Self-Care Deficit (6.5)

A state in which the individual experiences an impaired ability to perform or complete feeding, bathing, toileting, dressing, and grooming activities for himself or herself.

✹
Assessment Data

Defining Characteristics	• Disturbance of self-initiated, goal-directed activity • Poor personal hygiene • Inability to follow through with completion of daily tasks
Related Factors	• Hallucinations • Delusions • Apathy • Anergy

✹
Expected Outcomes

Initial	*The client will:* • Establish an adequate balance of rest, sleep, and activity • Establish nutritional eating patterns • Participate in self-care activities
Discharge	*The client will:* • Maintain adequate routines for physiologic well-being • Demonstrate independence in self-care activities

Therapeutic Aims

- Promote an adequate balance of rest, sleep, and activity.
- Promote adequate nutrition, hydration, and elimination.
- Facilitate adequate grooming, hygiene, and other activities of daily living.

Implementation

Nursing Interventions	Rationale
Be alert to the client's physical needs.	The client may be unaware of or unresponsive to his or her needs. Physical needs must be met to enhance the client's ability to meet emotional needs.
Observe the client's pattern of food and fluid intake; you may need to monitor and record intake, output, and daily weight.	The client may be unaware of or may ignore his or her needs for food and fluids.
Monitor the client's elimination patterns. You may need to use PRN medication to establish regularity.	Constipation frequently occurs with the use of major tranquilizers, decreased food and fluid intake, and decreased activity levels.
Explain any task in short, simple steps.	A complex task will be easier for the client if it is broken down into a series of steps.
Using clear, direct sentences, instruct the client to do one part of the task at a time.	The client may not be able to remember all the steps at once.
Tell the client your expectations directly. Do not ask the client to choose unnecessarily. Tell the client it is time to eat or get dressed rather than asking if he or she wants to eat or dress.	The client may not be able to make choices or may make poor choices.
Do not confuse the client with reasons as to why things are to be done.	Abstract ideas will not be comprehended and will interfere with task completion.
Allow the client ample time to complete any task.	It may take the client longer to dress or comb his or her hair because of a lack of concentration and short attention span.
Remain with the client throughout the task; do not attempt to hurry the client.	Trying to rush the client will frustrate him or her and make completion of the task impossible.
Assist the client as needed to maintain daily functions and adequate personal hygiene.	The client's sense of dignity and well-being is enhanced if he or she is clean, smells good, looks nice, and so forth.
Gradually withdraw assistance and supervise the client's grooming or other self-care skills. Praise the client for completed activities of daily living and for initiating self-care activities.	It is important for the client to gain his or her independence as soon as possible. Positive reinforcement increases the likelihood of recurrence.

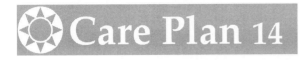

Chemical, Toxic, or Physical Damage or Critical Care Unit Psychosis

Psychotic behavior caused by chemical, toxic, or physical damage or sleep deprivation usually is acute and will subside in a short time with treatment of the underlying cause. Sometimes, however, residual damage remains after the psychotic behavior subsides, for example, Korsakoff syndrome or heavy metal ingestion, such as lead poisoning. In these instances long-term treatment related to the residual damage is required. The major types of psychoses in this category follow:

Korsakoff syndrome results from chronic alcoholism and the associated vitamin B_1 (thiamine) deficiency. It usually occurs after a minimum of 5 to 10 years of heavy alcohol intake. The brain damage it causes is irreversible, even when further alcohol consumption is eliminated.

Drug-induced psychosis occurs most commonly following massive doses or chronic use of amphetamines; it clears in 1 to 2 weeks when drug intake is discontinued. It also may result from use of hallucinogenic drugs (such as LSD); this lasts from 12 hours to 2 days. With repeated hallucinogen use, psychosis may occur briefly without recent drug ingestion. This psychosis is most common between the ages of 15 and 35.

Endocrine imbalances may produce psychotic behavior, such as the intake of large doses of steroids, resulting in toxic blood levels. The abrupt withdrawal of steroids also may produce psychotic behavior. Thyroid disturbances (for example, thyrotoxicosis) can produce psychotic behavior that subsides spontaneously when thyroxin is brought to a therapeutic level.

Sleep deprivation of rapid eye movement (REM) cycle sleep, which is associated with extreme stress, can produce psychotic behavior. The most common example is *critical care unit psychosis*. Clients in critical care units experience constant stimuli (lights, sounds), disruptions of diurnal patterns, interruption of sleep every 15 to 30 minutes, and so on and often exhibit psychotic behavior or symptoms.

The behaviors seen with these types of psychoses are clinically similar to those seen with schizophrenia. The major difference is that treatment of these psychoses is aimed at correcting the underlying cause. The client may improve quite rapidly and dramatically as the cause is treated or removed.

Nursing Diagnoses Addressed in this Care Plan

Sensory/Perceptual Alterations
High Risk for Injury

Related Nursing Diagnoses

Altered Health Maintenance
Self-Care Deficits
Impaired Verbal Communication

Nursing Diagnosis	*Sensory/Perceptual Alterations (Specify) (Visual, Auditory, Kinesthetic, Gustatory, Tactile, Olfactory) (7.2)*

A state in which an individual experiences a change in the amount or patterning of oncoming stimuli accompanied by a diminished, exaggerated, distorted, or impaired response to such stimuli.

Assessment Data

Defining Characteristics	• Hallucinations
	• Disorientation
	• Fear
	• Inability to concentrate
	• Inattention to personal hygiene or grooming

Related Factors	• Delusions
	• Disrupted diurnal patterns
	• Impaired sleep cycle
	• Disturbance of eating habits
	• Excessive environmental stimuli

Expected Outcomes

Initial	*The client will:*
	• Be oriented to person, time, place, and situation
	• Establish a balance of rest, sleep, and activity
	• Establish adequate nutrition, hydration, and elimination
	• Participate in self-care activities

Discharge	*The client will:*
	• Maintain adequate, balanced physiologic functioning
	• Communicate effectively with others
	• Demonstrate independence in self-care activities

Therapeutic Aims

• Restore balanced physiologic functioning.
• Promote reality orientation.
• Decrease fears, anxiety, and other psychiatric problems.

Implementation

Nursing Interventions	Rationale
Be alert to the client's physical needs.	The client's physical needs are crucial. He or she may not attend to hunger, fatigue, and so forth.
Observe the client's patterns of food and fluid intake; you may need to monitor and record intake, output, and daily weight.	Adequate nutrition is important for the client's well-being.
Monitor the client's elimination patterns. You may need to administer a medication to the client to maintain bowel regularity.	Constipation is a frequent side effect of major tranquilizers.
Institute relaxing, quieting activities before bedtime (tepid bath, warm milk, quiet environment).	Calming, pre-bedtime activities facilitate rest and sleep.
Spend time with the client to facilitate reality orientation.	Your physical presence is reality.
Reorient the client to person, place, and time as necessary, by using the client's name often and by telling the client your name, the date, the place and situation, and so forth.	Reminding the client of surroundings, people, and time increases his or her reality contact.
Evaluate the use of touch with the client.	Touch can be reassuring and may provide security for the client.
Be simple, direct, and concise when speaking to the client. Talk with the client about concrete or familiar things; avoid ideologic or theoretic discussions.	The client's ability to process abstractions or complexities is impaired.
Direct activities toward helping the client accept and remain in contact with reality; use recreational or occupational therapy when appropriate.	The greater the client's reality contact and involvement in activities, the less time he or she will deal in unreality.

Nursing Diagnosis

High Risk for Injury (1.6.1)
A state in which the individual is at risk of injury as a result of environmental conditions interacting with the individual's adaptive and defensive resources.

Risk Factors

- Feelings of hostility
- Fear
- Cognitive deficits
- Emotional impairment
- Integrative dysfunction
- Sensory or motor deficits
- History of combative or acting-out behavior
- Inability to perceive harmful stimuli

❊
Expected Outcomes

Initial	*The client will:*
	• Be free of injury
	• Not harm others or destroy property
	• Be free of toxic substances

Discharge	*The client will:*
	• Demonstrate adherence to the treatment regimen
	• Avoid toxic or chemical substances
	• Verbalize plans for further treatment, if indicated

❊
Therapeutic Aims

• Provide a safe environment.

• Decrease acting-out behavior.

❊
Implementation

Nursing Interventions	Rationale
Reassure the client that the environment is safe by briefly and simply explaining ward procedures, routines, and so forth.	The psychotic client frequently acts out based on fear as a means of protecting himself or herself.
Protect the client from self-destructive activities by restraining the client or removing items that could be used in self-destructive behavior. See Care Plan 52: Aggressive Behavior.	The client's physical safety is a priority.
Remove the client to a quiet area or withdraw your attention if the client acts out, provided there is no potential danger to the client or others.	Decreased attention from you and others may help to extinguish unacceptable behavior.
Set limits on the client's behavior when he or she is unable to do so if the behavior interferes with other clients or becomes self-destructive. Do not set limits to punish the client.	Limit setting is the positive use of external control to promote safety and security.

Section Five

Neuropsychiatric Illness

Clients who have a neurologic illness often exhibit behaviors that are commonly considered psychiatric or are often encountered with psychiatric illnesses, such as delusions, hallucinations, or inappropriate behaviors. The care plans in this section discuss a number of conditions in which neuropsychiatric problems occur and address nursing care for these clients and caregiver considerations related to these problems (for additional information on caregiver concerns, see Care Plan 5: Supporting the Caregiver).

Dementia

The primary feature of *dementia* is a global impairment of cognitive function, with changes in the affective, behavioral, or psychomotor domains as well. Dementia is a type of organic mental syndrome according to DSM-III-R classification (1987). It is not necessarily a component of the aging process. Some minor forgetfulness usually occurs in elderly clients, but this differs drastically from the changes seen in dementia. Do not assume that because a client is elderly he or she will be confused, forgetful, and so forth.

The major disorders that result in dementia are:

Cerebral arteriosclerosis results in a decreased blood supply to the brain, causing hypoxia of the cerebral cortex. Initial symptoms are simple forgetfulness, short attention span, and decreased ability to concentrate. It usually is progressive and may result in psychosis. It usually begins between the ages of 60 and 70.

Alzheimer disease has organic pathology that includes atrophy of cerebral neurons, plaque deposits, and enlargement of the third and fourth ventricles of the brain. It usually begins in people about 50 years old, may last 5 years or more, and includes progressive loss of speech, loss of motor function, and profound personality and behavioral changes, such as paranoia, delusions, hallucinations, inattention to hygiene, belligerence, and loss of sphinctor control.

Pick disease involves frontal and temporal lobe atrophy and results in a clinical picture similar to Alzheimer disease. Death occurs more rapidly, usually in 2 to 5 years.

Senile dementia (in clients over 65) or *presenile dementia* (in younger clients) is a general term referring to progressive changes resulting from diffuse, primary degeneration and loss of brain neurons. The client's behavior becomes uninhibited, socially inappropriate, or embarrassing due to cerebral lobe atrophy. Psychomotor deficits do not accompany this pathology, and death is not a direct result of the neural changes.

Acquired immunodeficiency syndrome (AIDS) is a disorder caused by infection with human immunodeficiency virus (HIV). Dementia and other neurologic problems result from direct invasion of nervous tissue by HIV and from other illnesses that can be present in AIDS, such as toxoplasmosis, cytomegalovirus, and others. This type of dementia often is called *AIDS dementia (AD), AIDS-dementia complex,* or *HIV encephalopathy*. AD can result in a wide variety of symptoms, ranging from mild sensory impairment to gross memory and cognitive deficits to severe muscle dysfunction. (See Basic Concepts: HIV Disease and AIDS.)

Parkinson disease is a progressive disease involving loss of neurons of the basal ganglia that produces tremor, muscle rigidity, and loss of postural reflexes. Bunting and Fitzsimmons (1991) report that "delirium, dementia, and depression are the most commonly reported psychiatric manifestations of Parkinson disease" (p. 158). The development of delirium, dementia, and depression as components of Parkinson disease has become more prevalent as successful treatment of individuals has extended life expectancy.

Nursing Diagnoses Addressed in this Care Plan

Self-Care Deficit
Altered Thought Processes
Impaired Social Interaction

Related Nursing Diagnoses

High Risk for Violence: Self-Directed or Directed at Others
High Risk for Injury
Sleep Pattern Disturbance
Altered Family Processes
Altered Role Performance

Nursing Diagnosis

Self-Care Deficit (6.5)

A state in which the individual experiences an impaired ability to perform or complete feeding, bathing, toileting, dressing, and grooming activities for himself or herself.

Assessment Data

Defining Characteristics	• Attention deficits • Apathy • Impaired performance of daily living activities
Related Factors	• Sleep pattern disturbance • Inadequate food and fluid intake • Sensorimotor deficits • Physical problems related to immobility

Expected Outcomes

Initial	*The client will:* • Be free of injury • Not injure others or destroy property • Establish adequate nutrition, hydration, and elimination • Establish an adequate balance of rest, sleep, and activity

(continued)
Expected Outcomes

Discharge   *The client will:*

- Remain free of injury
- Maintain balanced physiologic functions
- Attain his or her optimal level of functioning

Therapeutic Aims

- Promote homeostasis.
- Provide a safe environment.
- Facilitate adequate performance of daily living activities.
- Facilitate rest and sleep.
- Promote adequate nutrition, hydration, and elimination.

Implementation

Nursing Interventions	Rationale
Offer the client small amounts of food frequently, including juices, malts, and fortified liquids.	Use of fortified liquids will provide the maximum amount of nutrition without fatiguing the client.
Provide a quiet environment with decreased stimulation for meal times. Assist the client with eating (for example, feed the client) as necessary.	The client may be easily distracted by external stimuli.
Monitor the client's bowel movements; do not allow impaction to occur.	The client's inactivity, decreased food and fluid intake, and use of major tranquilizers can cause constipation and can lead to impaction if not monitored.
Provide activity and stimulation during the day. Do not allow the client to sleep all day.	The client will be wakeful at night, when confusion is worse, if he or she sleeps excessively during the day.
Provide a regular nightly routine, such as tepid bath and a quiet environment.	These measures facilitate readiness for sleep.
Use bedtime medication for sleep, if necessary. Closely observe the client for beneficial effects or potential side effects. Dosages may need to be decreased for the elderly.	Sedatives or hypnotics may be helpful to facilitate sleep. In some people, however, these drugs can cause restlessness and confusion, and their use should be discontinued. Slow metabolism or decreased liver or kidney function can result in toxicity in elderly clients.
Assess the client's ability to ambulate independently if he or she is elderly or physically disabled; assist the client until you are sure of physical safety and independence.	Independence is important for the client, but physical safety is a priority.
Observe the client to ascertain his or her whereabouts at all times.	The client may wander off and endanger himself or herself unknowingly.
Check the client frequently at night.	Confusion or disorientation may increase at night.

(continued)
Implementation

Nursing Interventions	Rationale
Provide adequate light in the environment, even at night (for example, a nightlight).	Adequate light decreases the client's misperceptions of shadows, and so forth.
Provide adequate restraints (Posey, vest, and so forth) if necessary for protection. *Note:* Side rails alone may prove dangerous if the client tries to climb over them.	Restraints can increase the client's agitation and fear but may be needed for his or her safety.
Explain any task in short, simple steps.	A complex task is easier for the client if it is broken down into a series of steps.
Use clear, direct sentences; instruct the client to do one part of the task at a time.	The client may not be able to remember all the steps at once.
Tell the client your expectations directly. Do not ask the client to choose unnecessarily (for example, tell the client it is time to eat rather than asking if he or she wants to eat).	The client may not be able to make choices or may make poor choices.
Do not confuse the client with reasons as to why things are to be done.	Abstract ideas will not be comprehended.
Allow the client an ample amount of time to perform any given task.	It may take the client longer to dress or comb his or her hair because of a lack of concentration or short attention span.
Remain with the client throughout the task; do not attempt to hurry the client.	Trying to rush the client will frustrate him or her and make completing the task impossible.
Assist the client as needed to maintain daily functions and adequate personal hygiene.	The client's sense of dignity and well-being is enhanced if he or she is clean, smells good, looks nice, and so forth.

Nursing Diagnosis

Altered Thought Processes (8.3)
A state in which an individual experiences a disruption in cognitive operations and activities.

Assessment Data

Defining Characteristics

- Disorientation
- Suspiciousness or mistrust
- Inability to concentrate
- Fear
- Lack of reasonable judgment
- Inability to deal with abstract thoughts or ideas

(continued)
Assessment Data

| Related Factors | • Inappropriate social behavior
• Delusions
• Hallucinations
• Combative behavior |

Expected Outcomes

| Initial | *The client will:* |

- Increase reality contact
- Demonstrate decreased agitation or restlessness
- Demonstrate decreased delusions or hallucinations

| Discharge | *The client will:* |

- Demonstrate accurate awareness of surroundings
- Attain his or her optimal level of functioning
- Live in the least restrictive environment possible

Therapeutic Aims

- Decrease delusions, hallucinations, and restlessness.
- Provide reality orientation.
- Facilitate memory.
- Decrease confusion and disorientation.

Implementation

Nursing Interventions	Rationale
Do not isolate the client. It may be helpful to place the client in a room near the nursing station to facilitate interaction.	Contact with others is reality. Hallucinations usually increase when the client is alone.
Assess the client's disorientation or confusion regularly.	The client's level of orientation may vary.
Refer to the date, time of day, and recent activities during your interactions with the client.	Reminders help to orient the client, and he or she does not have to ask.
Correct errors in the client's perceptions of reality in a matter-of-fact manner. Do not laugh at the client's misperceptions, and do not allow other clients to ridicule the client.	Failing to correct the client's errors in reality contact or laughing at the client undermines his or her sense of personal worth and dignity.
Encourage visits from the client's friends and family, and assess their effect on the client's confusion and memory. You may need to limit the visits if the client tolerates them poorly.	Family and friends usually enhance the client's reality contact. Increased agitation or confusion following visits may signal the need to limit frequency or duration of visits.

(continued)
Implementation

Nursing Interventions	Rationale
Allow the client to have familiar possessions in his or her room. Pictures and personal clothing usually are helpful.	Assign the same staff members to work with the client whenever possible to decrease his or her confusion.

Nursing Diagnosis

Impaired Social Interaction (3.1.1)

The state in which an individual participates in an insufficient or excessive quantity or ineffective quality of social exchange.

Assessment Data

Defining Characteristics	• Confusion with or without periods of awareness and lucidity • Feelings of frustration • Feelings of hopelessness • Impaired memory, particularly concerning recent events • Disinterest in surroundings
Related Factors	• Withdrawn behavior • Lack of social skills • Low self-esteem • Lack of or inaccessibility to support system

Expected Outcomes

Initial	*The client will:* • Interact with others in the immediate environment • Express feelings of frustration or hopelessness • Limit negative comments about self • Decrease socially inappropriate behavior
Discharge	*The client will:* • Engage in satisfactory interpersonal relationships within his or her limitations • Verbalize increased feelings or self-worth within his or her limitations

Therapeutic Aims

• Promote self-esteem.
• Promote interest in surroundings.
• Decrease inappropriate behavior.
• Facilitate socialization skills.

✱ Implementation

Nursing Interventions	Rationale
Do not allow the client to embarrass himself or herself in front of others. Intervene as soon as you observe embarrassing behavior (for example, undressing, advances toward others, urinating somewhere other than the bathroom).	You must protect the client's privacy and dignity when he or she is unable to do so.
Take a matter-of-fact approach; do not chastise or ridicule the client.	Scolding the client (as you might a child) is not helpful, because the client is not willfully misbehaving, and this is something the client can't understand.
Offer acceptable alternatives, and redirect the client's activities ("Mr. X, it is not appropriate to undress here, I'll help you to your room to undress").	Providing alternatives guides the client to appropriate behavior, of which he or she may be unaware.
Praise the client for appropriate behavior.	Positive feedback increases the frequency of desired behavior and lets the client know what is acceptable.
Determine what the client's interests, hobbies, and favorite activities were before hospitalization. (It may be necessary to obtain this information from the client's family or friends.)	It is easier to continue or resume previous interests and hobbies than to develop new ones.
Assess the client's current capability of engaging in former hobbies or activities. Make these activities available as much as possible.	Some former activities may not be feasible, depending on the client's physical and mental capabilities. The client may need to assume a role as a spectator rather than a participant for these activities.
Introduce the activities during a time of the day when the client seems most able to concentrate and participate.	This will maximize the client's ability to participate successfully.
Approach the client with a calm, positive attitude. Convey the idea that you believe he or she can succeed.	A positive approach enhances the client's confidence.
Begin with small, short-term activities, initially one-to-one with staff, and gradually progress to small groups.	Successful completion is more likely with simple, short activities that involve fewer people.
Increase the length or complexity of the activity or task gradually.	Gradually increasing the difficulty challenges the client to his or her maximum potential.
Evaluate the activities and approaches; determine those that are most successful, and continue to use them.	Consistency decreases the client's frustration and builds on his or her success.
Encourage small group activities or discussion of an activity with clients who share similar interests.	The client's social skills may be enhanced when discussing common interests with others.

⊛ *(continued)*

Implementation

Nursing Interventions	Rationale
Involve the client with people from the community, such as volunteers, for social interaction. Identify groups outside the hospital in which the client can participate in the future.	The client has an opportunity to become familiar with people in the community with whom he or she may continue to socialize after hospitalization.
Allow the client to ventilate feelings of despair or hopelessness. Do not merely try to cheer up the client or belittle his or her feelings by using pat phrases or platitudes.	It is important to remember that the client is an adult, and disability can be quite frustrating to him or her.

Organic Mental Syndromes

The essential feature of all *organic mental syndromes* is a psychologic or behavioral problem caused by permanent or transitory dysfunction of the brain.

The organic mental syndromes can be grouped into six categories:

Delirium involves disorganized thoughts and speech, the inability to attend appropriately to external stimuli, and a reduced level of consciousness. It is most common in children and in adults over age 60. The duration is usually 1 week, and it is medically managed by treatment of the underlying cause. The underlying pathology may include systemic infections, metabolic disorders, renal disease, postsurgical complications, or alcohol withdrawal. (See Care Plan 31: Alcohol Detoxification.)

Amnesic syndrome involves an impairment of memory not attributable to other organic syndromes. The client exhibits confabulation, lack of insight, shallow affect, and apathy. The most common cause is thiamine deficiency related to alcohol abuse. Additional etiologic factors include brain pathology from head trauma, surgery, infarction, or hypoxia. The incidence is relatively rare.

Organic delusional syndrome is characterized by delusions resulting from organic damage, with no other symptoms that indicate schizophrenia or delusional disorder.

Organic hallucinosis is characterized by persistent or recurrent hallucinations due to an organic factor. Clients may or may not recognize the hallucinations as such and may be either pleasantly entertained by the hallucinations, anxious, or frightened. Organic hallucinosis is relatively uncommon but does occur in some clients who are blind or deaf. It also is associated with alcohol detoxification.

Organic affective or *mood syndrome* involves widely ranging mood swings, both elevated and depressed, that are organically based. Head injuries are the most common cause of the syndrome.

Organic personality syndrome is characterized by outbursts of aggression, labile moods, apathy, impaired judgment, and socially inappropriate behavior. Head injury and temporal lobe epilepsy frequently are associated with this diagnosis. It also is seen in the beginning stages of some neurologic diseases, such as Huntington's chorea and multiple sclerosis.

Although some of the distinct symptoms may require varied interventions, basic interventions address the commonalities in these disorders. Disorders with an organic etiology do not respond to psychotropic medications as readily as major psychiatric disorders. The client or nurse must deal with symptoms recurrently, relying primarily on behavioral interventions. The goals and expected outcomes for a client with an organic disorder must be altered with the realization that in some cases the problems are due to permanent brain dysfunction, which may be a barrier to learning or behavior changes. Fluctuation of symptoms on a daily or more frequent basis is common and requires reassessment and evaluation on a continuous basis.

Nursing Diagnoses Addressed in this Care Plan

Impaired Social Interaction
Ineffective Individual Coping

Related Nursing Diagnoses

Altered Role Performance
Noncompliance
Altered Family Processes
Diversional Activity Deficit
Impaired Home Maintenance Management
Self-Esteem Disturbance

Nursing Diagnosis

Ineffective Individual Coping (5.1.1.1)
Impairment of adaptive behaviors and problem-solving abilities of a person in meeting life's demands and roles.

Assessment Data

Defining Characteristics	• Poor judgment
	• Cognitive impairment
	• Impaired memory
	• Lack of or limited insight

Related Factors	• Loss of personal control
	• Inability to perceive harm
	• Delusions
	• Hallucinations

Expected Outcomes

| Initial | *The client will:* |

• Engage in a trust relationship with staff and caregiver
• Be free of injury
• Increase reality contact
• Participate in treatment

| Discharge | *The client will:* |

• Establish or follow a routine for activities of daily living
• Demonstrate decreased delusions, hallucinations, or other symptoms

❋ *(continued)*
Expected Outcomes

Discharge	• Verbally recognize symptoms or validate perceptions with staff or caregiver before taking action
	• Live in the least restrictive environment that is safe

❋
Therapeutic Aims

- Provide a safe environment.
- Establish a trust relationship.
- Maximize the client's independence.
- Minimize the client's misperceptions.

❋
Implementation

Nursing Interventions	Rationale
Do not allow the client to assume responsibility for decisions or actions if he or she is unsafe.	The client's safety is a priority. He or she may be unable to discriminate accurately potentially harmful actions or situations.
If limits on the client's behavior or actions are necessary, explain limits, consequences, and reasons clearly, within the client's ability to understand.	The client has the right to be informed of any restrictions and the reasons limits are needed.
Involve the client in making plans or decisions as much as he or she is able to participate.	Compliance with treatment is enhanced if the client is emotionally invested in it.
Include a community contact person or caregiver in planning and treatment as soon as possible.	The sooner a person outside the hospital setting becomes involved, the sooner the client begins to form a relationship with him or her.
Give the client factual feedback on his or her misperceptions, delusions, or hallucinations.	The client must be aware of his or her behavior before he or she can take measures to modify that behavior.
In a matter-of-fact manner, convey to the client that others do not share his or her interpretations.	When given feedback in a nonjudgmental way, the client can feel validated for his or her feelings, while recognizing that others do not respond to similar stimuli in the same way.
Assess the client daily or more often if needed for his or her level of functioning.	Clients with organically based problems tend to fluctuate frequently in terms of their capabilities.
Allow the client to make decisions as much as he or she is able.	Decision making increases the client's participation and his or her independence and self-esteem.
Assist the client to establish a daily routine, including hygiene, activities, and so forth.	Activities that are routine or part of the client's habits do not require continual decisions about whether or not to perform a particular task.
Encourage the client to use a calendar or written schedule rather than verbal reminders, if possible.	Written schedules are concrete and allow the client to "remind" himself or herself, decreasing reliance on others.

Nursing Diagnosis

Impaired Social Interaction (3.1.1)

The state in which an individual participates in an insufficient or excessive quantity or ineffective quality of social exchange.

Assessment Data

Defining Characteristics	• Apathy
	• Emotional blandness
	• Irritability
	• Lack of initiative
	• Feelings of hopelessness or powerlessness
	• Recognition of lost capabilities

Related Factors	• Lack of leisure skills
	• Poor social skills
	• Ineffective or inaccessible support system
	• Mood swings

Expected Outcomes

Initial	*The client will:*
	• Verbalize feelings of hopelessness or powerlessness
	• Verbalize or express losses
	• Respond to social contacts in the structured environment

Discharge	*The client will:*
	• Demonstrate appropriate social interactions
	• Participate in leisure activities with others
	• Verbalize or demonstrate increased feelings of self-worth, if possible
	• Progress through stages of grieving within his or her limitations

Therapeutic Aims

• Promote involvement with social and leisure activities.
• Facilitate expression of feelings.

Implementation

Nursing Interventions	Rationale
Encourage the client to verbalize feelings, especially feelings of loss, anger, resentment, and so forth.	Expressing feelings is an initial step toward dealing with them constructively.
Give the client positive feedback when he or she is able to identify areas that are difficult for him or her.	Positive reinforcement of a desired behavior helps to increase the frequency of that behavior.
Ask the client to clarify any feelings that he or she expresses vaguely. Encourage the client to be specific.	Clarification can prevent a misunderstanding of what the client is trying to convey.

✹ *(continued)*
Implementation

Nursing Interventions	Rationale
If the client becomes agitated when discussing sensitive topics or seems unable to express himself or herself, redirect the client to a more neutral topic, or engage the client in a calming or pleasurable activity.	At times, the client will be overwhelmed by feelings or unable to express himself or herself in a way that is therapeutic or productive. This may be particularly true as the organic changes progress.
Encourage the client to interact with staff or other clients on topics of interest.	The client may be reluctant to initiate interaction and may need external stimulation to converse with others.
Encourage the client to reminisce about events in his or her past.	The client's long-term memory is more intact than short-term memory, so reminiscing often is within the client's capabilities when discussing current events is not.
Give the client positive feedback for engaging in social interactions and leisure activities.	Positive feedback increases the likelihood that the client will continue to interact and participate in activities.
Identify support systems outside the hospital that provide opportunities for social interaction after the client is discharged.	The client is not likely to maintain the level of interaction or participation in activities that he or she has achieved without continued stimulation.

Neurologic Illnesses

Degenerative neurologic illnesses may involve the premature senescence of nerve cells or a metabolic disturbance, or it may have an unknown etiology. The effects of these illnesses drastically alter the lives of clients, their families, and significant others. These illnesses are accompanied by a wide variety of physical symptoms and psychologic alterations, which result in the disruption of the client's life. The progressive nature of these disorders requires constant adaptation for the client and his or her family or significant others.

Major neurologic disorders include the following:

Huntington's chorea is an inherited, dominant gene disease primarily involving cerebral atrophy, demyelination, and ventricle enlargement. The initial symptom is *chorea,* or *choreiform movements.* These movements are continuous (except during sleep) and involve facial contortions, twisting, turning, and tongue movements. Personality changes are the initial psychosocial manifestations—the client is irritable, demanding, and suspicious. This is followed by memory loss and decreased intellectual ability, and the disease progresses like other dementias. (See Care Plan 15: "Dementia.") Incidence of psychosis and suicide is high. The disease may last 10 to 20 years before death occurs.

Multiple sclerosis (MS) is characterized by demyelination throughout the central nervous system. It usually begins with muscular weakness, visual impairment, and urinary bladder dysfunction. This disease usually is characterized by remissions and exacerbations, although as many as 30% of clients with MS worsen steadily from the onset. Between remissions, symptoms tend to become more severe with increasing permanent deficits. The disease usually is diagnosed between ages 20 and 40 and lasts approximately 20 years before death occurs, but this may vary greatly with individuals. Clients with MS range from being depressed and irritable to being neurotic, euphoric, and giddy. Inappropriate social behavior, belligerence, or apathy may be seen.

Amyotropic lateral sclerosis is a motor neuron disease that causes destruction of the myelin sheaths and the formation of scar tissue. This causes progressive muscle weakness, atrophy, and fasciculations. It affects men more frequently than women and appears in middle age. The client remains alert, and sensation is unaffected. Death usually occurs in 5 years due to respiratory complications.

Parkinson disease, also known as *paralysis agitans,* is a progressive disease involving loss of neurons of the basal ganglia. It is characterized by tremor, muscle rigidity, and loss of postural reflexes. The client may experience drooling, a shuffling gait that is propulsive, masklike facies, and slow, monotonous speech. It affects men and women equally, usually beginning at ages 50 to 60 but is not a primary cause of death.

Myasthenia gravis is a relatively rare disease in which nerve impulses fail to pass the myoneural junction. The etiology is unknown, and there are no observable structural changes in the muscles or nerves. The disease usually occurs in young adults, and it is characterized by remissions and exacerbations of muscular weakness and fatigability, ptosis of the eyelids, dysphagia, and respiratory difficulties.

In addition to the behavioral and psychologic changes that are manifested by clients with these neurologic diseases, many other problems are possible. This includes depression, withdrawn behavior, suicidal ideation, hostile or aggressive behavior, and disturbances in sleep patterns and nutritional intake. (See other care plans in this *Manual* as indicated.)

Nursing Diagnoses Addressed in this Care Plan

Body Image Disturbance
Altered Role Performance

Related Nursing Diagnoses

Impaired Adjustment
Altered Health Maintenance
Self-Esteem Disturbance
Social Isolation
Knowledge Deficit
Diversional Activity Deficit
Powerlessness
Hopelessness

Nursing Diagnosis

Body Image Disturbance (7.1.1)
Disruption in the way one perceives one's body image.

Assessment Data

Defining Characteristics

- Emotional lability
- Fear of rejection by others
- Inappropriate social behavior
- Denial of changes
- Distorted perceptions
- Loss of personal control
- Helplessness
- Anger about bodily changes resulting from disease
- Rejection of physical self as altered by disease

✸ *(continued*
Assessment Data

Related Factors	• Inadequate knowledge • Physical problems or limitations • Related emotional or psychiatric problems

✸
Expected Outcomes

Initial	*The client will:* • Acknowledge changes or losses in realistic terms • Verbalize feelings openly • Participate in planning and decision making • Demonstrate appropriate social interactions
Discharge	*The client will:* • Discuss future plans, incorporating the loss or change • Progress through stages of grief • Seek needed support from health professionals, caregivers, and significant others

✸
Therapeutic Aims

• Promote expression of feelings.
• Maximize independence.
• Facilitate grief work and integration of change in body image.

✸
Implementation

Nursing Interventions	Rationale
Encourage the client to discuss his or her feelings openly, particularly "negative" feelings, such as frustration, anger, grief, resentment, and hopelessness.	The client may tend to suppress "negative feelings" unless he or she knows expression of those feelings is encouraged.
Allow adequate time to sit with the client for discussion of feelings when physical care is not being provided.	This gives the client the message that discussing feelings is as important as physical care.
Include the client's family or significant others during some of the discussions to help them share feelings with each other.	The client and his or her family or significant others may be hesitant to openly discuss feelings, believing it is preferable always to be cheerful and optimistic.
Encourage the client (and his or her family or significant others) to discuss the client's loss in terms of things that are no longer possible and things that the client or family can still do.	The client (and his or her family or significant others) need to verbalize realistic changes in realistic terms before they can begin to cope with them successfully.
Do not attempt to cheer the client or change the subject when he or she is upset or verbalizing negative thoughts.	False cheerfulness belittles the client's real feelings and gives the message that it is unacceptable to discuss negative feelings and thoughts.
Do not falsely reassure the client. Answer all questions honestly and directly.	An attitude of false reassurance can be condescending to the client and a barrier to the client's adaptation to actual losses.

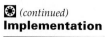 *(continued)*
Implementation

Nursing Interventions	Rationale
Give the client positive feedback for open expression of feelings.	Positive feedback can provide genuine reassurance for the client and encourage the continuing expression of feelings.

Nursing Diagnosis

Altered Role Performance (3.2.1)
Disruption in the way one perceives one's role.

Assessment Data

Defining Characteristics	• Apathy • Inability to continue pre-illness role • Loss of independence (current or anticipated) • Attention deficits • Low self-esteem • Fear of unknown • Inability to concentrate
Related Factors	• Inadequate problem-solving skills • Resentment of dependency • Financial concerns • Change in family structure and roles • Cognitive and perceptual impairment

Expected Outcomes

Initial	*The client will:* • Identify life areas that require alterations due to the illness • Maintain independence within his or her limitations • Verbalize abilities and limitations realistically
Discharge	*The client will:* • Verbalize increased feelings of self-worth • Discuss current or anticipated changes in family with significant others • Organize his or her affairs • Make a written list of future wishes to deal with anticipated situations

Therapeutic Aims

• Maximize independence and control.
• Assist the client to anticipate further changes.
• Facilitate planning with significant others.

Implementation

Nursing Interventions	Rationale
Allow the client to complete any tasks that are within his or her physical capabilities.	Completion of self-care and other responsibilities without assistance allows the client to retain as much independence as possible and enhances his or her self-esteem.
Provide ample time for task completion to avoid rushing the client.	The client will be slower with respect to psychomotor skills. Rushing the client increases frustration and is a barrier to successful task completion.
Provide rest periods at regular intervals. Do not wait until the client is too exhausted to continue.	Rest periods prevent overtiring. Once fatigue is present, the client's ability to recover is impaired.
Break complex tasks into small steps.	Accomplishing a number of small tasks allows the client to have an increased number of successful experiences. The client will be more likely to complete smaller steps because his or her concentration span or other abilities may be impaired.
As psychomotor skills diminish, allow the client to continue decision making about tasks, even if he or she is unable to perform the task.	Decision making allows the client to retain some personal control over his or her situation, even when he or she is dependent on others for physical care. Also, the client's cognitive abilities may remain intact longer than psychomotor skills.
Approach the client on an adult level, using a matter-of-fact approach regarding personal care.	A matter-of-fact attitude lessens the possibility that the client will become embarrassed or feel awkward.
When the client becomes frustrated, have him or her stop the task and try again later. Avoid doing the task for the client at these times.	Allowing the client to stop a frustrating situation, relax, and try again decreases his or her frustration and teaches the client to do this in the future. Performing the task for the client may convey your belief that he or she is unable to participate in care.
Involve the client in any discussion about how care is given, who will give care (when possible), and so forth.	This allows the client to remain included and, when possible, retain decision making and personal control.
If the client's energy is diminished, allow him or her to choose which tasks he or she would like to perform and to delegate other tasks to a caregiver.	Allowing the client choices within his or her ability enhances his or her sense of personal control.
Provide factual information to the client, family or significant others, and caregivers about what the client can expect as the disease progresses.	Facing unknown situations can increase anxiety. Reality may not be as frightening as what the client imagines.
Discuss with the client ways in which he or she might deal with future changes when they do occur.	Anticipatory planning can further alleviate the client's anxiety.

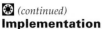 *(continued)*
Implementation

Nursing Interventions	Rationale
Assist the client and his or her caregivers to discuss situations involving the client's anticipated loss of abilities in the future. With input from the client, decisions can be made about how to handle problems when they arise.	The client and his or her caregivers can agree on pre-arranged solutions that may be more effective than trying to problem solve when the client is less able to participate.
If a designated caregiver is not available, help the client make decisions now for actions in the future, when he or she may not be capable of decision making.	Anticipating situations allows the client to retain some control over his or her future.
Assist the client to discuss his or her wishes with family or significant others about heroic measures for medical care, life support, funeral, and so forth. Encourage the client to have his or her wishes in writing as well.	Discussion of the client's wishes allows him or her to have input about crucial decisions that will have to be made eventually and lessens the burden of those decisions for family members.
Encourage the client to develop interests that will be appropriate for the time when physical stamina is diminished.	Stimulation and diversional activities that are suitable for his or her capabilities will enhance the client's quality of life and decrease frustration about disabilities.
Assist the client to begin enjoying these activities now, before they become medically necessary.	If the client has the opportunity to enjoy these activities now, he or she can develop real interest in them and not feel they are solely imposed by physical limitations.

Care Plan 18

Head Injury

Head injury is the third leading cause of neurologic disability in the United States. It primarily affects adolescents and adults under the age of 35. The long-term effects of head injury are behavioral, psychologic, and physical. Common residual problems (after physical rehabilitation is complete) include memory and sensory deficits, impaired cognition, impulsivity, and profound personality changes. As medical technology and trauma services have improved, many more people have survived head injuries (Pylar, 1989); as many as 50,000 new victims per year are left to cope with significant intellectual and physical impairment that can preclude their return to a normal life. Head injuries usually are caused by accidents (for example, falls, diving, vehicular accidents) or other trauma (for example, assault, physical abuse, combative sports).

Following physical recovery, few resources are available for long-term rehabilitation for head-injured clients. Families must cope with drastic changes in the individual's ability to earn a living, participate in social activities, or function in the roles of spouse, parent, partner, sibling, or child. Family members are forced to assume new roles as the family system attempts to reestablish equilibrium. Most head-injured clients are aware to some extent of their previous potential and the current level of impairment that has dramatically changed their lives.

The physical rehabilitation needs of head-injured clients are great. This care plan focuses on the behavioral and psychologic needs of these clients. Frequently, head injury is the basis for the diagnoses of Organic Personality Disorder and Organic Affective Disorder. (See Care Plan 16: Organic Mental Syndromes.)

Nursing Diagnoses Addressed in this Care Plan

High Risk for Injury
Impaired Adjustment

Related Nursing Diagnoses

Ineffective Individual Coping
Altered Family Processes
Self-Esteem Disturbance
Diversional Activity Deficit
Noncompliance
Impaired Social Interaction
High Risk for Violence: Self-Directed or Directed at Others

Nursing Diagnosis

High Risk for Injury (1.6.1)
A state in which the individual is at risk as a result of environmental conditions interacting with his or her adaptive and defensive resources.

Risk Factors

- Inappropriate or unacceptable social behavior
- Sensory or memory deficits
- Impulsive behavior
- Impaired cognition
- Inability to distinguish potentially harmful situations
- Lack of awareness of physical or cognitive impairment

Expected Outcomes

Initial

The client will:

- Be free of injury
- Respond to limits regarding safety
- Respond to cues from others regarding acceptable social behaviors

Discharge

The client will:

- Refrain from unnecessary risks
- Perform daily routine safely
- Demonstrate socially appropriate behavior

Therapeutic Aims

- Prevent injury.
- Promote safe behaviors.
- Decrease impulsivity.
- Promote socially acceptable behavior.

Implementation

Nursing Interventions	Rationale
Provide a safe environment.	The client's safety is a priority. The client may be unable to behave in a safe manner due to his or her impaired judgment or impulsivity.
Intervene if the client is exhibiting behavior that is unsafe or socially inappropriate.	The client lacks the ability to determine the appropriateness of his or her behavior.
Use a matter-of-fact approach. Do not scold or chastise the client or become angry with him or her.	The client's behavior is not willful and may be responsive to verbal corrections. The client may have a negative response to the tone of your voice yet miss the meaning of your words altogether. Being matter-of-fact decreases the client's embarrassment and avoids a power struggle.
Set and reinforce limits regarding safe behavior.	The client's ability to recognize unsafe actions is impaired.

(continued)
Implementation

Nursing Interventions	Rationale
Redirect the client to more socially appropriate behavior.	Redirection provides a socially appropriate alternative for the client.
Give positive feedback for appropriate behavior.	Positive feedback can increase the frequency of the desired behavior.
Provide the client with opportunities for release of tension that are safe (for example, using a punching bag or exercising in the gym).	Physical activity provides the client with a way to relieve tension in a healthy, safe manner.

Nursing Diagnosis

Impaired Adjustment (5.1.1.1.1)
The state in which the individual is unable to modify his or her life-style or behavior in a manner consistent with a change in health status.

Assessment Data

Defining Characteristics	• Irritability • Mood swings • Negativism • Apathy • Low self-esteem • Poor judgment
Related Factors	• Impaired cognition • Altered body image • Incomplete grieving • Resistance to or noncompliance with therapy • Impaired social skills • Lack of insight or understanding

Expected Outcomes

Initial	*The client will:* • Verbalize feelings openly and honestly • Participate in planning treatment • Demonstrate a daily routine, including self-care activities, responsibilities, and recreation • Comply with therapeutic regimen
Discharge	*The client will:* • Verbalize increased feelings of self-worth • Verbalize knowledge of neurologic condition and abilities, treatment, or safe use of medication, if any

(continued)
Expected Outcomes

Discharge

- Demonstrate progress with grief work
- Perform functional role within his or her limitations

Therapeutic Aims

- Promote expression of feelings.
- Facilitate grief work.
- Promote coping with deficits and role changes.
- Decrease apathy or negativism.
- Promote compliance with treatment.

Implementation

Nursing Interventions	Rationale
Encourage the client to verbalize feelings openly.	Identification and expression of feelings is an essential step toward dealing with those feelings.
Encourage appropriate expression of anger or resentment.	The client may benefit from permission to express negative feelings safely.
Do not attempt to cheer the client with statements such as "At least you're alive; that's something to be thankful for."	The client may not agree with your opinion or could feel that his or her real feelings are belittled.
Assist the client to specify his or her losses in concrete terms.	It is easier to deal with a loss stated in specific terms, rather than overwhelming, vague terms.
Give positive feedback for expression of honest feelings. Avoid reinforcing only hopeful or cheerful client statements.	The client must feel free to express actual feelings, not just those that are happy or optimistic.
Assist the client to rediscover old interests or identify new ones.	The client may have forgotten old interests or may lack motivation to pursue old or new interests.
Make needed adaptations to accommodate the client's physical limitations when possible.	Previous interests or hobbies may still be possible with adaptation or assistive devices.
Ask open-ended questions, rather than giving specific suggestions or asking questions that can be answered "yes" or "no." For example, ask "What shall we try today?" rather than "Do you want to . . . ?"	Negative responses are common when you ask "Do you want . . . ?" questions. Open-ended questions put responsibility on the client to respond more fully.
Give the client a list of potential activities from which he or she must make a selection for the day.	Allowing the client a choice from acceptable or recommended activities gives him or her a sense of control and responsibility.
Respond to negativism with validation for the client's feelings, but maintain positive expectations for the client's behavior or expectations. For example, if the client says "I don't know if I'll like . . ." re-	It often is unsuccessful to convince the client that he or she will like something new. It is more useful to validate his or her feelings, yet encourage the client to try something new.

✸ *(continued)*
Implementation

Nursing Interventions	Rationale
spond with "I don't know either. I guess you'll have to give it a try."	
Provide social skill teaching.	Social awareness and skills frequently are lost or impaired in head-injured clients.
Role play real life situations with which the client has demonstrated difficulty.	Role playing assists the client to relearn lost skills.
Coach the client toward the development of acceptable behaviors.	Coaching allows shaping the client's behavior toward successful completion of the behavior.
Provide reinforcement for successful use of social skills.	Reinforcement enhances the likelihood of recurring behavior.
Include the client in any aspects of daily care (for example, preference of time for therapy) in which he or she can have input.	The client is more likely to comply if he or she has had input in decision making.
Help the client to identify choices.	The client's cognitive impairment may prohibit him or her from seeing alternatives.
With the client, make a schedule of daily events or activities. It may be helpful to use a calendar.	Establishing a routine requires fewer changes and decision points for the client. Written materials provide a concrete visual reminder.
Encourage the client to mark off items as they are completed.	A sense of accomplishment or completion can be enhanced with a concrete activity like crossing off tasks.
Offer verbal reminders, if necessary, referring to the written schedule.	Reminders keep the client focused on the task.
Refer to the day, date, and upcoming events (for example, "Today is Wednesday; that means Occupational Therapy will be this afternoon.")	Orientation is enhanced, and memory loss is diminished with references to date, place, time, and situation.
Give direct, factual information about the injury and the client's deficits to the client, his or her family or significant others, and caregivers.	It usually is easier to deal with known facts, even if they are not optimistic, than to fear the unknown or struggle with the frustration of unknown expectations.
Reassure the client and his or her significant others that these changes are part of the head injury, not willful uncooperativeness.	Behavioral and personality changes that occur with head injuries often are baffling to the client and his or her significant others. It may help him or her to know that they are part of the pathology of the injury.
Encourage the client to anticipate mood swings, and help him or her to identify ways to manage them.	Mood swings are common sequelae of head injuries. Knowing what to expect and having a plan to manage moods increases the client's ability to cope with them.

✳ *(continued)*
Implementation

Nursing Interventions	Rationale
Inform the client about what to expect realistically from medications. Decrease the client's reliance on medications to solve problems.	Medications may provide some stabilization in the client's mood but may not be effective in eliminating fluctuations. Clients with head injuries tend to attempt self-medication to obtain relief.
Instruct the client not to drink alcohol, use drugs, or deviate from his or her prescribed medication regimen.	Alcohol, drugs, and undesired drug interactions can further impair the client's judgment and cognition.
Encourage the client to continue to express feelings about lost capabilities as new situations arise that make deficits apparent.	Dealing with the residual effects of a head injury is an ongoing process.
Respond to the client's statements with validating and reflecting communication techniques. For example, if the client says "I'll never be able to do . . . ", say "That's probably true. It must be frustrating . . . "	Validating statements acknowledge the reality of the client's situation, which may not change. Reflection channels the discussion to feelings, with which the client can work.
Refer the client or family or significant others to a head injury support group, if one is available in your area.	It often is helpful for clients (and significant others) to talk with others who have shared similar losses and problems, particularly with chronic conditions such as head injury.

Section Six

Loss

The care plans in this section address problems that may be encountered when the client suffers a loss. The first care plan, "Grief," describes possible behaviors and nursing care considerations that may be involved in any loss or grieving situation. The second plan, "Altered Body Image," discusses issues and nursing care specific to a loss that involves a change in body image for the client. Finally, Care Plan 21: Living with a Chronic or Terminal Illness, addresses the care of a client who must face an illness that is chronic or terminal, from which there is no hope of actual recovery.

Grief

Grief, or grieving, is a subjective state that occurs in response to a loss (Stuart and Sundeen, 1991). This loss may be of anything that is significant to the client, such as health (after learning of an illness, sudden injury or disability, or during a chronic illness), a job or status, a loved one (through death, termination of a relationship, or separation of some kind), a pet, or a role (such as the mother role when the last child leaves the parental home). The loss may be *anticipated* when the client is aware that a loss will take place (such as when the client or a significant other is diagnosed with an illness or is dying) or *actual,* when the loss has already occurred or is occurring. A loss may be *observable* to others or may be *perceived* only by the client (as with the loss of a fantasy or ideal the client has held). Grief may be in response to any *change,* because change involves loss.

Grief has been described by various authors as a process that includes a number of stages or characteristic feelings or experiences. These include shock, being stopped in one's life or functioning, denial, numbness, developing awareness of the loss, preoccupation with the loss; feelings such as yearning, anger, ambivalence, depression, despair, and guilt; disorganization; release, acceptance, and integration of the loss or reorganization (Beck, Rawlins, and Williams, 1988; Carter, 1989; Kubler-Ross, 1969; Martin, 1989). Progression through this process does not necessarily occur in a certain order, and it is characterized by "stress, pain, and suffering and an impairment of function" (Stuart and Sundeen, 1991). Moreover, skipping stages or going from one into another and back again is common, and the time spent in each phase and in the whole process varies considerably among individuals (from weeks to years).

Grief may be called *grief work,* because the client actually must work through these phases of the process, expressing and accepting the feelings involved (though much of this work often is not completed in the hospital). When the client does not do this work, *dysfunctional grieving* (also called *unresolved grief* or a *morbid grief reaction*) may result, in which conscious grieving may be absent or delayed, distorted or exaggerated, or prolonged (chronic). In dysfunctional grieving the client may deny the loss; deny feelings related to the loss; experience impaired social relationships and functioning; exhibit depressed, withdrawn, or self-destructive behavior; develop symptoms of a physical or psychiatric illness; or continue to experience intense grief long after the acute mourning period.

A number of factors can contribute to dysfunctional or unresolved grieving. Houseman and Pheifer (1988) suggest that traumatic losses early in life, inability to share grief with others, and a lack of interpersonal support and acceptance make unresolved grief more likely. Wolfelt (1991) described three factors that increase the likelihood of what he called "complicated grief": social learning (such as "being strong" or denying or repressing the pain and suffering of grief), a lack of knowledge of the grief process, and a lack of participation in rituals of grief that could help facilitate social support and the expression of feelings.

Discharge planning is extremely important in working with the grieving client. New methods of dealing with stress must be developed if the lost person or object was integral to previous coping strategies, and the client's life-style must be adapted to the loss and new life situation. Loss and grief work are significant stresses from which the (nonterminal) client must recuperate physically as well as emotionally and which can increase the client's vulnerability to illness and even death (Martin, 1989). Rest, exercise, nutrition, hydration, and elimination should be monitored during hospitalization and be included in the discharge plans.

The goal in grief work is not to avoid or eliminate painful feelings. Rather, it is to experience, express, and work through the painful or uncomfortable emotions involved, toward successful integration of the loss.

Nursing Diagnosis Addressed in this Care Plan

Dysfunctional Grieving

Related Nursing Diagnoses

High Risk for Violence: Self-Directed or Directed at Others
Altered Health Maintenance
Sleep Pattern Disturbance
Spiritual Distress

| **Nursing Diagnosis** | ***Dysfunctional Grieving (9.2.1.1)***
 A state in which an individual's response to a loss (actual, perceived, or anticipated) is prolonged, distorted, exaggerated, or delayed and which may impair the individual's functioning. |

Assessment Data

Defining Characteristics	• Difficulty in accepting significant loss
	• Denial of loss
	• Denial of feelings
	• Difficulty in expressing feelings
	• Fear of intensity of feelings
	• Rumination
	• Feelings of despair, hopelessness, disillusionment
	• Feelings of helplessness, powerlessness
	• Loss of interest in activities of daily living
	• Anhedonia (inability to experience pleasure)
	• Ambivalent feelings toward the lost person or object
	• Guilt feelings
	• Crying
	• Anxiety
	• Agitation

(continued)
Assessment Data

Defining Characteristics	• Fatigue
	• Sleep disturbance
	• Self-destructive behavior, accident proneness
	• Anger, hostility, or aggressive behavior
	• Depressive behavior
	• Withdrawn behavior

Related Factors	• Perceived or observable loss
	• Social isolation
	• Physical symptoms or illness
	• Substance abuse

Expected Outcomes

Initial

The client will:

- Be free of self-inflicted harm
- Identify the loss
- Verbalize or demonstrate decreased suicidal, aggressive, depressive, or withdrawn behaviors
- Express feelings, verbally and nonverbally
- Verbalize knowledge of the grief process
- Establish or maintain adequate nutrition, hydration, and elimination
- Establish or maintain an adequate balance of rest, sleep, and activity

Discharge

The client will:

- Verbalize acceptance of the loss
- Demonstrate initial integration of the loss into his or her life
- Verbalize changes in life-style and coping mechanisms incorporating the fact of the loss
- Verbalize realistic future plans integrating the loss
- Demonstrate physical recuperation from the stress of loss and grieving
- Progress through the grieving process
- Verbalize plans for continued therapy, if indicated
- Demonstrate reestablished relationships or social support outside the hospital

Therapeutic Aims

- Establish rapport and build trust.
- Promote adequate nutrition, hydration, and elimination.
- Promote an adequate balance of rest, sleep, and activity.
- Decrease depressive, withdrawn, aggressive, and self-destructive symptoms.
- Decrease secondary gain from depressive symptoms.
- Facilitate the client's progression through the stages of grieving:

  Decrease denial; help the client grasp the fact of the loss.

  Encourage identification of the loss and the expression of feelings about the lost person or object and the client's relationship with the person or object.

  Encourage the client to explore emotional changes as a result of the loss.

❋ (continued)
Therapeutic Aims

Facilitate the client's expression of ambivalent or angry feelings toward the lost person or object and toward himself or herself (anger, hatred, guilt, betrayal, resentment of grief work and the energy it takes, feelings of being deserted, and so forth).

Encourage the client to consciously adapt his or her life-style to the loss and to make concrete and realistic future plans.

• Facilitate a supportive environment.

• Encourage ventilation of feelings within the therapeutic milieu.

• Decrease the client's fears of being overwhelmed by feelings and of having feelings that are destructive, harmful, or undesirable.

• Discourage dependence on a particular staff member or on the therapeutic environment for expression of feelings.

• Facilitate growth in the client's ability to express and deal with feelings (in or out of the hospital).

• Facilitate relief of spiritual distress.

• Help the client recuperate from the stress caused by the loss (attain optimal level of health and functioning).

• Encourage early discharge planning.

❋
Implementation

Nursing Interventions	Rationale
Initially, assign the same staff members to the client, then gradually vary the staff people. See Care Plan 1: Building a Trust Relationship.	The client may be overwhelmed by loss and may fear facing the loss and his or her feelings. His or her ability to respond to others may be impaired. Limiting the number of new contacts initially will provide consistency and facilitate familiarity and trust. However, the number of people interacting with the client should increase as soon as possible to minimize dependency and to facilitate the client's ability to communicate with a variety of people.
After establishing rapport with the client, bring up the loss in a supportive manner; if the client refuses to discuss it, withdraw and state your intention to return. ("I can understand that you may not want to talk with me about this now. I will come to talk with you again at 11:00, maybe we can talk about it then.") Return at the stated time, then continue to be as supportive as possible rather than confronting the client.	Your presence demonstrates interest and caring. Telling the client you will return conveys your support. The client may need emotional support to face and express uncomfortable or painful feelings. Confronting the client or pushing him or her to express feelings may increase anxiety and lead to further denial or avoidance.
Talk with the client in realistic terms concerning his or her loss; discuss concrete changes that have occurred in his or her life as a result of the loss and changes that the client must now begin to make.	Discussing the loss on this level may help to make it more real for the client.

✽ *(continued)*
Implementation

Nursing Interventions	Rationale
Encourage the expression of feelings in ways with which the client is comfortable, for example, talking, writing, drawing, crying, and so forth. Convey your acceptance of these feelings and means of expression. Offer the client verbal support for attempts to express feelings.	Expression of feelings can help the client to identify, accept, and work through his or her feelings, even if these are painful or otherwise uncomfortable for the client.
Encourage the client to recall experiences, talk about what was involved in his or her relationship with the lost person or object, and so forth. Discuss with the client the changes in his or her feelings toward self, others, and the lost person or object as a result of the loss and grief process.	Discussing the lost object or person can help the client identify and express the loss, what the loss means to him or her, and his or her emotional response.
Encourage appropriate (that is, safe) expression of all feelings that the client has toward the lost person or object and convey acceptance. Assure the client that even "negative" feelings like anger and resentment are normal and healthy in grieving.	Feelings are not inherently bad or good. Giving the client support for expressing feelings may help the client accept uncomfortable feelings.
Note: If you feel uncomfortable with the client's expression of feelings (such as crying) or with your role in bringing up painful feelings, then withdraw temporarily. Examine and try to become comfortable with your own feelings or have the client speak with someone who is comfortable in that role. (See Basic Concepts: Nurse–Client Interactions.)	Your comfort with the client's feelings conveys support and acceptance. If you are uncomfortable, however, you may inadvertently convey disinterest or disapproval or may reinforce the client's avoidance of feelings.
Convey to the client that although feelings may be uncomfortable, they are natural and necessary to this process, that he or she can withstand having these feelings, and that the feelings will not harm him or her.	The client may fear the intensity of his or her feelings.
Discourage the client's using hospitalization or activities to avoid grieving ("to get my mind off it"); do not support avoidance of grief work. Convey that although the client does not have to think or talk about his or her feelings at all times, a part of each day should be spent dealing with or being aware of them. At least once per shift, invite the client to talk about his or her loss, feelings, plans, and so forth.	It is important to reinforce the client's grief work as necessary and healthy. Avoiding feelings may delay the client's progress through grieving.
Discourage rumination or stopping in one stage of grief work (if the client is ruminating on his or her own guilt, for example; after listening to the client's feelings, tell the client you will talk about other aspects of grief and feelings).	The client needs to identify and express the feelings that underlie the rumination and to proceed through the grief process.

(continued)
Implementation

Nursing Interventions	Rationale
Referral to the facility chaplain, clergy, or other spiritual resource person may be indicated.	The client may be more comfortable discussing spiritual issues with an advisor who shares his or her belief system.
Provide opportunities for the release of tension, anger, guilt, and so forth through physical activities. Promote regular exercise as a healthy means of dealing with stress and tension.	Physical activity provides a way to relieve tension in a healthy, nondestructive manner.
Limit times and frequency of therapeutic interactions with the client. Encourage independent, spontaneous expression of feelings (writing, initiating interactions with other clients or with other staff members, getting involved in a physical activity). Plan staff-initiated interactions at times that allow the client to fulfill responsibilities (activities, unit duties) and maintain personal care (sleeping, eating, hygiene).	The client needs to develop independent skills of communicating feelings and to integrate the loss into his or her daily life.
Expect the client to fulfill his or her own responsibilities, and support the client for doing so. Withdraw your attention when the client does not fulfill responsibilities (that is, do not have a therapeutic interaction when the client has refused to participate in an activity).	It is important to minimize secondary gain and to convey that the client can fulfill responsibilities and activities of daily living while grieving.
Encourage the client to talk with others, individually and in small groups (larger as tolerated), about the loss in terms of his or her own and others' feelings and about experiences and changes resulting from the loss.	The client needs to develop independent skills of communicating feelings and to integrate the loss into his or her daily life.
Facilitate sharing, communicating, ventilating feelings, and support among clients. Use larger groups (such as open report) for a general discussion of loss and grief (with or without focusing on this client's loss). However, help the client also realize that there are limits to sharing grief in a social context.	Sharing grief and experiences with others can help the client identify and express feelings and feel normal in grieving. Dwelling on grief in social interactions, however, can result in other people's discomfort with their own feelings and may lead to the client being avoided by friends and significant others.
Point out to the client that a major aspect of loss is a real physical stress. Encourage good nutrition, hydration, and elimination, as well as adequate rest and daily physical exercise (such as walking, running, swimming, or cycling), in the hospital and postdischarge.	The client may be unaware of the physical stress of the loss or may lack interest in the activities of daily living. Physical exercise can relieve tension or pent-up feelings in a healthy, nondestructive manner.
Teach the client (and his or her family or significant others) about the grief process.	The client and his or her family or significant others may have little or no knowledge of grief or the process involved in recovery.

✳ *(continued)*
Implementation

Nursing Interventions	Rationale
Point out to the client that time spent grieving can be a nurturing time, a time of learning and growth from which to gather the strength to go forward.	The grief process allows the client to adjust to a change in his or her life and to begin to move toward opportunities in the future.
Urge the client to identify and pursue his or her own strengths inside and outside the hospital. Facilitate activities that promote development of the client's strengths.	The client's own strengths are a major factor in his or her ability to deal with continuing grief work.
As much as possible, include in each interaction with the client some discussion of goals, the future, and discharge plans.	The client needs to integrate loss and grief into his or her life outside the hospital.
Help the client plan for the future with regard to changes made necessary by the loss, at whatever levels the loss affects (living arrangements, finances, social activities, vocation, recreation, and so forth). Use hospital and community resources.	Planning the future with regard to the loss may help the client integrate the loss and accept the continuation of his or her own life.

Altered Body Image

Body image is a person's perception of his or her physical self. This perception includes physical appearance, emotional reactions, and sensations and extends beyond the body to include objects such as clothing or items used in work (Wilson and Kneisl, 1988). A person's body image forms as he or she develops, beginning at birth and changing throughout life. It is closely tied to self-esteem and identity (McFarland and Thomas, 1991), both of which are threatened by an alteration in body image. A person's body image includes conscious and unconscious perceptions of the body's physical attributes and functioning, as well as attitudes and feelings about the body, its parts, and its functioning. Body image also is influenced by messages one receives from others (Bronheim, Strain, and Biller, 1991; Tomaselli, Jenks, and Morin, 1991; Wilson and Kneisl, 1988). Feelings of body image and the sense of self include those related to sexuality, femininity, masculinity, parenthood, youthfulness, maturity, health, strength, and ability.

Altered body image is a change in a person's perception of and attitudes about his or her physical self. This alteration often occurs in response to a major physical change and involves a loss (Wilson and Kneisl, 1988) and grieving. This loss may be the result of a burn or other trauma; the diagnosis of a chronic, debilitating, disfiguring, or terminal illness (see Basic Concepts: HIV Disease and AIDS and Care Plan 21: Living with a Chronic or Terminal Illness); surgery (especially radical or mutilating), stoma, or amputation; or stroke. The loss may be the result of changes in appearance, fitness, or abilities that occur as a result of growth, maturation, or aging in any stage of life, such as adolescence, adulthood, or growing old (see Care Plan 10: Adjustment Disorders of Adolescents, Care Plan 47: Adjustment Disorders of Adults, and Basic Concepts: The Aging Client). It may even be a part of a procedure the client has chosen, such as gender change, breast augmentation or reduction, or other reconstructive surgery.

An alteration in body image involves grief work, as in any loss. Grieving in response to a change in body image can include shock, denial or disbelief, fear, anger, depression, and acceptance or reorganization; it can be a functional adaptation, or it may be dysfunctional or unresolved (Newell, 1991). (See Care Plan 19: Grief.) However, grief related to a change in one's own body image differs from the grief that results from the loss of a person or thing outside oneself because a permanent change in body image or loss of physical function remains present and cannot be replaced. Thus, the resolution of the grief becomes adaptation to a change that does not get better or go away. Progression through the various stages of grieving is not necessarily orderly; these phases may overlap, and the client may vacillate among them. A change in body image is more traumatic when it is external and visible to the person and others; involves the face, genitals, or breasts;

occurs suddenly (Wilson and Kneisl, 1988); or is unforeseen, uncontrolled, or unwanted (Piotrowski, 1982).

The client's perception of his or her altered body image is more significant than the concrete or observable disability or loss. The removal of an internal portion of the body or any change in the client's health status may be as traumatic to the client as the loss of an extremity that is visible. The intensity of the client's reactions or feelings is not necessarily proportional to the actual loss or disability.

Health care personnel sometimes tend to minimize the change in a client's body and communicate to the client, directly or indirectly, that the loss is not as bad as the client feels it is. Nurses must try to maintain awareness of this possibility, because they may have become accustomed to seeing illness, surgery, and so forth and no longer experience strong feelings in response to these events. Medical and nursing staff may insulate themselves emotionally from such traumatic events as a defense mechanism; they may view these medical situations in a matter-of-fact, "clinical" way; or they may see them as positive events (such as having a stoma or an amputation versus dying), without recognizing or appreciating the emotional implications for the client.

An alteration in body image affects the client's need to feel normal, and it often involves embarrassment or social stigma. The client's significant others are affected by the change, and the client faces their responses, as well as the responses of each new person and new situation he or she encounters. It is essential to remember that this client is still a person, whatever the alteration in his or her body.

Note: The discussion of altered body image differs from body image *distortion,* such as occurs in anorexia nervosa, when a client perceives his or her body to be fat or much larger than it actually is. Such a distortion may be of delusional proportions and may occur in clients with neurologic or psychiatric illness. See other care plans as appropriate.

Nursing Diagnoses Addressed in this Care Plan

Body Image Disturbance
Self-Esteem Disturbance

Related Nursing Diagnoses

Dysfunctional Grieving
High Risk for Violence: Self-Directed or Directed at Others
Social Isolation
Anxiety
Altered Role Performance
Sexual Dysfunction
Knowledge Deficit regarding illness, treatment plan, or safe use of medications

---

Nursing Diagnosis	***Body Image Disturbance (7.1.1)***
	Disruption in the way one perceives one's body image.

Assessment Data

Defining Characteristics	• Actual or perceived physical change or illness
	• Verbal or nonverbal response to change in body structure or function
	• Denial of physical change or illness

✳ *(continued)*
Assessment Data

Defining Characteristics	• Anger, hostility, or rage

• Anger, hostility, or rage
• Guilt
• Resentment
• Confusion
• Anxiety or fear
• Feelings of hopelessness or worthlessness
• Depressive behavior
• Despair
• Withdrawn behavior
• Dissociation or depersonalization
• Grief
• Self-destructive behavior
• Regression
• Dependency
• Refusal to perform self-care activities or activities of daily living (when physically capable)
• Identity concerns (sexual role, role as wage-earner, parental role, and so forth)

Related Factors

• Physical problems related to surgery, injury, or illness
• Aging
• Weight loss or gain

✳
Expected Outcomes

Initial

The client will:

• Verbalize the physical change, loss, or disability
• Discuss altered body image with staff members
• Discuss altered body image with significant others
• Identify and express feelings, verbally and nonverbally
• Establish or maintain adequate nutrition, hydration, and elimination
• Establish or maintain an adequate balance of rest, sleep, and activity
• Participate in treatment program and activities
• Participate in self-care related to surgery, injury, or illness

Discharge

The client will:

• Progress through the grief process
• Verbalize knowledge of his or her physical condition, treatment, and safe use of medication, if any
• Demonstrate skills in activities of daily living and self-care
• Verbalize knowledge of the grief process and recovery
• Identify and use sources of support outside the hospital
• Participate in social activities or groups
• Verbalize changes in life-style and coping mechanisms incorporating the loss or change
• Verbalize realistic future plans integrating the loss or change

Therapeutic Aims

- Build a trust relationship.
- Help the client acknowledge the loss or change.
- Help the client progress through the grief process.
- Promote adequate nutrition, hydration, and elimination.
- Promote an adequate balance of rest, sleep, and activity.
- Decrease suicidal and depressive symtpoms.
- Promote interactions and relationships with others.
- Promote learning about the change and integration of new skills.
- Promote adaptation of the client's life-style, plans, and goals to the change.

Implementation

Nursing Interventions	Rationale
Initially, assign the same staff members to work with the client. Gradually increase the number of people interacting with the client. See Care Plan 1: Building a Trust Relationship.	The client's ability to respond to others may be impaired. The client may expect rejection from others due to the physical change or loss. Initially limiting the number of new contacts will facilitate familiarity and trust. Increasing the number of people interacting with the client will promote the client's ability to communicate with a variety of people.
Approach the client and initiate interaction; use silence and active listening to facilitate communication.	The client's ability to initiate interactions may be impaired due to low self-esteem, anger, and so on. Your presence will demonstrate interest, caring, and acceptance.
Be aware of your own feelings regarding the client's physical change and appearance. Talk with other staff members about feelings of discomfort, repulsion, disapproval, and so forth. Examine your own behavior with the client (such as not looking at or not touching the client or other avoidance behaviors).	Identifying and exploring your own feelings will allow you to be more comfortable with the client. You will be less likely to inadvertently communicate feelings of discomfort and so forth to the client.
In your interactions with the client, view him or her as a whole person, not only as a person with a disability (however, do not ignore or deny the disability or change).	The client needs to know that others will still respond to him or her as a person and that the physical change or loss is not all that others see. Ignoring the change or disability may reinforce the client's denial.
As the client is ready for it, encourage discussion of the physical change in simple, matter-of-fact, concrete terms. Ask for the client's perceptions, and begin teaching the client about the change or illness.	Acknowledgment of the change or loss is necessary to the grief process. Frank but sensitive discussion will convey your acceptance of the client's change and promote feelings of normalcy. Eliciting the client's perceptions may facilitate expression of feelings and help you identify areas in which information is needed.
Encourage expression of feelings, including anger, resentment, guilt, self-blame, envy of healthy people, fears of rejection and inadequacy, and feelings about the change itself (repulsion, fear, and so forth). See Care Plan 51: Hostile Behavior.	Identification and expression of these feelings is a part of grieving and can help the client work through the feelings, even if they are painful or otherwise uncomfortable. The client needs to know that feelings like these are normal and acceptable, not bad.

✳ *(continued)*
Implementation

Nursing Interventions	Rationale
Encourage discussion of what the change means to the client, changes in the client's perception of his or her abilities, feelings of helplessness or inadequacy, feelings of guilt, and so forth.	The client may be experiencing overwhelming feelings of fear, worthlessness, helplessness, and powerlessness. The client may feel burdensome to others, to the point that he or she may feel unable to survive having to depend on others for needs that were formerly met independently. The client may feel that he or she is being punished with the change or disability.
Allow the client quiet time alone to think and express feelings through writing, crying, and other outlets.	The client may need privacy to express certain feelings. He or she needs to develop independence in identifying and expressing feelings.
Referral to the facility chaplain, clergy, or other spiritual resource person may be indicated.	The client may be more comfortable discussing spiritual issues with an advisor who shares his or her belief system.
Teach the client and his or her significant others about the grief process.	The client and his or her family or significant others may have little or no knowledge of the grief process.
See Basic Concepts: The Aging Client, Nurse–Client Interactions, and Care Plan 19: Grief.	
Review with the client his or her strengths and abilities. Help the client identify abilities that are not affected by this physical change and that are changed in some way but not lost.	The client's body image includes feelings about abilities and is closely linked to self-esteem. The client may feel that this physical change has destroyed or changed all of his or her strengths and may need help in identifying those abilities retained.
Communicate realistic expectations of the client; do not expect *less* than the client is capable of doing.	Expecting less than the client is capable of will undermine the client's performance and growth. If the client perceives inability, however, he or she may indeed not be capable at this time.
See Care Plan 23: Depressive Behavior, Care Plan 24: Suicidal Behavior, Care Plan 28: The Client Who Will Not Eat, and Care Plan 48: Sleep Disturbances.	
Encourage the client to identify and express feelings of isolation and fears of rejection and the reactions of others.	The client may expect rejection from others and may project his or her own negative feelings about the change onto others.
Talk with the client's significant others; assess the impact of the client's change, encourage discussion of their feelings and response to the change. Family therapy may be indicated.	The client's significant others are affected by this change and may have feelings of fear, repulsion, inadequacy (in the client's care or with the client's grief), guilt, and so forth. Expression of these feelings (and your acceptance of them) may help the client's significant others work through them.

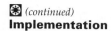 *(continued)*
Implementation

Nursing Interventions	Rationale
Use role playing and rehearsal techniques to help the client anticipate and prepare for the reactions of others, learn to ask for help, and learn to teach others about self.	Anticipatory guidance can increase the client's abilities and confidence in facing others. The client may have been relatively independent until this time and may not be comfortable asking others for help.
Help the client identify and use support systems outside the hospital.	Support groups of people who have experienced the same or a similar change can help the client adapt to the loss. Group or individual therapy may be indicated after hospitalization. Social support (family, friends, former social groups) can help the client feel normal and integrate the new self into his or her life as a whole.
Teach the client and his or her significant others about the physical change; teach skills needed to deal with the change, including self-care, caregiving skills, and safe use of medications, if any. Ask for the client's perceptions, return demonstrations, and so forth. Allow and encourage the client to practice skills and share them with others. Refer the client to a nurse practitioner or to occupational, physical, recreational, or vocational therapists as appropriate. Refer the client to a support group in the area (or by mail if there are no local groups).	The client needs to acquire information and skills related to the physical change to promote self-care and confidence. Information and skills can help the client develop and accept a new body image and integrate the change, prostheses, or other apparatus as necessary.
Discuss sexual concerns and information with the client as appropriate. Remain nonjudgmental and aware of the client's feelings in this area. Refer the client to a support group or a therapist if appropriate.	Sexuality is a basic need and concern to both female and male clients. The client may be afraid to discuss sexuality, may not know how, or may fear disapproval. The client may need to learn new ways to give and receive sexual pleasure and to perceive sexuality. If you are unaware of your own feelings in this area, you may inadvertently express discomfort or disapproval to the client. (See Basic Concepts: Sexuality.) Sexual assertiveness groups and other resources for the disabled are available.
Explore with the client ways of adapting his or her life-style and activities. Identify alternatives, resources, new or changed roles, goals, plans, and so forth.	The client needs to develop and integrate new or altered behaviors, perceptions of self, and goals to adapt to the change.
Help the client prepare to achieve and sustain his or her optimal level of functioning in the future.	It is important not to undermine or underestimate the client's abilities simply because he or she has a disability.
See Care Plan 2: Discharge Planning.	

Nursing Diagnosis	*Self-Esteem Disturbance (7.1.2)* *Negative self evaluation or feelings about self or self-capabilities, which may be directly or indirectly expressed.*

Assessment Data

Defining Characteristics	• Feelings of hopelessness or worthlessness • Self-deprecatory verbalization • Lack of self-confidence • Anxiety or fear • Depressive behavior • Despair • Withdrawn behavior • Self-destructive behavior • Regression • Dependency
Related Factors	• Loss of health, role, or status • Physical change or illness • Change in body image • Aging

Expected Outcomes

Initial	*The client will:* • Be free of self-inflicted harm • Demonstrate decreased suicidal and depressive symptoms • Verbalize increased feelings of self-worth
Discharge	*The client will:* • Be free of suicidal and depressive symptoms • Demonstrate increased feelings of self-worth

Therapeutic Aim

• Promote self-esteem and identification and use of strengths.

Implementation

Nursing Interventions	Rationale
Provide opportunities for the client to succeed at activities, tasks, and interactions. Give positive feedback, and point out the client's demonstrated abilities and strengths.	The client may feel incapable of succeeding at anything and may need help and encouragement to attempt activities. Activities within the client's abilities will provide opportunities for success. Positive feedback provides reinforcement for the client's growth and can enhance self-esteem.
Be realistic in your feedback to the client; do not flatter or be otherwise dishonest.	Clients with low self-esteem do not benefit from flattery or undue praise.

✺ (continued)
Implementation

Nursing Interventions	Rationale
Review with the client his or her strengths and abilities that are not affected by this physical change and those that are changed in some way but not lost.	The client's body image includes feelings about abilities and is closely linked to self-esteem. The client may feel that this physical change has destroyed or changed all of his or her strengths and may need help in identifying those abilities retained.

See Basic Concepts: Building Self-Esteem.

Living with a Chronic or Terminal Illness

Many people in the United States today live with a chronic or terminal illness. This situation results from many factors, including life-style (for example, being sedentary or having a high level of stress), chemical dependence (including cigarette smoking), increased longevity, infection with human immunodeficiency virus (HIV) and other diseases, and the availability of treatments (but not cures) for many diseases. People who are living with such an illness face many challenges and losses, which influence various aspects of their lives. Clients with acquired immunodeficiency virus (AIDS) or other chronic or terminal illnesses are at increased risk for suicide (Stuart and Sundeen, 1991). Clients who have a progressive or terminal illness, with little or no hope of recovery, face continual change and loss (see Care Plan 19: Grief). They must deal with an altered body image that involves the loss of health and may include loss of physical or mental abilities, loss of internal organs, or a change in appearance (see Care Plan 20: Altered Body Image). People with AIDS, for example, often experience severe acute illnesses that can cause extreme weight loss, hair loss, skin lesions, loss of abilities and independence, neurologic impairment, and many other problems.

The loss of a future, if a client has a terminal illness, can be devastating, especially if the client is relatively young or if the illness was sudden or unexpected. Social and economic factors also may be significant problems. Roles and relationships may change, and other people in the client's life may be uncomfortable or withdraw from the client.

In the case of AIDS or other HIV-related diseases, social sanctions against homosexuality or drug use may come into play. Often, for example, a client's family may have been unaware of the client's homosexuality until the client is diagnosed with AIDS. Revelation of the client's homosexuality or drug use may result in the loss of housing, employment, family, or children. For these reasons confidentiality issues are extremely important. The client may blame himself or herself for the illness or be told by others that he or she deserves to be ill because of his or her drug use or homosexuality. (See Basic Concepts: HIV Disease and AIDS.)

Whether the client has AIDS or another chronic or terminal illness, he or she may face the loss of work, income, insurance, housing, social support, and independence. The client may need assistance in obtaining care and in negotiating with social service agencies. The client's family or significant others may need teaching about the client's illness and needs for care, assistance in dealing with their own grief and changes resulting from the client's illness, or assistance with caregiving responsibilities. (See Care Plan 5: Supporting the Caregiver.)

Nursing Diagnoses Addressed in this Care Plan

Anticipatory Grieving
Hopelessness
Altered Health Maintenance

Related Nursing Diagnoses

Body Image Disturbance
Self-Esteem Disturbance
High Risk for Violence: Self-Directed or Directed at Others
Fear
Spiritual Distress
Social Isolation
Altered Role Performance
Knowledge Deficit regarding illness, treatment plan, or safe use of medications

Nursing Diagnosis **Assessment Data**	*Anticipatory Grieving (9.2.1.2)* *A state in which an individual grieves before an actual loss.*

Defining Characteristics	• Potential loss of health, abilities, or life • Expression of distress regarding potential loss • Anger, hostility, or rage • Guilt • Anhedonia (inability to experience pleasure) • Suicidal ideas or feelings • Depression • Sorrow • Despair • Denial of illness or potential loss • Resentment • Altered communication patterns • Changes in eating habits • Sleep disturbances
Related Factors	• Chronic illness • Terminal illness • Altered body image • Inability to perform self-care • Feelings of hopelessness or worthlessness • Feelings of helplessness or powerlessness • Anxiety or fear • Withdrawn behavior • Chemical dependence

Expected Outcomes

Initial	*The client will:*

- Verbalize awareness of his or her illness
- Discuss illness with staff members
- Discuss illness with significant others
- Identify and express feelings, verbally and nonverbally
- Be free of self-inflicted harm
- Demonstrate decreased suicidal, withdrawn, or depressive symptoms
- Participate in treatment program

Discharge	*The client will:*

- Identify and use sources of social support outside the hospital
- Verbalize plans for continued therapy if indicated
- Progress through the grief process

Therapeutic Aims

- Build a trust relationship.
- Help the client acknowledge his or her illness.
- Help the client progress through the grief process.
- Promote expression of feelings, especially anger, self-blame, anxiety, sadness, despair, spiritual distress, and so forth.
- Decrease suicidal, depressive, or withdrawn behavior.
- Promote self-esteem.

Implementation

Nursing Interventions	Rationale
Initially, assign the same staff members to the client. Gradually introduce new staff members.	The client's ability to relate to others may be impaired. Limiting the number of new contacts initially will promote familiarity and trust and decrease feelings of being overwhelmed.
Approach the client in a nonjudgmental way. Be sure to deal with your own feelings of discomfort, if any, related to the client's illness, drug use, or homosexuality.	The client may fear social sanctions or blame related to his or her illness (especially, but not only, with AIDS). All clients are entitled to nonjudgmental nursing care. Being aware of and dealing with your own feelings will help prevent those feelings from interfering in your relationships with the client and his or her significant others.
See Basic Concepts: HIV Disease and AIDS and Care Plan 1: Building a Trust Relationship.	
Approach the client and initiate interactions; use silence and active listening to facilitate communication.	The client may fear rejection from others if he or she talks about the illness. Your presence indicates caring and acceptance.

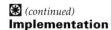 (continued)
Implementation

Nursing Interventions	Rationale
As the client tolerates, encourage discussion of the client's illness, first with staff members, then with the client's significant others and other clients. Be gentle in your approach to the client about his or her illness; talk about the illness in simple, matter-of-fact terms.	Acknowledgment of the illness is necessary to the grief process. Gentility demonstrates regard for the client's feelings. Being matter-of-fact about the illness can help separate the fact of the illness from emotional issues related to grieving or other problems.
Encourage the client to express his or her feelings verbally and nonverbally, in nondestructive ways.	Ventilation of feelings can help lessen feelings of despair and so forth and helps to progress through the grief process.
Referral to the facility chaplain, clergy, or other spiritual resource person may be indicated.	The client may be more comfortable discussing spiritual issues with an advisor who shares his or her belief system.
See Basic Concepts: The Aging Client and Spirituality and Care Plan 19: Grief.	
With the client, identify his or her strengths, resources, and sources of hope, pleasure, and support.	The client may feel so overwhelmed that he or she is unable to see anything positive about himself or herself.
Give the client honest praise for the things that he or she is able to do; acknowledge the client's efforts in the context of his or her illness, impaired abilities, or dying.	The client will not benefit from dishonesty or flattery. However, accomplishments that may seem small to a person without an illness may indeed merit praise in the context of a major illness.
Assure the client that his or her illness is not a form of punishment and that he or she does not deserve to have the illness.	The client may feel responsible for contracting the illness. Other people may state or imply that illness is a punishment or that the client is to blame.
Point out to the client that having a chronic or terminal illness and grieving are difficult tasks. Give the client positive feedback for his or her work in this area.	The client may not realize the work that he or she is doing to face and live with his or her illness.
Encourage the client to identify supportive personal relationships outside the hospital and to maintain those relationships after discharge.	The client may fear rejection from others in his or her life and may need encouragement to contact others.
Help the client to identify community resources, agencies, and groups for assistance after discharge. Referral to a social worker may be indicated.	The client may need continued support after discharge. Social workers can help the client to identify and contact resources. Many communities have support groups for clients who have chronic or terminal illnesses. There also are state and national associations related to many illnesses that provide information and services.
Encourage the client to continue therapy after discharge if indicated.	Grieving, chronic illness, or dying may require long-term therapy.

Nursing Diagnosis	*Hopelessness (7.3.1)* *A subjective state in which an individual sees limited or no alternatives or personal choices available and is unable to mobilize energy on his or her own behalf.*

Assessment Data

Defining Characteristics	• Anger, hostility, or rage • Anhedonia (inability to experience pleasure) • Suicidal ideas or feelings • Depression • Sorrow • Despair • Passivity • Decreased communication • Lack of initiative • Anergy • Impaired social interaction • Withdrawn behavior • Sleep disturbances • Changes in eating habits
Related Factors	• Terminal illness • Overwhelming loss • Physical problems related to the illness • Neurologic problems related to the illness • Inability to perform self-care • Altered body image • Feelings of helplessness or powerlessness • Guilt • Low self-esteem • Loss of spiritual faith • Chemical dependence

Expected Outcomes

Initial	*The client will:* • Be free of self-inflicted harm • Demonstrate decreased suicidal, withdrawn, or depressive symptoms
Discharge	*The client will:* • Demonstrate a maximum level of decision making in planning his or her own care • Be free of suicidal, withdrawn, and depressive symptoms • Demonstrate the ability to identify choices or alternatives • Demonstrate active participation in self-care and plans for life after discharge

Therapeutic Aims

- Provide a safe environment.
- Promote expression of feelings, especially anger, self-blame, anxiety, sadness, despair, spiritual distress, and so forth.
- Decrease suicidal, depressive, or withdrawn behavior.

Implementation

Nursing Interventions	Rationale
Assess the client's suicidal potential, and institute suicide precautions if indicated. See Care Plan 24: Suicidal Behavior.	Clients with a chronic or terminal illness are at increased risk for suicide. The client's safety is a priority.
Encourage the client to express his or her feelings verbally and nonverbally, in nondestructive ways. See Care Plan 23: Depressive Behavior.	Ventilation of feelings can help lessen feelings of despair and so forth and helps the client to progress through the grief process.
Teach the client the steps of the problem-solving process: Describe the problem, list and evaluate alternatives, select and implement an alternative, evaluate the effectiveness of the action.	The client may feel overwhelmed by his or her situation and may not know how to implement a systematic approach to solving problems.
Referral to the facility chaplain, clergy, or other spiritual resource person may be indicated.	The client may be more comfortable discussing spiritual issues with an advisor who shares his or her belief system.
Encourage the client to continue therapy after discharge if indicated.	Grieving, chronic illness, or dying may require long-term therapy.

Nursing Diagnosis

Altered Health Maintenance (6.4.2)
Inability to identify, manage, and/or seek help to maintain health.

Assessment Data

Defining Characteristics

- Inability to take responsibility for meeting basic self-care needs
- Inability to perform necessary self-care activities
- Lack of knowledge regarding self-care
- Lack of resources with which to meet self-care needs
- Impaired personal support system
- Lack of interest in caring for self

Related Factors

- Chronic illness
- Terminal illness
- Physical problems related to the illness
- Neurologic problems related to the illness
- Feelings of being overwhelmed, despair
- Chemical dependence

❋
Expected Outcomes

Initial	*The client will:*

- Establish or maintain adequate nutrition, hydration, and elimination within limits of illness
- Establish or maintain an adequate balance of rest, sleep, and activity
- Participate in self-care activities commensurate with physical ability

Discharge	*The client will:*

- Arrange for continued care after discharge
- Demonstrate maximum level of decision making in planning his or her own care
- Perform self-care activities commensurate with physical abilities
- Verbalize knowledge of his or her illness, treatment, self-care, and safe use of medications, if any

❋
Therapeutic Aims

- Provide nursing care for physical and neurologic problems related to the illness.
- Promote adequate nutrition, hydration, and elimination.
- Promote an adequate balance of rest, sleep, and activity.
- Help the client prepare for discharge.

❋
Implementation

Nursing Interventions	Rationale
Assess the client's level of self-care ability related to activities of daily living and to illness care.	The client may be physically unable to perform self-care activities or may be impaired due to feelings of despair of self-destructive feelings.
Encourage the client to be as independent as possible in self-care activities. See Care Plan 28: The Client Who Will Not Eat and Care Plan 48: Sleep Disturbances.	Achieving independence in self-care activities may help promote the client's self-esteem and sense of control.
Encourage the client to continue to make decisions about his or her care even after physical abilities decrease.	Decision making allows the client to continue to participate in his or her care and to maintain maximum control.
Teach the client and his or her family and significant others about the client's illness, treatment, safe use of medications if any, and the grief process.	The client and his or her significant others may have little or no knowledge of the client's illness, treatment, medications, or the grief process.
Help the client to identify community resources, agencies, and groups for assistance after discharge. Referral to a social worker may be indicated.	The client may need continued support after discharge. Social workers can help the client to identify and contact resources. Many communities have support groups for clients who have chronic or terminal illnesses. There also are state and national associations related to many illnesses that provide information and services.

Section Seven

Affect

Affect, or mood, can be described as an emotional tone, feeling, or reaction to experience. Disturbances in affect can be manifested by a wide range of behaviors, such as suicidal thoughts and behavior, withdrawn behavior, or a profound increase or decrease in the client's level of psychomotor activity. The care plans in this section address the behaviors and problems most directly related to affect, but the care plans in other sections of the *Manual* also may be appropriate in the planning of a particular client's care (for example, Care Plan 49: Withdrawn Behavior).

Problems related to affect may result from a psychiatric disorder (eg, bipolar affective disorder), a crisis or loss in a client's life, or some other condition (eg, depressive neurosis). Regardless of the specific cause of the client's problem, however, these clients often have great difficulty recognizing and expressing emotions. Encouraging and facilitating the expression of feelings is repeatedly suggested as a nursing intervention in this *Manual*, and can be most effective when nurses are aware of and work through their *own* feelings so they do not interfere with the nurse–client relationship (see Basic Concepts: Nurse–Client Interactions).

Manic Behavior

Manic behavior is characterized by an increased activity level and by an "elevated, expansive, or irritable" mood (Wilson and Kneisl, 1988). Manic behavior often occurs in *bipolar affective disorder* (previously known as *manic–depressive illness*), which is characterized by a history of high and low moods with periods of relatively normal and effective functioning in between.

The onset of bipolar affective disorder usually is between ages 20 and 40. Research indicates that there is a genetic component to this illness (McFarland and Thomas, 1991). The client often has a family history of alcoholism or other substance abuse. Frequently, the client also manifests substance abuse or alcoholism. This may be an attempt to self-medicate, or the client may have a *dual diagnosis*— bipolar affective disorder and substance abuse—each of which necessitates treatment. (See Care Plan 34: Dual Diagnosis.)

Lithium carbonate (Lithane) frequently is the drug of choice in the treatment of bipolar affective disorder; carbamazepine (Tegretol) is another drug that often is used. These drugs may be contraindicated in clients with impaired liver, renal, or cardiac functioning. Safe and effective use of these medications requires maintenance of a blood level within a therapeutic range; monitoring of this level at specified intervals is required. When the therapeutic level is exceeded, toxicity can result. See Appendix E for a listing of signs and symptoms that may indicate toxic or near-toxic blood levels.

Nursing Diagnoses Addressed in this Care Plan

High Risk for Violence: Self-Directed or Directed at Others
Defensive Coping
Altered Thought Processes
Altered Health Maintenance
Knowledge Deficit regarding illness, treatment plan, or safe use of medications

Related Nursing Diagnoses

High Risk for Injury
Sensory/Perceptual Alterations
Self-Esteem Disturbance
Ineffective Management of Therapeutic Regimen (individuals)
Impaired Social Interaction
Altered Nutrition: Less than Body Requirements
Sleep Pattern Disturbance

Nursing Diagnosis

High Risk for Violence: Self-Directed or Directed at Others (9.2.2)
A state in which an individual experiences behaviors that can be physically harmful either to the self or others.

Risk Factors

- Restlessness
- Hyperactivity
- Agitation
- Hostile behavior
- Threatened or actual aggression toward self or others

Expected Outcomes

Initial

The client will:

- Demonstrate decreased restlessness, hyperactivity, and agitation
- Demonstrate decreased hostility
- Not harm himself or herself or others

Discharge

The client will:

- Be free of restlessness, hyperactivity, and agitation
- Be free of threatened or actual aggression toward self or others

Therapeutic Aims

- Provide a safe environment.
- Prevent the client from harming himself or herself or others.
- Decrease hyperactivity, restlessness, and agitation.

Implementation

Nursing Interventions	Rationale
Provide a safe environment for the client.	Physical safety of the client and others is a priority. The client may use many common items and environmental situations in a destructive manner.
See Care Plan 24: Suicidal Behavior, Care Plan 51: Hostile Behavior, and Care Plan 52: Aggressive Behavior.	
Decrease environmental stimuli whenever possible. Respond to cues of increased restlessness or agitation by removing stimuli and perhaps isolating the client; a single or private occupancy room may be beneficial.	The client's ability to deal with stimuli is impaired.
Administer chemotherapy (probably lithium or antipsychotic medications initially). Use PRN medication judiciously, preferably before the client's behavior becomes destructive.	Chemical control can help the client regain self-control. However, medications should not be used to control the client's behavior for the convenience of the staff or as a substitute for working with the client's feelings and problems.

(continued)
Implementation

Nursing Interventions	Rationale
Provide a consistent, structured environment. Let the client know what is expected of him or her. Set goals with the client as soon as possible.	Consistency and structure can reassure the client. The client must know what is expected before he or she can work toward meeting those expectations.
Give simple, direct explanations for routine actions, procedures, tests, and so forth. Do not argue with the client.	The client is limited in his or her ability to perceive and respond to complex stimuli. Stating a clear limit tells the client what is expected. Arguing with the client interjects doubt and undermines the limit.
Encourage the client to verbalize his or her feelings of anxiety, anger, or fear. Explore ways to relieve stress and tension with the client as soon as possible.	Ventilation of feelings may help relieve anxiety, anger, and so forth.
Encourage supervised physical activity.	Physical activity can diminish tension and hyperac-

Nursing Diagnosis

Defensive Coping (5.1.1.1.2)

The state in which an individual repeatedly projects falsely positive self evaluation based on a self protective pattern which defends against underlying perceived threats to positive self-regard.

Assessment Data

Defining Characteristics	• Denial of problems
	• Exaggeration of achievements
	• Grandiose schemes, plans, or stated self-image
	• Buying sprees
	• Inappropriate, bizarre, or flamboyant dress or use of make-up or jewelry
	• Flirtatious, seductive behavior
	• Sexual acting-out
Related Factors	• Low self-esteem
	• Bipolar Affective Disorder
	• Other psychiatric problems

Expected Outcomes

Initial	*The client will:*
	• Demonstrate increased feelings of self-worth
	• Demonstrate more appropriate appearance (dress, use of make-up, and so forth)
Discharge	*The client will:*
	• Verbalize increased feelings of self-worth
	• Demonstrate appropriate appearance and behavior

Therapeutic Aims

- Decrease bizarre appearance and behavior, sexual acting out, and so forth.
- Provide emotional support.
- Promote self-esteem.

Implementation

Nursing Interventions	Rationale
Ignore or withdraw your attention from bizarre appearance and behavior and sexual acting out, as much as possible.	It is important to minimize attention given to unacceptable behaviors. Withdrawing attention can be more effective than negative reinforcement in decreasing unacceptable behavior.
Give the client positive feedback whenever appropriate.	Positive feedback provides reinforcement for the client's growth and can enhance self-esteem. It is essential to support the client in positive ways and not to give attention only for unacceptable behaviors.
Initially, structure tasks at which the client will succeed (short-term, simple projects or responsibilities, occupational or recreational therapy activities). Gradually increase the number and complexity of activities and responsibilities expected of the client. Give feedback at each level of accomplishment.	The client may be limited in his or her ability to deal with complex tasks or stimuli. Any task that the client is able to complete provides an opportunity for positive feedback to the client.

Nursing Diagnosis

Altered Thought Processes (8.3)
A state in which an individual experiences a disruption in cognitive operations and activities.

Assessment Data

Defining Characteristics	• Disorientation
	• Decreased concentration, short attention span
	• Loose associations (loosely and poorly associated ideas)
	• Push of speech (rapid, forced speech)
	• Tangentiality of ideas and speech
	• Hallucinations
	• Delusions
Related Factors	• Psychotic process
	• Sleep deprivation
	• Psychiatric illness

❋ Expected Outcomes

Initial	*The client will:*

- Demonstrate decreased restlessness, hyperactivity, and agitation
- Demonstrate orientation to person, place, and time
- Demonstrate decreased hallucinations or delusions
- Demonstrate an increased attention span
- Talk with others about present reality
- Demonstrate decreased push of speech, tangentiality, loose associations

Discharge	*The client will:*

- Be free of delusions or hallucinations
- Demonstrate orientation to person, place, and time
- Demonstrate adequate cognitive functioning

❋ Therapeutic Aims

- Establish rapport and build a trust relationship.
- Decrease disorientation, hallucinations, delusions, and other psychotic symptoms.
- Decrease hyperactivity, restlessness, and agitation.
- Provide treatment for associated psychiatric problems.
- Prepare the client for discharge.
- Promote safety and compliance with medication therapy.

❋ Implementation

Nursing Interventions	Rationale
Show acceptance of the client as a person.	The client is acceptable as a person regardless of his or her behaviors, which may or may not be acceptable.
Use a firm yet calm, relaxed approach.	Your presence and manner will help to communicate your interest, expectations, and limits, as well as your self-control.
Make only promises you can realistically keep.	Breaking a promise will result in the client's mistrust and is detrimental to a therapeutic relationship.
Initially, assign the client to the same staff members when possible (keep in mind the staff member's ability to work with a manic client for extended periods of time).	The client's ability to respond may be impaired. Consistency can reassure the client. Working with this client may be difficult and tiring due to his or her agitation, hyperactivity, and so on.
See Care Plan 1: Building a Trust Relationship.	
Reorient the client to person, place, and time as indicated (call the client by name, tell the client your name, tell the client where he or she is and the date, and so forth).	Repeated presentation of reality is concrete reinforcement for the client.
Spend time with the client.	Your physical presence is reality.

❋ *(continued)*
Implementation

Nursing Interventions	Rationale
Set and maintain limits on behavior that is destructive or adversely affects others.	Limits must be established by others when the client is unable to use internal controls effectively. The physical safety and emotional needs of other clients are important.
See Care Plan 11: Delusions, Care Plan 12: Hallucinations, and Care Plan 51: Hostile Behavior.	
Decrease environmental stimuli whenever possible. Respond to cues of increased restlessness or agitation by removing stimuli and perhaps isolating the client; a single or private occupancy room may be beneficial.	The client's ability to deal with stimuli is impaired.
Limit group activities in terms of size of group and frequency of activities based on the client's level of tolerance.	The client's ability to respond to others and to deal with increased amounts and complexity of stimuli is impaired.
Provide a consistent, structured environment. Let the client know what is expected of him or her. Set goals with the client as soon as possible.	Consistency and structure can reassure the client. The client must know what is expected before he or she can work toward meeting those expectations.
Help the client plan activities within his or her scope of achievement.	The client's attention span is short, and his or her ability to deal with complex stimuli is impaired.
Avoid highly competitive activities.	Competitive situations can exacerbate the client's hostile and aggressive feelings or can reinforce the client's low self-esteem.
Evaluate how much stimuli and responsibility the client can tolerate with respect to group activities, interactions with others, or visitors, and attempt to limit these accordingly.	The client is unable to provide limits and may be unaware of his or her impaired ability to deal with others.
Encourage the client's appropriate expression of feelings regarding future treatment plans or discharge plans. Support any realistic goals and plans the patient proposes.	Positive support can reinforce the client's healthy expression of feelings, realistic plans, and responsible behavior after discharge.
See Care Plan 34: Dual Diagnosis.	Substance abuse often is a problem in clients with bipolar affective disorder.

Nursing Diagnosis	*Self-Care Deficit (6.5)*

Nursing Diagnosis

Self-Care Deficit (6.5)

A state in which the individual experiences an impaired ability to perform or complete feeding, bathing, toileting, dressing, and grooming activities for oneself.

Assessment Data

Defining Characteristics	• Inability to take responsibility for meeting basic health and self-care needs • Inadequate food and fluid intake • Inattention to personal needs • Impaired personal support system
Related Factors	• Lack of awareness of personal needs • Lack of ability to make judgments regarding health and self-care needs • Altered thought processes • Sensory-perceptual alterations • Ineffective individual coping • Lack of material resources • Hyperactivity • Insomnia • Fatigue

Expected Outcomes

Initial	*The client will:* • Establish adequate nutrition, hydration, and elimination • Establish an adequate balance of rest, sleep, and activity
Discharge	*The client will:* • Maintain adequate nutrition, hydration, and elimination • Maintain an adequate balance of rest, sleep, and activity

Therapeutic Aims

• Promote rest and sleep.
• Encourage a nutritious diet.
• Assist the client in meeting his or her basic needs and carrying out necessary activities of daily living.

Implementation

Nursing Interventions	Rationale
Provide time for a rest period, nap, or quiet time during the client's daily schedule.	The client's increased activity increases his or her need for rest.
Observe the client closely for signs of fatigue. Monitor his or her sleep patterns.	The client may be unaware of fatigue or may ignore the need for rest.
Decrease stimuli before the client retires (dim lights, turn down television, provide a warm bath).	Limiting noise and other stimuli will help encourage rest and sleep.

(continued)
Implementation

Nursing Interventions	Rationale
Use comfort measures or sleeping medication if needed.	Comfort measures and sleeping medications can enhance the client's ability to rest and sleep.
Encourage the client to follow a routine of sleeping at night (limit interaction with the client at night) rather than during the day (allow only a short nap during the day).	Talking with the client for long periods during night hours will interfere with the client's sleep by stimulating the client, giving the client attention for not sleeping, and not expecting the client to sleep. Sleeping excessively during the day hours may decrease the client's need for and ability to sleep at night.
See Care Plan 48: Sleep Disturbances.	
Monitor the client's eating patterns and food and fluid intake. You may need to record intake and output and calorie and protein intake.	The client may be unaware of physical needs or may ignore feelings of thirst and hunger.
The client may need a high-calorie diet with supplemental feedings.	The client's increased activity level increases his or her need for nutrients.
Provide foods that the client can carry with him or her (fortified milkshakes, sandwiches, "finger foods"). See Care Plan 28: The Client Who Will Not Eat.	If the client is unable or unwilling to sit and eat, highly nutritious foods that require little effort to eat may be effective.
Monitor the client's elimination patterns.	The client may be unaware of or ignore the need to defecate. Constipation is a frequent adverse effect of antipsychotic medications.
If necessary, assist the client with personal hygiene, including mouthcare, bathing, dressing, and laundering clothes.	The client may be unaware of or lack interest in personal hygiene. Good personal hygiene and grooming can foster feelings of well-being and self-esteem.
Encourage the client to meet as many of his or her own needs as possible.	The client must be encouraged to be as independent as possible to promote self-esteem.

Nursing Diagnosis

Knowledge Deficit Regarding Illness, Treatment Plan, and Safe Use of Medications (8.1.1)

A state in which the client and/or his or her significant others lack specific knowledge necessary to self-care or care of the client.

Assessment Data

Defining Characteristics

- Inappropriate behavior related to self-care
- Inadequate retention of information presented
- Inadequate understanding of information presented

(continued)
Assessment Data

Related Factors	• No prior teaching or learning • Lack of interest in learning • Altered thought processes • Psychiatric illness • Cognitive impairment

Expected Outcomes

Initial	*The client will:* • Participate in learning about his or her illness, treatment, and safe use of medications
Discharge	*The client will:* • Verbalize knowledge of his or her illness • Demonstrate knowledge of adverse and toxic effects of medications • Demonstrate continued compliance with chemotherapy • Verbalize knowledge and acceptance of the need for continued therapy, chemotherapy, regular blood tests, and so forth

Therapeutic Aim

• Teach the client and his or her significant others about the client's illness, treatment, and safe use of medications.

Implementation

Nursing Interventions	Rationale
Teach the client and his or her family or significant others about manic behavior, bipolar affective disorder, and other problems as indicated.	The client and his or her family or significant others may have little or no knowledge of disease process(es) or need for continued treatment.
Inform the client and his or her family or significant others about chemotherapy: dosage, the need to take the medication only as prescribed, the toxic symptoms (see Appendix E), the need to monitor blood levels, and other considerations.	Severe toxic effects are possible in therapy with lithium or carbamazepine. Regular blood tests are necessary to monitor the serum levels.
Explain information in clear, simple terms. Reinforce teaching with written material as indicated. Ask the client and his or her family or significant others to state their understanding of the material as you explain. Encourage the client to ask questions and to express feelings and concerns.	The client and his or her significant others may have little or no understanding of medications and toxicity. Asking for the client's perception of the material and encouraging questions will help to eliminate misunderstanding and miscommunication.
Stress to the client and to the client's family or significant others that medications must be taken regularly and continually to be effective; just because the client feels better or because his or her mood is level is not sufficient cause to discontinue the drug.	A relatively constant blood level, within the therapeutic range, is necessary for successful maintenance treatment with lithium or carbamazepine.

Depressive Behavior

Depression is an affective state characterized by feelings of sadness, guilt, and low self-esteem, often related to loss. This loss may or may not be recent and may be observable to others or perceived only by the client, such as disillusionment or loss of a dream. Depression may be manifested by a slowing of activity or by agitation and may be accompanied by physical changes due to the slowing of physiologic processes (Wilson and Kneisl, 1992).

Depressive behavior may be seen in the following:

Grief, the process of a normal response to a loss.

Psychotic depression, a depression so profound that the client loses contact with reality, develops delusions and hallucinations, and is frequently suicidal.

Postpartum depression, which occurs after childbirth; symptoms may range from mild depressive feelings to acute psychotic behavior.

Premenstrual syndrome (PMS), a complex of symptoms that begins the week prior to menstrual flow and often recurs with each menstrual cycle. Symptoms differ in severity among individuals and may include depression, anxiety, tension, irritability, and mood swings.

Bipolar affective disorder, depressed type, in which apprehension, perplexity, uneasiness, and agitation are manifested. Hallucinations and delusions (usually of guilt or of hypochondriacal or paranoid ideas) may occur.

Depressive behavior frequently occurs in clients during alcohol or other drug withdrawal and may be seen in a number of other disorders or behaviors, such as anorexia nervosa, schizophrenia, and so forth.

Nursing Diagnoses Addressed in this Care Plan

Ineffective Individual Coping
Impaired Social Interaction
Chronic Low Self-Esteem
Self-Care Deficit

Related Nursing Diagnoses

Social Isolation
Altered Thought Processes
High Risk for Violence: Self-Directed or Directed at Others
Sexual Dysfunction
Dysfunctional Grieving
Spiritual Distress
Sleep Pattern Disturbance
Hopelessness

Nursing Diagnosis	**Ineffective Individual Coping (5.1.1.1)**

The state in which an individual demonstrates an impairment in adaptive behaviors and problem-solving abilities in meeting life's demands and roles.

Assessment Data

Defining Characteristics

- Suicidal ideas or behavior
- Slowed mental processes
- Disordered thoughts
- Feelings of despair, hopelessness, and worthlessness
- Guilt
- Anhedonia (inability to experience pleasure)
- Disorientation
- Generalized restlessness or agitation
- Sleep disturbances: early awakening, insomnia, or excessive sleeping
- Anger or hostility (may not be overt)
- Rumination
- Delusions, hallucinations, or other psychotic symptoms
- Sexual dysfunction: diminished interest in sexual activity, inability to experience pleasure
- Fear of intensity of feelings
- Anxiety

Related Factors

- Bipolar affective disorder
- Adjustment disorders
- History of traumatic stress
- History of abuse
- Substance abuse
- Lack of support system
- Phobias

❋
Expected Outcomes

Initial	*The client will:*
	• Be free of self-inflicted harm • Engage in reality-based interactions • Be oriented to person, place, and time • Express feelings directly with congruent verbal and nonverbal messages • Express anger or hostility outwardly in a safe manner
Discharge	*The client will:*
	• Be free of psychotic symptoms • Demonstrate functional level of psychomotor activity • Demonstrate an increased ability to cope with anxiety, stress, or frustration • Verbalize or demonstrate acceptance of loss or change, if any • Identify a support system in the community

❋
Therapeutic Aims

- Prevent self-harm.
- Build a trust relationship.
- Decrease disorientation, rumination, hallucinations, or delusions.
- Promote expression of feelings.
- Alleviate feelings of depression.

❋
Implementation

Nursing Interventions	Rationale
Provide a safe environment for the client.	Physical safety of the client is a priority. Many common items and environmental situations may be used by the client in a self-destructive manner.
Continually assess the client's potential for suicide.	Depressed clients may have a potential for suicide that may or may not be expressed and that may change with time. You must remain aware of this suicide potential at all times.
Observe the client closely, especially under the following circumstances:	You must be aware of the client's activities at all times when there is a potential for suicide or self-injury:
After antidepressant medication begins to raise the client's mood	Risk of suicide increases as the client's energy level is increased by medication.
After any sudden dramatic behavioral change (sudden cheerfulness, relief, freedom from guilt, or giving away personal belongings)	These changes may indicate that the client has come to a decision to commit suicide.
Unstructured time on the unit	Risk of suicide increases when the client's time is unstructured.
Times when the number of staff on the unit is limited	Risk of suicide increases when observation of the client decreases.

✸ *(continued)*
Implementation

Nursing Interventions	Rationale
Reorient the client to person, place, and time as indicated (call the client by name, tell the client your name, tell the client where he or she is, and so forth).	Repeated presentation of reality is concrete reinforcement for the client.
Spend time with the client.	Your physical presence is reality.
If the client is ruminating, tell him or her that you will talk about reality or about the client's feelings, but limit the attention given to repeated expressions of rumination.	Minimizing attention and reinforcement may help decrease rumination. Providing reinforcement for reality orientation and expression of feelings will encourage these behaviors.
Initially, assign the same staff members to work with the client whenever possible.	The client's ability to respond to others may be impaired. Limiting the number of new contacts initially will facilitate familiarity and trust. However, the number of people interacting with the client should increase as soon as possible to minimize dependency and to facilitate the client's abilities to communicate with a variety of people.
When approaching the client, use a moderate, level tone of voice. Avoid being overly cheerful.	Being overly cheerful may indicate to the client that other feelings are not acceptable—that being cheerful is the goal or the norm.
Use silence and active listening when interacting with the client. Let the client know that you are concerned and that you consider the client a worthwhile person.	Your presence and use of active listening will communicate your interest and concern. The client may not communicate if you are talking too much. Your silence will convey your expectation that the client will communicate and your acceptance of the client's difficulty with communication.
When first communicating with the client, use simple, direct sentences; avoid complex sentences or directions.	The client's ability to perceive and respond to complex stimuli is impaired.
Avoid asking the client many questions, especially questions that require only brief answers.	Asking questions and requiring only brief answers may discourage the client from communicating or taking responsibility for expressing his or her feelings.
Interact with the client on topics with which he or she is comfortable. Do not probe for information.	Topics that are uncomfortable for the client and probing may be threatening and initially may discourage communication. When trust has been established, the client may be encouraged to discuss more difficult topics.
Teach the client about the problem-solving process: Explore possible options, examine the consequences of each alternative, select and implement an alternative, and evaluate the results.	The client may be unaware of a systematic method for solving problems. Successful use of the problem-solving process facilitates the client's confidence in the use of coping skills.

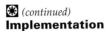 *(continued)*
Implementation

Nursing Interventions	Rationale
Provide positive feedback at each step of the process. If the client is not satisfied with the chosen alternative, assist the client to select another alternative.	Positive feedback at each step will give the client many opportunities for success and encourage him or her to persist in problem solving, as well as enhance the client's confidence. The client also can learn to "survive" making a mistake.

Nursing Diagnosis

Impaired Social Interaction (3.1.1)
The state in which an individual participates in an insufficient or excessive quantity or ineffective quality of social exchange.

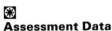
Assessment Data

Defining Characteristics	• Withdrawn behavior
	• Verbalization diminished in quantity, quality, or spontaneity
	• Rumination
	• Low self-esteem
	• Unsatisfactory or inadequate interpersonal relationships
	• Verbalizing or exhibiting discomfort around others
	• Social isolation
	• Inadequate social skills
	• Poor personal hygiene
Related Factors	• Absence of available significant others
	• Lack of support system
	• History of abuse

Expected Outcomes

Initial	*The client will:*
	• Communicate with others
	• Participate in activities
Discharge	*The client will:*
	• Assume responsibility for dealing with feelings and finding others with whom to talk
	• Reestablish or maintain relationships and a social life
	• Establish a support system

Therapeutic Aims

- Decrease withdrawn behavior.
- Promote leisure skills.
- Encourage socialization.

❋
Implementation

Nursing Interventions	Rationale
Encourage the client to ventilate feelings in whatever way is comfortable—verbal and nonverbal. Let the client know you will listen and accept what is being expressed.	Ventilation of feelings may help relieve feelings of despair, hopelessness, sadness, and so forth. Feelings are not inherently good or bad. You must remain nonjudgmental about the client's feelings and directly express this to the client.
Be comfortable sitting with the client in silence. Let the client know you are available to converse, but don't require the client to talk.	Your presence and use of active listening will indicate your interest and concern. Your silence will convey your expectation that the client will communicate and your acceptance of the client's difficulty with communication.
Allow (and encourage) the client to cry. Stay with and support the client if he or she desires. Provide privacy if the client desires and it is safe to do so.	Crying is a healthy way of expressing feelings of sadness, hopelessness, and despair. The client may not feel comfortable crying and may need encouragement or privacy.
Do not cut off interactions with cheerful remarks or platitudes (for example, "No one really wants to die," "Of course life is worth living," or "You'll feel better soon."). Do not belittle the client's feelings. Accept the client's verbalizations of feelings as real, and give support for this ventilation of feelings, especially for expressions of emotions that may be difficult for the client to accept in himself or herself (like anger).	You may be uncomfortable with certain feelings the client expresses. If this is true, it is important for you to recognize this and discuss it with another staff member rather than directly or indirectly communicating your discomfort to the client. Proclaiming the client's feelings to be inappropriate or wrong or otherwise belittling them is detrimental.
Teach the client social skills, and encourage him or her to practice these skills with staff members and other clients. Give the client feedback regarding social interactions.	The client may lack social skills and confidence in social interactions; this may contribute to the client's depression and social isolation.
Encourage the client to pursue personal interests, hobbies, and recreational activities. Consultation with a recreational therapist may be indicated.	Recreational activities can help the client's social interactions and provide enjoyment.
Encourage the client to identify supportive people outside the hospital and to develop these relationships.	Increasing the client's support system may help decrease future depressive behavior and social isolation.

Nursing Diagnosis	*Self-Care Deficit (6.5)*

A state in which an individual experiences an impaired ability to perform or complete feeding, bathing, toileting, dressing, and grooming activities for oneself.

Assessment Data

Defining Characteristics	• Anergy (overall lack of energy for purposeful activity) • Decreased motor activity • Lack of awareness or interest in personal needs • Self-destructive feelings • Withdrawn behavior • Psychologic immobility • Feelings of worthlessness
Related Factors	• Sleep disturbances • Disturbances of appetite or regular eating patterns • Constipation • Fatigue

Expected Outcomes

Initial	*The client will:* • Establish adequate nutrition, hydration, and elimination • Establish an adequate balance of rest, sleep, and activity • Establish adequate personal hygiene
Discharge	*The client will:* • Maintain adequately balanced physiologic functioning • Maintain adequate personal hygiene independently

Therapeutic Aims

• Promote adequate nutrition, hydration, and elimination.
• Promote an adequate balance of rest, sleep, and activity.
• Promote improved personal hygiene and appearance.

Implementation

Nursing Interventions	Rationale
Closely observe the client's food and fluid intake. Record intake, output, and daily weight if necessary.	The client may not be aware of or interested in meeting physical needs. Physical needs must be met in conjunction with psychological needs.
Offer the client foods that are easily chewed, fortified liquids such as orange juice with nutritional supplement, and high-protein malts.	If the client has little interest in eating, highly nutritious foods that require little effort to eat may be effective in meeting nutritional needs.
Try to find out what foods the client likes, and make them available at meals and for snacks.	The client may be more apt to eat foods he or she likes.

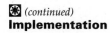 *(continued)*
Implementation

Nursing Interventions	Rationale
Do not tell the client that he or she will get sick or die from not eating or drinking.	The client may hope to become ill or die from not eating or drinking.
If the client is overeating, limit access to foods and the kitchen; schedule meals and snacks; serve limited portions. Give the client positive feedback for adhering to the prescribed diet.	The client may need limits to maintain a healthful diet.
Observe and record the client's pattern of bowel elimination.	Depressed clients may become severely constipated as a result of the depression, inadequate exercise, inadequate food or fluid intake, or the effects of some medications.
Encourage good fluid intake.	Constipation may be the result of inadequate fluid intake.
Be aware of PRN laxative orders and the possible need to offer medication to the client.	The client may be unaware of constipation and may not ask for medication.
Provide the client with his or her own clothing and personal grooming items when possible.	Familiar items will decrease the client's confusion and promote task completion.
Initiate dressing and grooming tasks in the morning.	Clients with depression may have the most energy and feel best in the morning; therefore, he or she may have a greater chance for successful completion of tasks at that time.
Maintain a routine for dressing, grooming, and hygiene.	A routine eliminates needless decision making, such as whether or not to dress or perform personal hygiene.
The client may need physical assistance to get up, dress, and spend time on the unit.	The client's ability to arise, increase activity, and join in the milieu is impaired.
Be gentle but firm in setting limits regarding time spent in bed. Set a specific time when the client must be up in the morning and when and for how long the client may rest.	Specific limits let the client know what is expected of him or her and indicate genuine caring and concern for the client.
Provide a quiet, peaceful time for resting. Decrease environmental stimuli (loud conversation, bright lights) in the late evening.	Limiting noise and other stimuli will encourage rest and sleep.
Provide a nighttime routine or comfort measures (backrub, tepid bath, warm milk) just before bedtime.	Use of a routine may help the client expect to sleep.
Talk with the client for only brief periods during night hours to help alleviate anxiety and to provide reassurance before the client returns to bed.	Talking with the client for long periods during night hours will interfere with the client's sleep by stimulating the client, giving the client attention for not sleeping, and not expecting the client to sleep.

⊛ *(continued)*
Implementation

Interventions	Rationale
Do not allow the client to sleep for long periods during the day.	Sleeping excessively during the day may decrease the client's need for and ability to sleep at night.
Use PRN medications as indicated to facilitate sleep. *Note:* Some medications used for sleep may worsen depression or cause agitation in depressed persons.	Medications may be helpful in facilitating sleep.

Nursing Diagnosis
Assessment Data

Chronic Low Self-Esteem (7.1.2.1)
Long-standing negative self evaluation/feelings about self or self capabilities.

Defining Characteristics

• Feelings of inferiority
• Defeatist thinking
• Self-criticism
• Lack of involvement
• Minimizing of own strengths
• Guilt
• Feelings of despair, worthlessness

Related Factors

• Life-style or role losses
• Physical losses
• Unrealistic evaluation of self
• Medical or psychiatric problems
• Poor personal hygiene
• Delusions
• Adjustment disorders
• History of traumatic stress
• History of abuse

⊛
Expected Outcomes

Initial

The client will:

• Verbalize increased feelings of self-worth
• Express feelings directly and openly
• Evaluate own strengths realistically

Discharge

The client will:

• Demonstrate behavior consistent with increased self-esteem
• Make plans for the future consistent with personal strengths

◈
Therapeutic Aims

- Promote feelings of self-worth.
- Promote expression of feelings.
- Facilitate realistic self-evaluation.

◈
Implementation

Nursing Interventions	Rationale
Encourage the client to become involved with staff and other clients in the milieu through interactions and activities.	When the client can focus on other people or interactions, cyclic, negative thoughts are interrupted.
Give the client positive feedback for completion of responsibilities, such as self-care activities and interactions with others.	Positive feedback increases the likelihood that the client will continue the behavior.
Involve the client in activities that are pleasant or recreational as a break from self-examination.	The client needs to experience pleasurable activities that are not related to self and problems.
If negativism predominates the client's conversations, it may be helpful to structure the content of the client's interactions. For example, make an agreement to listen to 10 minutes of "negative" interaction after which the client agrees to interact on more neutral topics.	The client will feel you are really hearing his or her feelings yet will begin practicing the conscious interruption of negativistic thought and feeling patterns.
At first, provide simple activities that can be accomplished easily and quickly. Begin with a project on the unit with the client alone; progress to group occupational and recreational therapy sessions.	The client may be limited in his or her ability to deal with complex tasks or stimuli. Any task that the client is able to complete provides an opportunity for positive feedback to the client.
Give the client honest praise for the accomplishment of small activities or ward or individual responsibilities by realizing how difficult it can be for the client to perform these tasks.	Clients with low self-esteem do not benefit from flattery or undue praise. Positive feedback provides reinforcement for the client's growth and can enhance self-esteem.
Gradually increase the number and complexity of activities or responsibilities expected of the client; give positive feedback at each level of accomplishment.	As the client's abilities increase, he or she can accomplish more complex activities and receive more feedback.
It may be necessary to stress to the client that he or she should begin doing things to feel better, rather than waiting to feel better before doing things.	The client will receive positive feedback for accomplishments and will have the opportunity to recognize his or her own achievements. Without this stimiuli, the client may lack motivation to attempt activities.
Explore with the client his or her personal strengths. Making a written list is sometimes helpful.	You can help the client discover his or her strengths. It will not be useful, however, for you to list the client's strengths. He or she needs to identify them but may benefit from your supportive expectation that he or she will do so.

Suicidal Behavior

Suicide is a significant cause of death worldwide: In 1986 suicide was the eighth leading cause of death in the United States and the third leading cause of death among people aged 15 to 24. Suicide is broadly defined as "a conscious act of self-induced annihilation" (Stillion, McDowell, and May, 1989). Suicidal behavior is considered to be *direct self-destructive behavior. Indirect self-destructive behavior* includes activities that are harmful to the client but are not overt, conscious, suicidal actions (such as addictive behaviors, psychosomatic disorders, self-mutilating behaviors, and nonadherence to prescribed medical regimens) (Farberow, 1980).

Speculation about reasons for suicide include different situational factors and different theories. Suicide may be the culmination of self-destructive tendencies that have resulted from the client's internalizing his or her anger, or the client may be asking for help by attempting suicide. Many people who commit suicide have given a verbal warning or clue. (*Note:* It is not true that "anyone who talks about suicide doesn't actually commit suicide." However, not everyone who attempts or commits suicide has given any warning at all.) Depressed clients may certainly be suicidal, but many suicidal clients are not depressed; the client may view suicide as an escape from extreme despair or from a (perceived) intolerable life situation, such as a terminal illness (see Care Plan 21: Living with a Chronic or Terminal Illness.) *Remember:* Threatening suicide may be an effort to bring about a fundamental change in the client's life situation or to elicit a response from a significant person, but it may indeed be an indication of real intent to commit suicide.

Suicidal ideation is defined as thoughts of committing suicide or thoughts of methods to commit suicide.

Suicidal gesture is a behavior that is self-destructive in nature as though it were a suicide attempt but is not lethal (for example, writing a suicide note and taking 10 aspirin tablets). This often is considered to be manipulative behavior, but the nonlethality of the behavior may be a result of the client's ignorance of the effects of such behavior or methods; the client may indeed be sincere in his or her wish to die.

Suicide attempt is a self-destructive behavior that is potentially lethal.

Suicide precautions are specific actions taken by the nursing staff to protect a client from suicidal gestures and attempts and to ensure close observation of the client.

Statistically, rates of suicide vary among different groups. Men commit suicide more often than women; white people commit suicide more than African Americans; men aged 55 and older, women older than 75 years of age, and men between 25 and 34 years have the highest suicide rates in the United States (Stillion, McDowell, and May, 1989). The risk of suicide is increased in the following circumstances:

When a plan is formulated
When there is a history of suicide attempts
When there is a family history of suicide
When suicide attempts become more painful, more violent, or lethal
When the client is white, male, adolescent, or older than 55 years
When the client is divorced, widowed, separated, or living without family
When the client is terminally ill, addicted, or psychotic (Stuart and Sundeen, 1991)
When the client gives away personal possessions, settles accounts, ties up loose ends, and so forth
When the client is in an early stage of treatment with antidepressant medications, and his or her mood and activity level begin to elevate (Coggins, 1990)
When the client's mood or activity level suddenly changes

Many in-hospital suicides occur during unstructured time and when staff members are few (for example, nights and weekends). There may be legal ramifications associated with the suicidal client who is hospitalized, especially if the client successfully commits suicide. It is especially important to observe the client closely, to document his or her behavior carefully, and to communicate *any* pertinent information to others who are making decisions about the client (especially if the client is to go on activities, on pass, or be discharged). The specific actions or precautions taken by nursing staff to protect a client from suicidal gestures and attempts will vary with each client's needs.
Remember: Every client has the potential for suicide.

Nursing Diagnoses Addressed in this Care Plan

High Risk for Violence: Self-Directed or Directed at Others
Ineffective Individual Coping
Self-Esteem Disturbance

Related Nursing Diagnoses

Hopelessness
Powerlessness
Impaired Social Interaction

**Nursing
Diagnosis**

Risk Factors

High Risk for Violence: Self-Directed or Directed at Others (9.2.2)
A state in which an individual experiences behaviors that can be physically harmful to the self or others.

- Suicidal ideas, feelings, ideation, plans, gestures, or attempts
- Lack of impulse control
- Lack of future orientation

❋ *(continued)*
Risk Factors

- Self-destructive tendencies
- Feelings of anger or hostility
- Agitation
- Aggressive behavior
- Feelings of worthlessness, hopelessness, or despair
- Guilt
- Anxiety
- Sleep disturbance
- Substance use
- Perceived or observable loss
- Social isolation
- Problems of depression, withdrawn behavior, eating disorders, psychotic behavior, personality disorder, manipulative behavior, posttraumatic stress, or other psychiatric problems

❋
Expected Outcomes

Initial

The client will:

- Not harm himself or herself or others
- Identify alternative ways of dealing with stress and emotional problems

Discharge

The client will:

- Not harm himself or herself or others
- Demonstrate use of alternative ways of dealing with stress and emotional problems
- Verbalize knowledge of self-destructive behavior(s), other psychiatric problems, and safe use of medication, if any

❋
Therapeutic Aims

- Provide a safe environment, and protect the client from self-destructive tendencies.
- Decrease suicidal behavior.
- Maintain close supervision of the client in keeping with the facility's policies and regulations.
- Be alert to possible signs that might indicate imminent suicidal behavior.
- Decrease rumination or excessive talk about suicide.
- Decrease feelings of depression, spiritual distress, and withdrawal.
- Help the client develop insight and increase his or her ability to express and deal with feelings in a healthy manner.
- Help the client identify and decrease self-destructive behavior.
- Attempt to alleviate anxiety related to the client's feelings of guilt, religious concerns regarding suicide, and so forth.
- Help the client prepare for discharge by increasing the client's ability to deal with possible suicidal feelings or urges that arise in the future.

Implementation

Nursing Interventions	Rationale
Determine the appropriate level of suicide precautions for the client. Institute these precautions immediately on admission (may be by nursing order or by physician order). Some suggested levels of precautions follow:	Physical safety of the client is a priority.
1. The client has one-to-one contact with a staff member at all times, even when going to the bathroom and sleeping. The client is restricted to the unit and is permitted to use nothing that may cause harm to him or her (for example, sharp objects, a belt).	1. A client who is at high risk for suicidal behavior needs constant supervision and limitation of opportunities to harm himself or herself.
2. The client has one-to-one contact with a staff member at all times but may attend activities off the unit (maintaining one-to-one contact).	2. A client at a somewhat lower risk of suicide may be permitted to join in activities and use potentially harmful objects (such as sharp objects) but still must have close supervision.
3. Special attention—the client's whereabouts and activities on the unit should be known at all times. The client must be accompanied by a staff member while off the unit but may be in a staff–client group.	3. A client with a lower level of suicide risk still requires observation, though one-to-one contact may not be necessary at all times when the client is on the unit.
Assess the client's suicidal potential, and evaluate the level of suicide precautions daily.	The client's suicidal potential varies; the risk may increase or decrease at any time.
In your initial assessment, note any previous suicide attempts and methods, as well as family history of mental illness or suicide. Obtain this information in a matter-of-fact manner; do not discuss at length or dwell on details.	Information on past suicide attempts, ideation, and family history is important in assessing suicide risk. The client may be using suicidal behavior as a manipulation or to obtain secondary gain. It is important to minimize reinforcement given to these behaviors.
Ask the client if he or she has a plan for suicide. Attempt to ascertain how detailed and feasible the plans are.	Risk of suicide increases when the client has formulated a plan, especially one that is possible for the client to carry out or is lethal.
Explain suicide precautions to the client.	The client is a participant in his or her care. Suicide precautions demonstrate your caring and concern for the client.
Be especially alert to sharp objects and other potentially dangerous items (glass containers, ashtrays, vases, matches, and lit cigarettes); items like these should not be in the client's possession.	The client's determination to commit suicide may lead him or her to use even common objects in self-destructive ways. Many seemingly innocuous items can be used, some lethally.
The client's room should be centrally located, preferably near the nurses' station and within view of the staff. Avoid placing the client in a room at the end of a hallway or near an exit, elevator, or stairwell.	The client at high risk for suicidal behavior requires close observation.
Make sure that windows are locked so that the client cannot open them (in a general hospital the maintenance department may have to seal or otherwise secure the windows).	The client may attempt to open and jump out of a window or throw himself or herself through a window if it is locked.

❀ *(continued)*
Implementation

Nursing Interventions	Rationale
If it is necessary for the client to use sharp objects, sign out all such objects to the client, and stay with the client during their use.	The client may use a sharp object to harm himself or herself or may conceal it for later use.
Have the client use an electric shaver if possible.	Even disposable razors can be quickly disassembled and the blade(s) used in a self-destructive manner.
It may be necessary to restrain the client or to place him or her in seclusion with no objects that can be used to self-inflict injury (electric outlets, silverware, and even bed clothing).	Physical safety of the client is a priority.
Know the whereabouts of the client at all times. Designate a specific staff person to be responsible for the client at all times. If this person must leave the unit for any reason, information and responsibility regarding supervision of the client must be transferred to another staff person.	The client at high risk for suicidal behavior needs close supervision. Designating responsibility for observation of the client to a specific person minimizes the possibility that the client will have inadequate supervision.
Stay with the client when he or she is meeting hygienic needs such as bathing, shaving, and cutting nails.	A staff member's presence and supervision may prevent self-destructive activity, or the staff member can immediately intervene to protect the client.
Check the client at frequent, *irregular* intervals during the night to ascertain the client's safety and whereabouts.	Checking at irregular intervals will minimize the client's ability to predict when he or she will (or will not) be observed.
Maintain especially close supervision of the client at any time there is a decrease in the number of staff, the amount of structure, or the level of stimulation (nursing report at the change of shift, mealtime, weekends, nights). Also, be especially aware of the client during any period of turmoil or distraction and when clients are going to and from activities.	Risk of suicide increases when there is a decrease in the number of staff, the amount of structure, or the level of stimulation. The client may use times of turmoil or distraction to slip away or to engage in self-destructive behavior.
Observe the client, and note behavior patterns; use this information to plan nursing care and the client's activities (for example, observe when the client is more animated or withdrawn). Note behaviors with regard to the time of day, structured versus unstructured time, interactions with others, tasks, activities, responsibilities, and attention span.	Assessment of the client's behavior can help to determine unusual behavior and may help to identify times of increased risk for suicidal behavior.
Be aware of the relationships the client is forming with other clients; note who may become his or her confidant. Be alert to any manipulative or attention-seeking behavior (see Care Plan 36: Passive–Aggressive or Manipulative Behavior).	The client may warn another client about a suicide attempt or may use other clients to elicit secondary gain.

✴ *(continued)*
Implementation

Nursing Interventions	Rationale
Be alert to the possibility of the client saving up his or her own medications or obtaining medications or dangerous objects from other clients or from visitors. You may need to check the client's mouth after medication administration or use liquid medications to ensure that they are ingested.	The client may accumulate medication to use in a suicide attempt. The client may manipulate or otherwise use other clients or visitors to obtain medications or other dangerous items.
Observe, record, and report any changes in the client's mood (elation, withdrawal, sudden resignation).	Risk of suicide increases when mood or behavior suddenly changes. *Remember:* As depression decreases, the client may have the energy to carry out a plan for suicide.
Note: The client may ask you not to tell anyone something he or she tells you. Avoid promising the client to keep secrets in this way; make it clear to the client that you must share all information with the other staff members on the treatment team, but assure the client of confidentiality with regard to anyone outside the treatment team.	The client may be attempting to manipulate you in this way or may be seeking attention for having a "secret" that may be a suicide plan. You must not assume individual responsibility for keeping secret a suicide plan the client may announce to you. If the client has a plan that he or she hints at but will not reveal, it is important to minimize attention given to this behavior, but suicide precautions may need to be used.
Tell the client that although you are willing to discuss emotions or other topics, you will not discuss prior suicide attempts or the details of such attempts repeatedly. (Discourage such conversations with other clients also.) Encourage the client to talk about his or her feelings, relationships, or life situation.	Reinforcement given to suicidal ideas and rumination must be minimized. However, the client needs to identify and express the feelings that underlie the suicidal behavior.
Convey that you care about the client and that you believe the client is a worthwhile human being.	The client is acceptable as a person regardless of his or her behaviors, which may or may not be acceptable.
Watch for behavior patterns, such as decreased communication, conversations about death or the futility of life, disorientation, low frustration tolerance, dependency and dissatisfaction with dependence, disinterest in surroundings, concealing articles that could be used to harm self.	These behaviors may indicate the client's decision to commit suicide.
Do not joke about death, belittle the client's wishes or feelings, or make insensitive remarks, such as "Everybody really wants to live."	The client's ability to understand and use abstractions such as humor is impaired. The client's feelings are real to him or her. The client may indeed not want to live; remarks such as this may further alienate the client or contribute to his or her low self-esteem.
Do not belittle the client's prior suicide attempts, which other staff members may deem "only" attention-seeking gestures.	People who make suicidal gestures are gambling with death and need help.
Do not make moral judgments about suicide or reinforce the client's feelings of guilt or sin.	Feelings such as guilt may underlie the client's suicidal behavior.

❀ *(continued)*
Implementation

Nursing Interventions	Rationale
Examine and remain aware of your own feelings regarding suicide. Talk with other staff members to deal with these feelings if necessary.	Many people have strong feelings about taking one's own life. Being aware of and working through your own feelings of disapproval, fear, seeing suicide as a sin, and so forth will diminish the possibility that you will inadvertently convey these feelings to the client.
Involve the client as much as possible in planning his or her own treatment.	The client's participation in his or her plan of care can help to increase a sense of responsibility and control.
Referral to the facility chaplain, clergy, or other spiritual resource person may be indicated.	The client may be more comfortable discussing spiritual issues with an advisor who shares his or her belief system. Referral to someone with expertise in religion may increase the client's trust and alleviate guilt.
Convey your interest in the client. Seek out the client for interaction at least once per shift. If the client says, "I don't feel like talking," "I don't want to talk to you," or "Leave me alone," remain with the client in silence or state that you will be back later to talk or be with the client, and then withdraw. You may tell the client that you will return at a specific time.	Your presence demonstrates interest and caring. The client may be testing your interest or pushing you away to isolate himself or herself. Telling the client you will return conveys your continued caring.
Give the client support for efforts to remain out of his or her room, to interact with other clients, or to attend activities.	The client's ability to interact with others is impaired. Positive feedback gives the client recognition for his or her efforts.
Encourage and support the client's expression of anger. (*Remember:* Do not take the anger personally.) Help the client deal with the fear of expressing anger, the fear of subsequent consequences and feelings, and so forth. Support the client in expressing anger or making plans to directly express anger when it occurs.	Self-destructive behavior can be seen as the result of anger turned inward. Verbal expression of anger can help to externalize these feelings.
Examine with the client his or her home environment and relationships outside the hospital. What, if any, changes should occur to decrease the likelihood of future suicidal behavior? Include the client's family or significant others in teaching, skill development, and therapy, if indicated.	The client's significant others may be reinforcing the client's suicidal behavior, or the suicidal behavior may be a symptom of a problem involving others in the client's life.
Plan with the client how he or she will recognize and deal with feelings and situations that have precipitated suicidal feelings or behavior in the past. Include whom the client will contact (ideally, identify someone in the home environment), where to go, what things may alleviate suicidal feelings (identify what has worked in the past).	Concrete plans may be helpful in averting a crisis or suicidal behavior. Recognition of feelings that lead to suicidal behavior may help the client seek help before reaching a critical point.

Nursing Diagnosis

Ineffective Individual Coping (5.1.1.1)
Impairment of adaptive behaviors and problem-solving abilities of a person in meeting life's demands and roles.

Assessment Data

Defining Characteristics

- Dysfunctional grieving
- Feelings of worthlessness or hopelessness
- Inability to problem-solve
- Feelings of anger or hostility
- Difficulty identifying and expressing emotions
- Guilt
- Self-destructive behavior
- Anxiety
- Lack of trust

Related Factors

- Depression
- Withdrawn behavior
- Sleep disturbance
- Substance use
- Low self-esteem
- Fatigue
- Perceived or observable loss
- Perceived crisis in life, situation, or relationship(s)
- Social isolation
- Posttraumatic stress
- Problems of eating disorders, psychotic behavior, personality disorder, manipulative behavior, or other psychiatric problems

Expected Outcomes

Initial

The client will:

- Participate in the treatment program
- Express feelings in a non–self-destructive manner
- Identify alternative ways of dealing with stress and emotional problems

Discharge

The client will:

- Demonstrate use of the problem-solving process
- Verbalize plans for using alternative ways of dealing with stress and emotional problems when they occur after discharge
- Verbalize plans for continued therapy after discharge if appropriate

Therapeutic Aims

- Decrease withdrawal; increase communication with others.
- Help the client develop insight and increase his or her ability to express and deal with feelings in a healthy manner.
- Help the client identify and decrease self-destructive behavior.

❄ *(continued)*
Therapeutic Aims

- Decrease feelings of depression.
- Relieve spiritual distress.
- Promote social skills and development of a support system outside the hospital.
- Help the client prepare for discharge by increasing his or her ability to deal with possible suicidal feelings or urges that arise in the future.

❄
Implementation

Nursing Interventions	Rationale
Encourage the client to ventilate his or her feelings; convey your acceptance of the client's feelings.	Ventilation of feelings can help the client to identify, accept, and work through his or her feelings, even if these are painful or otherwise uncomfortable for the client. Feelings are not inherently bad or good. You must remain nonjudgmental about the client's feelings and express this attitude to the client.
Involve the client as much as possible in planning his or her own treatment.	The client's participation in his or her plan of care can help to increase a sense of responsibility and control.
Convey your interest in the client. Seek out the client for interaction at least once per shift. If the client says, "I don't feel like talking," "I don't want to talk to you," or "Leave me alone," remain with the client in silence or state that you will be back later to talk or be with the client, and then withdraw. You may tell the client that you will return at a specific time.	Your presence demonstrates interest and caring. The client may be testing your interest or pushing you away to isolate himself or herself. Telling the client you will return conveys your continued caring.
Give the client support for efforts to remain out of his or her room, to interact with other clients, or to attend activities.	The client's ability to interact with others is impaired. Positive feedback gives the client recognition for his or her efforts.
Encourage and support the client's expression of anger. (*Remember:* Do not take the anger personally.) Help the client deal with the fear of expressing anger, the fear of subsequent consequences and feelings, and so forth. Support the client in expressing anger or making plans to directly express anger when it occurs.	Self-destructive behavior can be seen as the result of anger turned inward. Verbal expression of anger can help to externalize those feelings.
Encourage the client to express fears and emotions. Help the client identify situations in which he or she would feel more comfortable expressing feelings; use role playing to practice expressing emotions.	Ventilation of feelings can help the client identify, accept, and work through those feelings, even if they are painful or otherwise uncomfortable for him or her. Role playing allows the client to try out new behaviors in a supportive environment.
Provide opportunities for the client to express emotions and release tension in a non–self-destructive way, such as individual and group discussions, activities, and physical exercise.	The client needs to develop skills with which to replace self-destructive behavior.

❀ (continued)
Implementation

Nursing Interventions	Rationale
Teach the client about depression, self-destructive behavior, or other psychiatric problems (see other care plans as appropriate).	The client may have very little knowledge of or insight into his or her behavior and emotions.
Referral to the facility chaplain, clergy, or other spiritual resource person may be indicated.	The client may be more comfortable discussing spiritual issues with an advisor who shares his or her belief system. Referral to someone with expertise in religion may increase the client's trust and alleviate guilt.
Discuss the future with the client; consider hypothetical situations, emotional concerns, significant relationships, and future plans.	Anticipatory guidance can help the client prepare for future stress, crises, and so forth. *Remember:* Although the client is no longer suicidal (or is not suicidal at the moment), he or she is not necessarily ready for discharge.
Plan with the client how he or she will recognize and deal with feelings and situations that have precipitated suicidal feelings or behavior in the past. Include whom the client will contact (ideally, identify someone in the home environment), where to go, and what things may alleviate suicidal feelings (identify what has worked in the past).	Concrete plans may be helpful in averting a crisis or suicidal behavior. Recognition of feelings that lead to suicidal behavior may help the client seek help before reaching a critical point.
Teach the client about the use of the problem-solving process: identifying the problem, identifying and evaluating alternative solutions, choosing and implementing a solution, and evaluating its success.	The client may never have learned a logical, step-by-step approach to problem resolution.
Teach the client social skills, and encourage him or her to practice these skills with staff members and other clients. Give the client feedback regarding social interactions.	The client may lack skills and confidence in social interactions; this may contribute to the client's anxiety, depression, or social isolation.
Encourage the client to pursue personal interests, hobbies, and recreational activities. Consultation with a recreational therapist may be indicated.	Recreational activities can help increase the client's social interaction and provide enjoyment.
Encourage the client to identify supportive people outside the hospital environment and to develop those relationships. See Care Plan 2: Discharge Planning.	Increasing the client's support system may help decrease future suicidal behavior. The risk of suicide is increased when the client is socially isolated.

Nursing Diagnosis

Self-Esteem Disturbance (7.1.2)

Negative self-evaluation/feelings about self or self capabilities, which may be directly or indirectly expressed.

Assessment Data

Defining Characteristics	• Verbalization of low self-esteem, negative self-characteristics, or low opinion of self • Verbalization of guilt or shame • Feelings of worthlessness, hopelessness, or rejection
Related Factors	• Social isolation • Posttraumatic stress

Expected Outcomes

Initial	*The client will:* • Express feelings related to self-esteem and self-worth issues • Identify personal strengths and weaknesses realistically
Discharge	*The client will:* • Demonstrate behavior congruent with increased self-esteem • Verbalize plans to continue therapy regarding self-esteem issues if needed

Therapeutic Aims

• Promote feelings of self-worth.
• Help the client prepare for discharge.

Implementation

Nursing Interventions	Rationale
Convey that you care about the client and that you believe the client is a worthwhile human being.	The client is acceptable as a person regardless of his or her behaviors, which may or may not be acceptable.
Encourage the client to ventilate his or her feelings; convey your acceptance of the client's feelings.	Ventilation of feelings can help the client identify, accept, and work through his or her emotions, even if these are painful or otherwise uncomfortable for the client. Feelings are not inherently bad or good. You must remain nonjudgmental about the client's feelings and express this attitude to the client.
Initially, provide opportunities for the client to succeed at activities that are easily accomplished; give positive feedback even for very small accomplishments. *Note:* The client's self-esteem may be so low that he or she may feel able, for example, to make things only for others at first, not for his or her own personal use.	Positive feedback provides reinforcement for the client's growth and can enhance self-esteem. The client's ability to concentrate, complete tasks, and interact with others may be impaired.

❄ (continued)
Implementation

Nursing Interventions	Rationale
Encourage the client to take on progressively more challenging and rewarding activities. Give the client positive support for any efforts made to participate in activities or interact with others.	As the client's abilities to accomplish activities increase, he or she may be able to feel increasing self-esteem related to these accomplishments. Your direct verbal feedback can help the client recognize his or her active role in accomplishments and take credit for them.
Help the client identify positive aspects about himself or herself and his or her behavior or activities. You may point out positive aspects of the client as observations, without arguing with the client about his or her feelings.	The client may see only his or her negative self-evaluation; his or her ability to recognize the positive may be impaired. The client's feelings of low self-esteem are very real and valid to him or her. Your positive observations, however, present a different point of view that the client can examine and begin to integrate.
Give the client acknowledgment and support for his or her efforts to interact with others, participate in the treatment program, and express emotions.	Regardless of the level of accomplishment or "success" of a given activity, the client is making an effort and can benefit from acknowledgment of his or her efforts.
Do not flatter the client or be otherwise dishonest. Give honest, genuine, positive feedback to the client whenever possible.	The client will not benefit from insincerity; dishonesty undermines trust and the therapeutic relationship.
Encourage the client to pursue personal interests, hobbies, and recreational activities. Consultation with a recreational therapist may be indicated.	Recreational activities can help increase the client's social interaction and provide enjoyment.
Referral to a clergy member or spiritual advisor of the client's own faith may be indicated.	The client's feelings of shame or guilt may be related to his or her religious beliefs.
Encourage the client to pursue long-term therapy for self-esteem issues if indicated.	Self-esteem problems can be deeply rooted and require long-term therapy.

Section Eight

Physical Symptoms

Clients may manifest various physical symptoms that are related to emotional or psychiatric problems. Although these symptoms may or may not have a demonstrable organic cause, they are nevertheless real to the client and should not be minimized or dismissed. The care plans in this section differentiate the kinds of problems encountered in these situations and give suggestions for use in individual care plans.

It is important to remember that although a client has emotional problems, not all of the physical complaints that the client voices are necessarily caused by or related to those problems. A client's complaint or perception should never be disregarded because you think he or she is "just faking it," or because he or she has made many complaints. Some physical problems do indeed have a base in organic physiology as well as in stress or emotional difficulties (*psychosomatic illnesses*). Other behaviors or problems do not have a demonstrable organic cause but are real to the client and must be treated as such (*hypochondriacal behavior*). Symptoms also may be due to an unconscious process through which the client is attempting to deal with a conflict (*conversion reaction*) and, again, these symptoms are very real to the client.

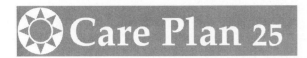

Psychosomatic Behavior

The term *psychosomatic* is derived from the Greek words *psyche,* meaning mind, and *soma,* meaning body. Psychosomatic illnesses often are common physical ailments that the client or the nurse may see as having been caused or exacerbated by stress or emotional illness. Physical illnesses that may be construed as having psychosomatic or *psychophysiologic* components or origins may involve any organ system. Some commonly accepted examples of these are psoriasis, ulcers, ulcerative colitis, headaches, rheumatoid arthritis, asthma, hyperventilation, palpitations, and anorexia nervosa.

Theories about psychosomatic illness range from the belief that all physical problems are organic in nature, having nothing to do with the psyche, to the belief that all physical problems are manifestations of or result from emotional ills. Theories also vary with regard to how symptoms or disease states are related to particular emotional problems. Certain *target organs* may be seen as symbolic of specific anxieties or stresses in all clients, or an individual client may be thought to subconsciously direct stress to particular body parts in that client. Perhaps the target organ was genetically weak in the client; therefore, it reacts with extra sensitivity to stress or anxiety.

Psychosomatic disorders are distinct from *hypochondriacal* behaviors in that psychosomatic disorders are real physical diseases or symptom complexes that have organic pathology, though they are related to stress or psychiatric problems. Hypochondriacal disorders have no organic pathology (see Care Plan 26: Hypochondriacal Behavior). Psychosomatic disorders may result in structural or organic changes in the body and may become life-threatening illnesses. Treatment of psychosomatic illness includes treatment of the physical illness and the underlying stress or psychiatric problem.

Nursing Diagnoses Addressed in this Care Plan

Ineffective Individual Coping
Ineffective Denial

Related Nursing Diagnoses

Anxiety
Knowledge Deficit regarding illness, treatment plan, or safe use of medications

Nursing Diagnosis

Ineffective Individual Coping (5.1.1.1)

Impairment of adaptive behaviors and problem-solving abilities of a person in meeting life's demands and roles.

Assessment Data

Defining Characteristics	• Inadequate coping skills • Inability to problem-solve • Stress-related physical complaints, symptoms, or disease complex(es) • Resistance to therapy or to the role of a psychiatric client • Anger or hostility • Resentment or guilt • Difficulty with interpersonal relationships • Dependency needs • Secondary gain (attention, evasion of responsibilities) due to illness • Use of alcohol or other chemicals for self-medication (to alter feelings or mood) • Inability to express feelings • Repression of feelings of guilt, anger, or fear • Patterns of coping through physical illness with resulting secondary gains
Related Factors	• Anxiety or fear • History of trauma or abuse • High level of stress • Low self-esteem • Depression

Expected Outcomes

Initial

The client will:

• Verbally express feelings of stress, anxiety, fear, or anger
• Acknowledge emotional or stress-related problems
• Verbalize the relationship between emotional problems and physical illness
• Increase his or her willingness to relinquish the "sick role"

Discharge

The client will:

• Verbalize understanding of the relationship between emotional stress and physical illness
• Decrease unnecessary use of medications
• Continue to verbally express feelings of stress, anxiety, fear, or anger
• Demonstrate increased satisfaction in interpersonal relationships
• Verbalize or demonstrate use of the problem-solving process
• Verbalize or demonstrate alternative ways to deal with life stresses and the anxiety or other feelings that occur in response to them
• Decrease use of alcohol or other chemicals
• Be physically well or achieve management of a continuing disorder
• Verbalize knowledge of psychosomatic illness, stress management techniques, therapeutic regimen(s), and medication use, if any

Therapeutic Aims

- Accurately assess and treat acute physical problems (actual physical condition).
- Promote the client's acceptance of and participation in his or her care.
- Promote the identification and expression of feelings.
- Decrease denial, anxiety, and anger.
- Decrease secondary gains.
- Help the client identify and develop alternative ways to deal with his or her feelings and stress.

Implementation

Nursing Interventions	Rationale
In the initial interview, do a thorough systems review for physical problems, complaints, history of diseases, treatment, surgeries, and hospitalizations. Be aware that the client may attempt to minimize or maximize his or her physical problems.	An adequate data base is necessary, because this client does have pathophysiology.
Develop a nursing care plan regarding the client's physical health, and implement it as soon as possible. Be matter-of-fact in your approach and treatment. Do not overemphasize physical problems or treatment or give undue attention or sympathy for physical illness.	Optimal physical health facilitates achievement of emotional health. You must consider the client's physical care but not as the primary focus. Remember that the client's problems are physically real and not hypochondriac or imaginary.
Talk with the client directly regarding a possible correlation between emotions or stress and physical symptoms or disease states.	The client's chance for health is enhanced if the interrelatedness of physical and emotional health is recognized.
Ask for the client's perceptions regarding his or her hospitalization and physical problems. However, do not argue with the client or put the client on the defensive.	The client's perceptions will tell you how he or she feels about the health problem. Arguing will damage your trust relationship.
Ask the client to identify his or her expectations of his or her hospitalization, including expectations of himself or herself and of the hospital staff. Try to involve the client in care planning, identifying problems, setting goals, and choosing actions to work toward those goals.	If the client is involved and invests energy in his or her care, the chances for positive outcomes increase.
Assess the client's life-style (activities and interactions with others) with regard to stress, support systems, dependency needs, and expression of emotions.	Stress-related factors are important in the dynamics of psychosomatic illnesses.
Talk with the client about your observations and assessment. Ask for the client's perceptions regarding stress, sources of satisfaction and dissatisfaction in his or her daily life, significant relationships, work, and so forth.	You are focusing on emotional issues. The client may have spent minimal time considering those aspects of health.

✲ *(continued)*
Implementation

Nursing Interventions	Rationale
Give the client positive feedback for focusing on emotional and interpersonal issues rather than on physical symptoms or disease.	Positive feedback increases the likelihood that the client will continue to express feelings and deal with interpersonal issues.
Without always connecting the client's physical problems with the client's emotions, encourage the client to identify and express feelings to himself or herself (perhaps in writing), to staff members (in individual conversations), and to groups (small and informal, progressing to larger and more formal).	It is less threatening for the client to begin expressing feelings to one person and work his or her way up to talking with more people about emotional issues.
Teach the client and his or her family or significant others about the concept of psychosomatic illness, stress, and stress management skills (for example, progressive relaxation and deep breathing).	The client may have little or no knowledge of stress or of stress management techniques.
Gradually attempt to identify with the client the connections between anxiety or stress and the exacerbation of his or her physical symptoms.	Acknowledging the interrelatedness of physical health and emotional health provides a basis for the client's future life-style changes.
Encourage the client to identify his or her own strengths; making a written list may be helpful.	It may be very difficult for the client to see his or her own strengths. Identifying personal strengths can promote an increased sense of self-worth.
Talk with the client and his or her significant others about the concept of secondary gains, and together develop a plan to reduce these gains for the client. Identify the needs the client is attempting to meet (for example, need for attention, means of dealing with perceived excess responsibilities or stress). Help the client plan to meet these needs in more direct ways.	Significant others may be unaware of how they reward the client for physical illness. Their participation in treatment is essential so the client can give up the sick role and deal with emotional problems.
Conferences with only the client's family or significant others may be helpful in identifying their attitudes and behaviors about the client. For example, they unknowingly may be giving the client the message that emotional problems are a sign of weakness and that only physical illness is acceptable.	Unless significant others make changes in their relationship with the client, chances for positive client changes are diminished.
Encourage the client to continue to identify stresses after his or her discharge from the hospital and to attempt to deal with them directly. Encourage the client to continue with therapy on an outpatient basis, if indicated.	Long-term change depends on how the client continues to progress after hospitalization.
Support the client's continued ventilation of feelings, and encourage the client to develop an outside support system to continue to talk about feelings after discharge (with significant others, with an ongoing support group, or through group therapy, if indicated).	The client needs to continue to express feelings to avoid returning to coping through physical illness.

☸ *(continued)*
Implementation

Nursing Interventions	Rationale
Give the client positive feedback for focusing on emotional and interpersonal issues rather than on physical symptoms or disease.	Positive feedback increases the likelihood that the client will continue to express feelings and deal with interpersonal issues.
If the client denies that he or she experiences stress or certain feelings, the discussion may need to be less direct. For example, point out possible or apparent stresses or feelings of the client, and ask the client for feedback about them.	Directly confronting the client's denial can make the denial stronger if the client is not ready to deal with issues.
Without always connecting the client's physical problems with his or her emotions, encourage the client to identify and express feelings to himself or herself (perhaps in writing), to staff members (in individual conversations), and to groups (small and informal, progressing to larger and more formal).	It is less threatening for the client to begin expressing feelings to one person and work his or her way up to talking with more people about emotional issues.
Teach the client and his or her family or significant others about the concept of psychosomatic illness, stress, and stress management skills (for example, progressive relaxation and deep breathing).	The client may have little or no knowledge of stress or of stress management techniques.
Gradually attempt to identify with the client the connections between anxiety or stress and the exacerbation of his or her physical symptoms.	Acknowledging the interrelatedness of physical health and emotional health provides a basis for the client's future life-style changes.
Encourage the client to continue to identify stresses after his or her discharge from the hospital and to attempt to deal with them directly. Encourage the client to continue with therapy on an outpatient basis, if indicated.	Long-term change depends on how the client continues to progress after hospitalization.
Support the client's continued ventilation of feelings, and encourage the client to develop an outside support system to continue to talk about feelings after discharge (with significant others, with an ongoing support group, or through group therapy, if indicated).	The client needs to continue to express feelings to avoid returning to coping through physical illness.

Hypochondriacal Behavior

Hypochondriasis is an exaggerated preoccupation the client has with his or her state of health, accompanied by various physical complaints that are not based on demonstrable organic pathology (Stuart and Sundeen, 1991). The client may feel real symptoms, such as pain, even though an organic basis for the symptoms cannot be found. As a nurse, you must carefully assess the client's physical condition and refer all somatic complaints to the medical staff for evaluation (at least the first time the client makes the specific complaint). Do *not* assume a complaint is hypochondriacal until after it has been evaluated medically.

By exhibiting hypochondriacal behavior, the client may be successfully avoiding certain responsibilities (vocational, educational, familial), receiving attention, or manipulating others by exhibiting symptoms or expressing complaints (all forms of *secondary gain*). It may be helpful to work with the client's family or significant others to decrease or eliminate secondary gains and to support the client's development of healthy ways to receive attention, deal with responsibilities, and so on. Somatic complaints may be a mechanism that the client has learned to deal with feelings, anxieties, or conflicts. The client may not be able to relinquish hypochondriacal behavior until his or her anxiety decreases or until he or she develops other behaviors to deal with these feelings. (See Section 12: Stress and Anxiety.)

Hypochondriacal symptoms may be found in clients who have difficulty expressing anger satisfactorily, including those with several types of psychiatric disorders, such as depression, schizophrenia, neurosis, or personality disorders (see other care plans as appropriate). The client may be using defense mechanisms and attempting subconsciously to turn emotions like anger into physical ailments.

It can be very frustrating to work with clients who exhibit hypochondriacal behavior. As a nurse, you must identify and work through personal feelings that arise while working with these clients to avoid acting out these feelings in nontherapeutic ways (such as avoiding the client). The prognosis for this type of client often is poor because they often deny emotional problems, exhibit other neurotic symptoms, and reject treatment by changing hospitals or physicians.

Nursing Diagnoses Addressed in this Care Plan

Ineffective Individual Coping
Anxiety

Related Nursing Diagnoses

Ineffective Family Coping
Altered Health Maintenance
Ineffective Denial

Nursing Diagnosis

Ineffective Individual Coping (5.1.1.1)
Impairment of adaptive behaviors and problem-solving abilities of a person in meeting life's demands and roles.

Assessment Data

Defining Characteristics

- Denial of emotional problems
- Difficulty identifying and expressing feelings
- Lack of insight
- Self-preoccupation, especially with physical functioning
- Fears of or rumination on disease
- Numerous somatic complaints (may involve many different organs or systems)
- Sensory complaints (pain, loss of taste sensation, olfactory complaints)
- Reluctance or refusal to participate in psychiatric treatment program or activities
- Reliance on medications or physical treatment (such as laxative dependence)
- Extensive use of over-the-counter medications, home remedies, enemas, and so forth
- Ritualistic behaviors (such as exaggerated bowel routines)
- Tremors
- Limited gratification from interpersonal relationships
- Lack of emotional support system

Related Factors

- Secondary gains (attention, evasion of responsibilities) received for physical problems
- History of repeated visits to physicians or hospital admissions
- History of repeated medical evaluations with no findings of abnormalities
- Delusions
- Fatigue
- Sleep disturbances
- Anxiety
- Loss of appetite
- Weight changes

Expected Outcomes

Initial	*The client will:*

- Participate in the treatment program
- Decrease the number and frequency of physical complaints
- Demonstrate compliance with medical therapy and medications
- Express feelings verbally
- Identify life stresses and anxieties
- Identify the relationship between stress and physical symptoms
- Demonstrate adequate energy, food, and fluid intake
- Identify alternative ways to deal with stress, anxiety, or other feelings

Discharge	*The client will:*

- Eliminate overuse of medications or physical treatments
- Decrease ritualistic behaviors
- Decrease physical attention-seeking complaints
- Demonstrate alternative ways to deal with stress, anxiety, or other feelings
- Verbalize increased insight into the dynamics of hypochondriacal behavior, including secondary gains
- Verbalize an understanding of therapeutic regimens and medications, if any

Therapeutic Aims

- Accurately assess and treat somatic complaints.
- Decrease the number and frequency of physical and sensory complaints.
- Decrease ritualistic physical behaviors, ruminations, or excessive fears of disease.
- Help the client identify life stresses or problems.
- Promote insight into the disorder.
- Promote expression of feelings.
- Decrease secondary gains.
- Decrease reliance on and use of medications and physical treatments.
- Help the client develop alternative ways of dealing with stress and anxiety.

Implementation

Nursing Interventions	Rationale
The initial nursing assessment should include a complete physical assessment, a history of previous complaints and treatment, and a consideration of each current complaint.	The nursing assessment provides a baseline from which to begin planning care.
The nursing staff should note the medical staff's assessment of each complaint on the client's admission.	Genuine physical problems must be noted and treated.
Each time the client voices a new complaint (or claims injury), the client should be referred to the medical staff for assessment (and treatment if appropriate).	It is unsafe to assume that all physical complaints are hypochondriacal—the client could really be ill or injured. The client may attempt to establish the legitimacy of complaints by being genuinely injured or ill.

✳ (*continued*)
Implementation

Nursing Interventions	Rationale
Minimize the amount of time and attention given to complaints. When the client makes a complaint, refer him or her to the medical staff (if it is a new complaint) or follow the team treatment plan; then tell the client you will discuss something else but not bodily complaints. Tell the client that you are interested in the client as a person, not just in his or her physical complaints. If the complaint is not acute, ask the client to save the complaint until a regular appointment with the medical staff.	If physical complaints are unsuccessful in gaining attention, they should decrease in frequency over time.
Withdraw your attention if the client insists on making complaints the sole topic of conversation. Tell the client your reason for withdrawal and that you desire to discuss other topics or will interact at a later time.	It is important to make clear to the client that attention is withdrawn from physical complaints, not from the client as a person.
Allow the client a specific time limit (like 5 minutes per hour) to discuss physical complaints with one person. The remaining staff will discuss only other issues with the client.	Because physical complaints have been the client's primary coping strategy, it is less threatening to the client if you limit this behavior initially rather than forbid it. The client's hypochondriacal behavior may exacerbate if he or she is denied this coping mechanism abruptly before new skills can be developed.
Do not argue with the client about his or her somatic complaints. Acknowledge the complaint as the client's feeling or perception and then follow the previous approaches.	Arguing with the client still constitutes attention, even though it is negative. The client is able to avoid discussing feelings.
Use the interventions suggested previously, as well as minimal objective reassurance in conjunction with questions (or other techniques) to explore the client's feelings. ("Your tests have shown that you have no lesions. Do you still feel that you do? What are your feelings about this?")	This approach helps the client make the transition to discussing feelings.
Encourage the client to discuss his or her feelings about the fears rather than the fears themselves.	The focus is on feelings of fear, not fear of physical problems.
Explore the client's feelings of lack of control over stress and life events.	The client may have helpless feelings but may not recognize this independently.
See Care Plan 45: Obsessive Thoughts or Compulsive Behavior.	
Initially, carefully assess the client's self-image, social patterns, and ways of dealing with anger, stress, and so forth.	This assessment provides a knowledge base regarding hypochondriacal behaviors.

⊕ *(continued)*
Implementation

Nursing Interventions	Rationale
Talk with the client about sources of satisfaction and dissatisfaction in his or her daily life, family and other significant relationships, employment, and so forth.	Open-ended discussion usually is nonthreatening and helps the client begin self-assessment.
After some discussion of the above and the continued strengthening of your trust relationship, talk more directly with the client, and encourage the client to talk more openly about specific stresses, recent and ongoing. What does the client perceive as stressful?	The client's perception of stressors usually is more significant than others' perception of those stressors. The client will operate on the basis of what he or she believes.
If the client is using denial as a defense mechanism, the discussion of stresses may need to be less direct, while you point out to the client apparent, probable, or possible stresses (in a nonthreatening way) and ask the client for feedback.	If the client is in denial, more direct approaches may produce anger or hostility and threaten the trust relationship.
Gradually, help the client identify possible connections between stress and anxiety and the occurrence or exacerbation of physical symptoms. Points you might assess are: What makes the client more or less comfortable? What is the client doing or what is going on around the client when he or she feels more or less comfortable or is experiencing symptoms?	The client can begin to see the relatedness of stress and physical problems at his or her own pace. Self-realization will be more acceptable to the client, as opposed to the nurse telling the client the problem.
Encourage the client to keep a diary of events or situations, stresses, and occurrence of symptoms. This diary can then be used to identify relationships between stresses and symptoms.	Reflecting on written items may be more accurate and less threatening to the client.
Talk with the client at least once per shift, focusing on the identification and expression of the client's feelings.	Continued, regular interest in the client facilitates the relationship. It also can desensitize the client regarding discussion of feelings and emotional issues.
Encourage the client to ventilate feelings by talking or crying, through physical activities, and so forth.	The client may have difficulty identifying and expressing feelings directly. Your encouragement and support may help him or her develop these skills.
Teach the client, his or her family, or significant others about the dynamics of hypochondriacal behavior and the treatment plan, including plans after discharge.	The client and his or her family or significant others may have little or no knowledge of stress, interpersonal dynamics, hypochondriacal behavior, and so on. Knowledge of the treatment plan will promote long-term behavior change.
Talk with the client and his or her significant others about the concept of secondary gains, and together develop a plan to reduce those gains. Identify the needs the client is attempting to meet with secondary gains (such as attention or escape from perceived responsibilities or from stress).	Maintaining limits to reduce secondary gain requires everyone's participation to be successful. The client's family and significant others must be aware of the client's needs if they want to be effective in helping to meet those needs.

❋ (continued)
Implementation

Nursing Interventions	Rationale
Help the client plan to meet his or her needs in more direct ways. (Show the client that attention and support are available when he or she is not exhibiting symptoms or complaints and when he or she deals with responsibilities directly or asserts himself or herself in the face of stress or discomfort.)	Positive feedback and support for healthier behavior tends to make that behavior recur more frequently. The client's family and significant others also must use positive reinforcement.
Reduce the benefits of illness as much as possible. Do not allow the client to avoid responsibilities by voicing somatic discomfort; do not excuse the client from activities; do not allow special privileges, such as staying in bed or dressing in night clothes.	If physical problems do not get the client what he or she wants, the client is less likely to cope in that manner.
Work with the medical staff to limit the number, variety, strength, and frequency of medications, enemas, and so forth that are made available to the client.	A team effort helps to discourage the client's manipulation of some staff members to obtain additional medication. See Care Plan 36: Passive–Aggressive or Manipulative Behavior.
When the client requests a medication or treatment for a complaint, encourage the client to identify what precipitated the complaint and to deal with the discomfort in other ways.	If the client can obtain stress relief in a nonchemical, nonmedical way, he or she is less likely to use the medication or treatment.
Observe and record the circumstances surrounding the occurrence or exacerbation of complaints; talk about your observations with the client.	Alerting the client to situations surrounding the complaint helps him or her see the relatedness of stress and physical symptoms.
Help the client identify and use nonchemical methods of pain relief, such as relaxation techniques.	Learning nonchemical pain relief techniques will shift the focus of coping away from physical means and increase the client's sense of control.
Teach the client more healthful daily living habits with regard to diet, sleep, comfort measures, stress management techniques, daily fluid intake, daily exercise, decreased stimuli, rest, possible connection between caffeine and anxiety symptoms, and so forth. See Care Plan 48: Sleep Disturbances.	Optimal physical wellness is especially important with clients using physical symptoms as a coping strategy.
Encourage the client to identify and express feelings directly in interpersonal relationships or stressful situations, especially feelings with which the client is uncomfortable (such as anger or resentment).	Direct expression of feelings will minimize the need to use physical symptoms to express them.
Notice the client's interactions with others (other clients, staff members, visitors, significant others, yourself), and give positive feedback for self-assertion and the direct expression of feelings, especially anger, resentment, and other so-called negative emotions. See Basic Concepts: Nurse–Client Interactions.	The client can gain confidence in dealing with stress. The client needs to know that appropriate expressions of anger or other negative emotions are acceptable and that he or she can feel better physically as a result of these expressions.

Nursing Diagnosis	*Anxiety (9.3.1)*
	A vague uneasy feeling whose source is often nonspecific or unknown to the individual.

Assessment Data

Defining Characteristics	• Self-preoccupation, especially with physical functioning
	• Fears of or rumination on disease
	• History of repeated visits to physicians or hospital admissions
	• Tremors

Related Factors	• Situational or maturational crisis
	• Ineffective coping mechanisms
	• Delusions
	• Sleep disturbances
	• Loss of appetite

Expected Outcomes

Initial	*The client will:*
	• Express feelings verbally
	• Identify life stresses and anxieties.
	• Identify alternative ways to deal with stress, anxiety, or other feelings

Discharge	*The client will:*
	• Demonstrate alternative ways to deal with stress, anxiety, or other feelings

Therapeutic Aims

• Help the client identify life stresses or problems.
• Promote expression of feelings.
• Help the client develop alternative ways of dealing with stress and anxiety.

Implementation

Nursing Interventions	Rationale
Encourage the client to discuss his or her feelings about the fears rather than the fears themselves.	The focus is on feelings of fear, not fear of physical problems.
Help the client explore his or her feelings of lack of control over stress and life events.	The client may have helpless feelings but may not recognize this independently.
Talk with the client at least once per shift, focusing on the identification of and expression of the client's feelings.	Continued, regular interest in the client facilitates the relationship. It also can desensitize the client regarding discussion of feelings and emotional issues.
Encourage the client to ventilate feelings by talking or crying, through physical activities, and so forth.	The client may have difficulty identifying and expressing feelings directly. Your encouragement and support may help the client develop these skills.

✳ *(continued)*
Implementation

Nursing Interventions	Rationale
Encourage the client to identify and express feelings directly in interpersonal relationships or stressful situations, especially feelings with which the client is uncomfortable (such as anger or resentment).	Direct expression of feelings will minimize the need to use physical symptoms to express them.
Notice the client's interactions with others (other clients, staff members, visitors, significant others, yourself), and give positive feedback for the direct expression of feelings, self-assertion, and especially for the expression of anger, resentment, and other so-called negative emotions.	The client can gain confidence in dealing with stress. The client needs to know that appropriate expressions of anger or other negative emotions are acceptable and that he or she can feel better physically as a result of those expressions.

Conversion Reaction

A *conversion reaction* is a change in or loss of physical functioning, without a demonstrable organic problem (Stuart and Sundeen, 1991). The physical symptom(s) manifested in a conversion reaction is considered to be the translation of conflict or repressed, unresolved feelings into a physical manifestation. Conversion reactions are not within the conscious control of the client; he or she is not faking the physical symptoms and feels that symptoms are not in his or her control. Symptoms can be manifested in sensory or motor function. Common sensory symptoms include impaired vision, blindness, deafness, and loss of sensation of the extremities. Common motor symptoms include mutism, paralysis of the extremities, dizziness, and ataxia. Often, only a single physical symptom is present; the symptom frequently is directly related to the underlying conflict, as illustrated by the following situations.

The physical symptom may give the client a "legitimate reason" to avoid the conflict. For example, a young man wishes to attend college, but his father wants him to remain at home to help on the farm. The young man develops a paralysis of his legs, rendering him unable to do farm work. His conflict is therefore resolved by a physical disability beyond his control.

The physical symptom may represent "deserved punishment" for behavior about which the client has guilt feelings. For example, a young woman gains pleasure from seeing movies and watching television, which are specifically forbidden by her family's religious beliefs. She feels guilty because she has violated those beliefs and develops blindness, which she perceives as punishment and which relieves her guilt.

The physical symptom is very real; the client actually cannot walk or see (if paralysis or blindness, respectively, is the symptom). The focus of therapeutic work, however, is on the resolution of the conflict and conflicting feelings, rather than on the physical symptom per se. Removal from the conflict (as occurs when the client is hospitalized) frequently produces gradual relief or remission of the physical symptom. As the client approaches discharge, however, the physical symptom may return.

Conversion reactions also are classified as *hysterical neuroses, conversion type* (DSM-III-R, 1987), and the client may experience other problems related to hysterical, or histrionic, behavior. For example, the client may receive *secondary gains* related to the symptom or disability he or she is experiencing. The client also may be unconcerned about the severity of the symptom ("la belle indifference"); unconsciously, the client instead may be relieved that the conflict is resolved.

Nursing Diagnoses Addressed in this Care Plan

Ineffective Individual Coping
Ineffective Denial

Related Nursing Diagnoses

Ineffective Family Coping (Compromised or Disabling)
Altered Health Maintenance
Altered Role Performance
Anxiety
Impaired Physical Mobility
Altered Health Maintenance

Nursing Diagnosis	*Ineffective Individual Coping (5.1.1.1)* *Impairment of adaptive behaviors and problem-solving abilities of a person in meeting life's demands and roles.*

Assessment Data

Defining Characteristics	• Inability to identify and resolve conflict or ask for help • Inability to meet role expectations • Inability to cope with present life situation • Inability to problem solve • Guilt and resentment • Anxiety • Feelings of inadequacy • Difficulty with feelings of anger, hostility, or conflict • Decreased ability to express needs and feelings • Secondary gain related to the physical symptom or disability (avoidance of dealing with a conflict, avoidance of responsibilities) • Unsatisfactory or inadequate interpersonal relationships
Related Factors	• Unresolved conflict • Situational or maturational crisis • Adjustment disorder • Low self-esteem • Physical limitation or disability (eg, blindness, paralysis, loss of voice) • Inability to perform self-care tasks or activities of daily living

Expected Outcomes

Initial	*The client will:* • Experience relief from acute stress or conflict • Be free of actual physical impairment • Identify the conflict underlying the physical symptom

❊ *(continued)*
Expected Outcomes

Initial	• Identify feelings of fear, anger, guilt, anxiety, or inadequacy • Be free of injury • Experience adequate nutrition, hydration, rest, and activity
Discharge	*The client will:* • Successfully cope with the conflict without recurrence of the conversion reaction • Verbalize feelings of fear, guilt, anxiety, or inadequacy • Express anger in a direct, nondestructive manner • Verbalize increased feelings of self-worth • Demonstrate interpersonal and intrapersonal strategies to deal with life stresses • Verbalize knowledge of illness, including concept of secondary gain • Verbalize plans to continue with therapy after discharge if indicated

❊
Therapeutic Aims

- Identify the source of conflict or stress.
- Determine the basis of the symptom.
- Relieve the client's stress or conflict.
- Promote adequate nutrition, hydration, and elimination.
- Promote rest and exercise.
- Prevent injury.
- Encourage expression of feelings and discussion of the conflict.
- Facilitate recognition of the relationship between the conflict and the physical symptom.
- Promote self-esteem.
- Help the client resolve the conflict or deal with it in ways other than by developing physical symptoms.
- Prepare the client for discharge.
- Prevent recurrence of the conversion reaction after discharge.

❊
Implementation

Nursing Interventions	Rationale
Obtain the client's thorough history on admission. Contact his or her family or significant others if necessary to complete the history. Send for records from prior hospitalizations, if possible.	A complete data base is essential to the validity of the diagnosis.
Talk with the client about his or her life, what is important to the client, and his or her usual environment, work, significant others, and so forth.	General leads or open discussion is a nonthreatening approach to discover the nature of the conflict.
Observe the client's behavior, especially in relation to the symptom. Document all observations, including precipitating events, if any; effects of the environment (such as the presence of others); and changes in the severity of the symptom(s).	Observational data will provide clues to the client's perception of stress, the effect of stress on the client, and his or her reliance on the conversion symptom to deal with that stress.

✳ *(continued)*
Implementation

Nursing Interventions	Rationale
The physician may order various tests to rule out a physical (organic) basis of the symptom. Assist or prepare the client as necessary.	Organic pathophysiology must be ruled out.
Approach the client with the attitude that you expect improvement in the physical symptom.	Hospitalization may relieve the conflict a great deal by removing the client from his or her usual environment. Communicating your expectation of improvement may help the client expect improvement.
Initially, avoid making demands on or requiring decisions of the client that are similar to the client's pre-hospitalization conflict or situation.	Such demands would recreate or intensify the client's conflict, which could result in exacerbation of the symptom or in the client clinging to the physical symptom longer.
Initially, if the stress is in relation to a particular person (or people) in the client's life, visits from that person or people may need to be discouraged, restricted, or prevented.	Temporary limitations of visits could help alleviate the client's stress.
As the client's physical symptom improves, gradually allow stressful situations to occur or increase visits by others, as tolerated. Monitor the client's response to stress.	The client can gradually begin to experience increased stresses as his or her skills develop in a supportive environment. However, too much stress may exacerbate the symptom.
Assess the client's food and fluid intake, elimination, and amount of rest as unobtrusively as possible.	You must be aware of the client's well-being, without giving excessive attention to it.
Any intervention regarding the client's physical state (poor food or fluid intake or lack of sleep) must be planned by the treatment team. All staff members must be unified and consistent in their approach.	A team approach provides consistency, which decreases opportunities for manipulation.
Provide the necessary nursing care in a matter-of-fact manner.	A matter-of-fact approach will minimize secondary gain and can help separate emotional issues from physical issues or symptoms.
Supervise the client unobtrusively for his or her ability to perform activities of daily living, ambulate independently, and so on. Intervene if the client is risking injury to himself or herself, but minimize the attention given to the client's physical supervision.	Often clients with histrionic types of behavior will not experience physical injuries.
Focus nursing interactions on discussions of the client's feelings, his or her home or work situation, and relationships with others.	Increased attention to emotional issues will help the client shift his or her attention to these issues.
Encourage the client to express his or her feelings directly, verbally or in writing. Support the client's efforts to express feelings.	Direct expression of feelings can relieve tension and conflict, diminishing the need for physical symptoms.
Explore with the client his or her personal relationships and related feelings.	Conversion reaction symptoms often are related to interpersonal conflicts or situations.

✳ (*continued*)
Implementation

Nursing Interventions	Rationale
Teach the client and his or her family or significant others about conversion reaction, stress, stress management, and conflict resolution strategies.	The client and his or her family or significant others may have little or no knowledge of stress, stress management, interpersonal dynamics, or the dynamics of the illness. Increasing their knowledge can promote understanding, motivation for change, and support for the client.
Praise the client if and when he or she is able to discuss the physical symptom as a method used to cope with conflict.	Positive feedback can reinforce the client's insight.
Provide opportunities for the client to succeed at activities, tasks, and interactions. Give positive feedback, and point out the client's demonstrated strengths and abilities.	Activities within the client's abilities will provide opportunities for success. Positive feedback provides reinforcement for the client's growth and can enhance self-esteem.
Help the client set goals for his or her behavior; give positive feedback when the client achieves these goals.	Achieving goals can foster self-confidence and self-esteem. Allowing the client to set goals promotes the client's sense of control and teaches goal-setting skills.
Explore alternative methods of expressing feelings related to the identified conflict.	The client has the opportunity to practice unfamiliar behavior with you in a nonthreatening environment.
Teach the client about the problem-solving process, and encourage him or her to use it to examine the conflict.	The client may have few or no problem-solving skills or knowledge of the problem-solving process.
Encourage the client to identify some strategies with which to deal or resolve the conflict. Together, evaluate the effectiveness of the alternative methods.	The client must actively seek new strategies because they are unfamiliar.
Give the client positive feedback for expressing his or her feelings about the conflict or for trying conflict resolution strategies.	Positive feedback can increase desired behavior.
Refer the client and his or her family or significant others for continuing therapy if appropriate.	The client may need long-term therapy to continue to develop skills for dealing with feelings, conflict, or interpersonal relationships.
Encourage the client to increase his or her support system outside the hospital. See Care Plan 2: Discharge Planning.	Extended support in the community strengthens the client's ability to cope more effectively.

Nursing Diagnosis

Ineffective Denial (5.1.1.1.3)

The state of a conscious or unconscious attempt to disavow the knowledge or meaning of an event to reduce anxiety or fear to the detriment of health.

Assessment Data

Defining Characteristics	• Indifference or lack of concern about the severity of the physical symptom • Refusal to seek health care for the physical symptom • Difficulty with feelings of anger, hostility, or conflict • Decreased ability to express needs and feelings
Related Factors	• Physical limitation or disability (eg, blindness, paralysis, loss of voice) • Anxiety • Low self-esteem • Secondary gain related to the physical symptom or disability (eg, avoidance of dealing with a conflict, avoidance of responsibilities) • Adjustment disorder • Unsatisfactory or inadequate interpersonal relationships

Expected Outcomes

Initial	*The client will:* • Identify the conflict underlying the physical symptom • Identify feelings of fear, anger, guilt, anxiety, or inadequacy • Verbalize steps of the problem-solving process
Discharge	*The client will:* • Verbalize feelings of fear, guilt, anxiety, or inadequacy • Verbalize knowledge of illness, including the concept of secondary gain • Demonstrate use of the problem-solving process

Therapeutic Aims

• Diminish the client's focus on the physical symptom.
• Prevent secondary gain related to the symptom.
• Encourage expression of feelings and discussion of the conflict.
• Facilitate recognition of the relationship between the conflict and the physical symptom.

Implementation

Nursing Interventions	Rationale
Involve the client in the usual activities, self-care, eating in the dining room, and so on as you would other clients.	Expecting the client to participate will enhance the likelihood that he or she will do so and will diminish secondary gain.

✿ *(continued)*
Implementation

Nursing Interventions	Rationale
After the symptom has been medically evaluated, withdraw attention from the client's physical status except for necessary care. Avoid long discussions of the physical symptom; withdraw your attention from the client if necessary.	Lack of attention to expression of physical complaints will help decrease that behavior.
Expect the client to participate in activities as fully as possible. Make your expectations clear to the client. Do not give the client special privileges or totally excuse him or her from all expectations due to physical limitations.	Granting special privileges to the client or excusing him or her from responsibilities or activities are forms of secondary gain. The client may need to become more uncomfortable with the physical conversion to risk relinquishing it as a coping strategy.
Do not argue with the client. Withdraw your attention if necessary.	Arguing with the client undermines limits. Withdrawing attention may be effective in diminishing secondary gain.
Focus nursing interactions on discussions of the client's feelings, his or her home or work situation, and relationships with others.	Increased attention to emotional issues will help the client shift his or her attention to these feelings and issues.
Explore with the client his or her personal relationships and related feelings.	Conversion reaction symptoms often are related to interpersonal conflicts or situations.
Teach the client and his or her family or significant others about conversion reaction, stress, stress management, and conflict resolution strategies.	The client and his or her family or significant others may have little or no knowledge of stress, stress management, interpersonal dynamics, or the dynamics of the illness. Increasing their knowledge can promote understanding, motivation for change, and support for the client.
Praise the client if and when he or she is able to discuss the physical symptom as a method used to cope with conflict.	Positive feedback can reinforce the client's insight.
Give the client positive feedback for expressing his or her feelings about the conflict or for trying conflict resolution strategies.	Positive feedback can increase desired behavior.

Section Nine

Eating

Behaviors and problems related to eating are seen in many different disorders and are briefly addressed in many of the care plans found in other sections of this *Manual*. The client's nutritional state is directly related to his or her physical health and often influences, or is influenced by, emotional or psychiatric problems as well.

The first care plan in this section primarily deals with an inadequate nutritional intake that is short term. Because the client's nutritional deficits are usually related to other emotional problems, this care plan may be most effective when integrated with (an)other care plan(s) in the *Manual* when planning for a particular client.

The second and third care plans deal with maladaptive eating patterns that are long term. Clients with anorexia nervosa, bulimia nervosa, or excessive eating patterns are often mistakenly believed to be well-adjusted, successful, and happy. Underlying that facade, however, the person attempts to deal with conflicts and emotions through destructive food-related behaviors. Eating disorders are complex problems that may require inpatient and outpatient treatment, family therapy, and years of work to overcome.

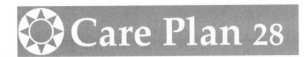

Care Plan 28

The Client Who Will Not Eat

Clients may not eat for a number of reasons, both physiologic and psychologic. A client may refuse to eat, be uninterested in eating, or be unaware of the need or desire to eat. A client may be experiencing physical problems that interfere with appetite (eg, nausea) or that make it difficult for the client to eat (eg, poor dentition or trouble swallowing).

Psychiatric problems that may underlie a client's not eating include the following (see related care plans as indicated):

Eating disorders
Depression
Withdrawal
Grief
Self-destructive behavior
Confusion
Agitation
Anger and hostility
Manic behavior
Delusions or other psychotic symptoms
Stress, anxiety, or phobias
Guilt
Low self-esteem
Manipulative behavior
Personality disorders

Physical problems that may contribute to a client's not eating include the following:

Effects of medications, such as altered taste sensation
Effects of acute or chronic physical illness, such as nausea or decreased appetite
Poor dentition or gum disease
Poorly fitting dentures
Difficulty swallowing or chewing
Difficulty feeding self
Physical disability, such as hemiplegia

Nursing Diagnoses Addressed in this Care Plan

Altered Nutrition: Less than Body Requirements
Ineffective Individual Coping

Related Nursing Diagnoses

Fluid Volume Deficit
Impaired Swallowing
Feeding Self-Care Deficit
Constipation
Noncompliance with treatment plan or prescribed medications

Nursing Diagnosis

Assessment Data

Altered Nutrition: Less than Body Requirements (1.1.2.2)

The state in which an individual experiences an intake of nutrients insufficient to meet metabolic needs.

Defining Characteristics	
	• Lack of appetite
	• Lack of interest in eating
	• Aversion to eating
	• Weight loss
	• Body weight 20% or more under ideal body weight
	• Refusal to eat
	• Difficulty eating
	• Malnutrition
	• Inadequate hydration
	• Electrolyte imbalance
	• Starvation
	• Disturbance in elimination
	• Difficulty swallowing

Related Factors

- Inability to ingest food
- Lack of awareness of need for food and fluids
- Delusions, other psychotic symptoms, or other psychiatric problems
- Anorexia nervosa

Expected Outcomes

Initial

The client will:

- Establish adequate nutrition, hydration, and elimination
- Demonstrate adequate fluid and electrolyte balance
- Eliminate signs and symptoms of malnutrition
- Demonstrate weight gain, if appropriate

(continued)
Expected Outcomes

Discharge	*The client will:*
	• Demonstrate independence in food and fluid intake
	• Maintain regular, adequate, nutritional eating habits
	• Maintain adequate or normal body weight

Therapeutic Aims

- Accurately assess the client's present physical and nutritional state and his or her recent and normal eating habits.
- Accurately observe and record intake and output.
- Promote physical health.
- Promote adequate elimination.
- Increase intake of food and liquids.
- Promote homeostasis.
- Promote the establishment or strengthening of independent nutritional eating habits.
- Promote the client's optimal level of health.

Implementation

Nursing Inverventions	Rationale
On the client's admission do a thorough assessment using physical assessment and interviews with the client and his or her family or significant others. Obtain detailed information regarding the client's eating patterns prior to the illness; familiar or liked foods and snacks; special diets, such as religious or vegetarian; recent changes in eating habits; gastro-intestinal (GI) or other physical complaints and disorders (medical evaluation may be indicated); circumstances that affect the client's appetite; other physical or psychiatric problems that may affect eating; and so forth.	Accurate baseline information is essential in planning and providing nursing care.
Strictly monitor intake and output. (Do not call the client's attention to intake and output notation; try to make unobtrusive observations.) Note and record the type and amount of food, the times and circumstances of eating. (For example, was the client alone? Was eating encouraged? What was the level of stimuli?)	Information on intake and output is necessary to assess the client's nutritional state. Unobtrusive observations minimize the client's secondary gain.
Weigh the client regularly. (The client should consistently wear only a hospital gown or pajamas when being weighed.)	The client may conceal weights under his or her clothing to appear to have gained weight.
Weight measurement should occur at the same time every day and should be taken in a matter-of-fact manner.	Treating weight measurement in a matter-of-fact manner will help to separate issues of weight and eating from emotional issues.

Implementation

Nursing Interventions	Rationale
Provide nursing care (and facilitate medical treatment) for physical problems that contribute to or result from the client's not eating.	The client's physical health is a priority. Many physical problems can contribute to or result from the client's not eating.
Provide fruit juices and foods high in fiber.	Fruit juices and foods high in fiber content promote adequate elimination.
Keep a record of the client's elimination. Record the color, amount, consistency, and frequency of stools.	The client may use laxatives, enemas, or suppositories to promote elimination. If the client is consuming little or no food or liquids only, stools may be less frequent or loose.
Have some food and liquids available for the client at all times.	The client may be interested in eating at times other than mealtimes.
Offer food, nutritious liquids, and water to the client frequently in small amounts.	The client may be overwhelmed by or may not tolerate large amounts of foods.
Discourage the intake of nonnutritional substances (eg, coffee, tea, or diet soda) except water. Encourage the use of milk or sugar (rather than a nondairy creamer or artificial sweetner) in coffee or tea.	It is important to maximize nutrition when the client can or will eat or drink.
Encourage the intake of liquids highest in nutritional value and calories. (Fruit juice is high in nutritive value; chocolate milk has 50 more calories per serving than white milk; whole milk can be ordered rather than nonfat or low-fat milk.)	If the client will not eat solid foods, liquids can provide many calories and nutrients.
Make fortified shakes available. These can be made by blending ice cream, milk, and powdered milk together (be sure to stir before giving to the client) or from dietary supplements (eg, fortified liquid meals or beverages).	Fortified liquids can be effective in providing maximal nutrition to a client who will not eat solid foods.
Offer foods that require little effort to eat (that is, are easily chewed and swallowed) and are visually and aromatically pleasant.	The client may feel that he or she does not have much energy to eat. Foods that are appealing can stimulate the client's interest and appetite.
If the client has GI complaints (eg, nausea), offer light, bland foods; clear soups; and clear carbonated beverages. Avoid fried foods, gravy, or spicy foods.	Light, bland foods or clear liquids may be more easily tolerated by (and more appealing to) the client with GI complaints.
If the client will take only liquids, gradually attempt to introduce solid foods into his or her diet (begin with cream soups, crackers, cooked cereal, and light foods).	Gradual introduction of solid foods may be effective in overcoming the client's resistance.
Try to accommodate the client's normal or previous eating habits as much as possible.	Reinforcing previous or current normal eating habits increases the likelihood that the client will eat.

❇️ *(continued)*
Implementation

Nursing Interventions	Rationale
When offering foods, *tell* the client you have something for him or her to eat; do not *ask* if he or she wants to eat or feels like eating. (However, do not order the client to eat; this approach is meant as a firm suggestion rather than an open opportunity for the client to respond by saying no.)	The client's ability to make decisions may be impaired, or the client may refuse to eat if asked. However, he or she may eat in response to your expectation that he or she will eat.
It may be necessary for you to get food and feed the client, get food and offer it to the client, accompany the client to get food, or sit with the client through meal time. Nasogastric (NG) tube feedings or intravenous therapy also may be necessary.	The client's physical health is a priority.
Gradually change from feeding the client to offering food to suggesting that the client get food for himself or herself. Observe and record changes in the frequency of eating and the amount eaten.	The client needs to develop independent eating habits.
Gradually decrease the frequency of suggestions, and allow the client to take responsibility for eating; again, record changes.	The transition from feeding the client to independent eating is more likely to be successful if it is gradual.

Nursing Diagnosis

Ineffective Individual Coping (5.1.1.1)
Impairment of adaptive behaviors and problem-solving abilities of a person in meeting life's demands and roles.

❇️
Assessment Data

Defining Characteristics	• Inability to meet basic needs for nutrition • Inability to ask for help • Inability to problem solve • Self-destructive behavior (refusal to eat) • Difficulty identifying and expressing feelings • Ineffective expression of emotional needs and conflicts
Related Factors	• Delusions, other psychotic symptoms, or other psychiatric problems • Low self-esteem • Anorexia nervosa

❇️
Expected Outcomes

Initial	*The client will:* • Demonstrate beginning ability to meet basic needs or ask for help • Demonstrate decreased delusions, phobias, guilt, or other related psychiatric problems

(continued)
Expected Outcomes

Discharge	*The client will:*
	• Demonstrate non–food-related coping mechanisms
	• Demonstrate improvement in related psychiatric problems
	• Verbalize plans to continue with therapy after discharge if indicated

Therapeutic Aims

- Prevent the client from obtaining secondary gain from not eating.
- Decrease manipulation of the staff.
- Decrease the association of food or not eating with guilt, depression, or punishment.
- Promote the development of non–food-related coping mechanisms.
- Prepare the client for discharge.

Implementation

Nursing Interventions	Rationale
Do not tell the client that he or she will get sick, weak, or may die from not eating.	The client may hope to become ill or die from not eating or drinking.
Do not threaten the client. (For example, "If you don't eat, you'll have to have an intravenous line.") However, use limits, consequences, consistency, and the giving and withdrawing of attention as appropriate. See Care Plan 29: Anorexia Nervosa and Care Plan 36: Passive–Aggressive or Manipulative Behavior.	Threatening the client will undermine trust and is not therapeutic. The effective use of limits and consistency of care will be helpful in reinforcing positive behaviors and minimizing secondary gain, refusal to eat, and so forth. Remember: Intravenous and tube feeding therapy are medical treatments, not punishments.
Give positive support and attention when the client eats; withdraw your attention when he or she refuses to eat.	Positive feedback provides reinforcement for the client's growth. It is essential that the client be supported in positive ways and that attention for unacceptable behaviors is minimized.
Talk with the client's family or significant others about the client's behavior and the concept of secondary gain; explain the client's treatment program, and enlist their cooperation.	The client's significant others may be unaware of the dynamics of secondary gain and may unwittingly reinforce the client's not eating.
If necessary, ask other clients to minimize attention given to the client for not eating.	Other clients may be unaware of the dynamics of secondary gain and may unwittingly reinforce the client's not eating.
Set up structured times and limits regarding eating. (For example, try to feed the client for 10 minutes, then withdraw for half an hour.) Be consistent in your approach and behavior.	Consistency and limits minimize the possibility of manipulation. Limiting meal times decreases the amount of time the client is dealing with issues of food and eating.
Assess or explore the client's history, particularly his or her attitudes and feelings regarding food and eating.	The client may associate food or eating with stress, pleasure, reward, guilt, resentment, religion, or morality. The client's family may emphasize food or

⊛ *(continued)*
Implementation

Nursing Interventions	Rationale
	use eating (or not eating) as a means of manipulation, control, and so forth.
Allow the client to have food only at specified snack and meal times. Encourage the client to eat at appropriate meal and snack times.	This can prevent the client from eating or not eating when he or she feels anxious, guilty, or depressed and will help to decrease these associations.
Encourage the client to express his or her feelings at times other than meal times.	Focusing on feelings without food present can help decrease associations between emotions and food.
Discourage (withdraw your attention from) rituals or other emotional associations with meals, food, and so forth.	Withdrawing attention from undesired behaviors will minimize reinforcement and may help decrease or eliminate these behaviors.
Teach the client (and his or her family or significant others) about stress, stress management, and disorders related to the client's not eating. Observe and record the client's perceptions of and responses to stress; encourage the client to approach a staff member when experiencing stress.	The client and his or her family or significant others may have little or no knowledge of stress. The client may need to learn to recognize stress and his or her responses to it, as well as techniques for stress management.
Talk with the client to identify others in his or her environment with whom the client can talk and to identify activities that might decrease stress or anxieties (eg, hobbies, physical activities).	The client can learn to ask for help, express feelings, and learn other ways to deal directly with emotions and stress rather than using food.
Work with the client regarding psychiatric problems that may be related to eating behaviors.	Psychiatric problems that contribute to the client's not eating must be resolved to ensure the client's independence in healthful eating patterns.

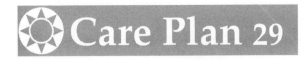

Anorexia Nervosa

Anorexia nervosa is an eating disorder characterized by "a refusal to maintain weight above a safe level, a weight fifteen percent or more below ideal body weight," fear of becoming obese, and a distortion of body image (Powers, 1990). More than 90% of clients with anorexia nervosa (called *anorexics*) are female, though the disorder does occur in males. Anorexia nervosa most commonly occurs in the adolescent and young adult years but has been reported in children and the elderly as well. The prevalence of anorexia nervosa has been reported as being as high as 1% in adolescent and young adult females (Kennedy and Goldbloom, 1991).

This disorder may be a lifelong chronic illness or may be restricted to an acute episode; it also can occur with bulimia nervosa. Anorexics have been described as restrictive (those who lose weight using self-starvation only) or bulimic (those who use starvation and purging behavior, with or without binging, to lose weight) (Palmer, 1990).

Anorexia nervosa can have grave physical consequences; mortality related to anorexia nervosa (malnutrition, complications, and suicide) has been reported as 18% to 20%. Success in treatment varies, but early recognition and treatment of the disorder increase chances for recovery (Powers, 1990).

The following characteristics have been noted in anorexics: achievement orientation, conformity, above average intelligence, excellent scholarship, perfection, high personal standards, immaturity, dependency, eagerness to please, and approval seeking. In addition, anorexics have been described as helpful, obedient, and dependable (Carino and Chmelko, 1983). Anorexic clients have been said to lack a sense of identity and to feel helpless and ineffectual in their lives. They may be using weight loss as a means of controlling their bodies (which gives a sense of control in their lives) or avoiding maturity (Palmer, 1990).

The cause of anorexia remains unknown, although several theories have been developed, including biologic, psychologic, familial, and sociocultural. A precipitating factor often can be identified that involves a major change in the client's life related to maturing (puberty, first sexual encounter, or sexual interest in the client by another person), leaving the family home (going to college or camp), or loss. These events may be seen as requiring a degree of maturity or social skills that the client has not yet developed (Palmer, 1990). Only approximately 20% of anorexics were found to have been overweight before developing anorexia nervosa (Powers, 1990), and the disorder is much more complex than a diet taken too far.

Family dynamics appear to play a significant role in the development of anorexia nervosa in a client. Families of anorexic clients have been described as being enmeshed (having intense relationships and a lack of boundaries), overprotective, rigid, and lacking conflict resolution (Palmer, 1990). In addition, a history of sexual abuse is reported in 30% of anorexic clients (Powers, 1990).

Cultural factors also may play a prominent role in anorexia nervosa. Thinness, especially in women, is highly valued in American society, and women often internalize the societal message that they will be judged on their appearance rather than their abilities. The socialization of women and changing expectations may be confusing and overwhelming to adolescent and young adult women (eg, conflicting messages regarding dependence versus independence, competing with others versus pleasing others, achieving in a career versus nurturing a family, and so forth). Many of the characteristics noted in anorexic women are ascribed to the female role in American society (dependency, pleasing others, helpfulness, and sensitivity).

Anorexia nervosa often requires long-term treatment and follow-up, including inpatient hospitalization, outpatient treatment, individual psychotherapy, and family therapy (Powers, 1990). Despite a substantial amount of research regarding pharmacologic treatment, no drug therapy has been particularly effective in treating anorexia (Kennedy and Goldbloom, 1991).

Nursing Diagnoses Addressed in this Care Plan

Altered Nutrition: Less than Body Requirements
Ineffective Individual Coping

Related Nursing Diagnoses

Ineffective Denial
Self-Esteem Disturbance
Sensory/Perceptual Alterations
Noncompliance with treatment plan
Ineffective Family Coping
High Risk for Violence: Self-Directed or Directed at Others
Powerlessness
Altered Health Maintenance
Fluid Volume Deficit
High Risk for Impaired Skin Integrity
Fatigue
Activity Intolerance

Nursing Diagnosis	***Altered Nutrition: Less than Body Requirements (1.1.2.2)***
	The state in which an individual experiences an intake of nutrients insufficient to meet metabolic needs.

Assessment Data

Defining Characteristics	• Weight loss
	• Body weight 20% or more under ideal body weight
	• Refusal to eat
	• Denial or loss of appetite
	• Inability to perceive accurately and respond to internal stimuli related to hunger or nutritional needs
	• Epigastric distress
	• Vomiting
	• Difficulty swallowing
	• Use or abuse of laxatives

Related Factors	• Intense fear of becoming obese
	• Dread or dislike of certain foods or types of foods (such as carbohydrates)
	• Disgust at the thought of eating
	• Preoccupation with food
	• Hiding and hoarding of food
	• Retaining feces and urine, eating large amounts of salt, or concealing weights on body to increase weight measurement
	• Denial of illness or resistance to treatment
	• Denial of being (too) thin
	• Excessive exercise
	• Anxiety
	• Physical problems or changes (may be life threatening), which include malnutrition; starvation; pale, dry skin; poor skin turgor; little subcutaneous tissue; lanugo (soft, downy body hair); edema; constipation; amenorrhea; cardiac arrhythmias, bradycardia, mitral and tricuspid valve prolapse; low basal metabolic rate; hypothermia; decreased mental acuity and concentration; hypotension; poor muscle tone and function; osteoporosis and fractures; absent secondary sexual characteristics; anemia and leukopenia; hypoglycemia; hypercholesterolemia; reduced serum immunoglobulins, increased susceptibility to infection and sepsis; impaired renal function; diabetes insipidus; decreased urinary 17-ketosteroids, estrogens, testosterone, and gonadotropins; fluid and electrolyte imbalance

Expected Outcomes

Initial	*The client will:*
	• Increase caloric and nutritional intake
	• Be free of complications of malnutrition
	• Develop an adequate nutritional state
	• Maintain skin integrity

• Demonstrate weight gain
• Demonstrate improvement in physical status related to the physical complications of anorexia nervosa

| Discharge | *The client will:* |

• Demonstrate regular, independent, nutritional eating habits
• Maintain a healthy weight level
• Demonstrate continued improvement in nutritional status

Therapeutic Aims

• Increase nutritional and caloric intake.
• Protect the client from complications of malnutrition.
• Promote physical health.
• Promote healthful eating habits.
• Promote weight gain.

Implementation

| Nursing Interventions | Rationale |

Note: It is especially important to use the following interventions selectively in developing an individual care plan for the client. The care plan presented here suggests several different kinds of interventions that can be used with different approaches to the care of the anorexic client. Some measures may be appropriate for clients whose nutritional state is severely compromised (total parenteral nutrition or nasoduodenal tube feedings), while others may be more effective in decreasing the attention given to food per se (eg, to focus only on weight, not on intake and output) with a client whose nutritional state is not as severely compromised. You may want to develop a specific protocol for each client, with nursing interventions (eg, tube feedings, supervision at and after meals) and client privileges based on compliance with calorie consumption or weight gain.

If the client is critically malnourished:

Nursing Interventions	Rationale
Parenteral nutrition (hyperalimentation or total parenteral nutrition) may be indicated through central venous or right atrial catheter. Monitor the client closely for signs and symptoms of infection.	Adequate nutrition, electrolytes, and so forth can be provided parenterally. The client has no opportunity to vomit this kind of nutritive substance. The client's immune system may be compromised related to malnutrition.
Tube feedings may be used alone or with oral or parenteral nutrition. Use of a nasoduodenal tube may be effective.	Fortified liquid diets can be provided through tube feedings. The use of a nasoduodenal tube decreases the chance of vomiting or siphoning feedings.
Supervise the client for a specified time (initially 90 minutes, decreasing gradually to 30 minutes) after tube feeding, or remove nasogastric tube after feeding.	Supervision decreases the client's opportunity to vomit or siphon feedings.
Offer the client the opportunity to eat food orally. Use tube feedings if the client consumes insufficient calories or loses weight or if indicated by medical condition (electrolytes and acid–base balance). Decrease tube feedings as oral consumption becomes adequate.	The client may prefer to eat food orally rather than have a tube feeding; however, the client's physical health is a priority.

(continued)
Implementation

Nursing Interventions	Rationale
When tube feeding is indicated (see above), insert the tube immediately in a matter-of-fact, nonpunitive manner, and administer feeding. Do not use tube feeding as a threat, and do not allow bargaining.	Limits and consistency are essential in avoiding power struggles and decreasing manipulative behavior. Remember, tube feedings are medical treatment, not punishment.
You may want to administer parenteral nutrition or tube feedings at night.	Using these methods at night may decrease attention or sympathy given to the client by others and will interfere less in the client's daytime activities.
If the client is not critically malnourished:	
Establish a contract with the client regarding his or her treatment, if the client will agree.	Contracting can promote the client's sense of control and self-responsibility and help establish goals. A contract is ineffective, however, if the client is not in agreement with its terms.
Initially, do not allow the client to eat with other clients or with visitors present.	Sanger and Cassino (1984) report that other clients repeat family patterns in urging the client to eat, giving attention to the client for not eating, and so forth.
Provide structure and limits to the client's meal times. Be consistent and matter-of-fact. Tell the client when it is time to eat, present the food, and state the limit(s) regarding meal time.	Clear limits let the client know what is expected of him or her.
Do not coax the client to eat. Do not use bribes or threats or focus on eating at all; withdraw your attention if the client refuses to eat. When the meal time is over, take the food away without discussing it with the client.	It is important to minimize the client's secondary gain from not eating. Issues of control (especially regarding eating) are central to the client's problem and must not be reinforced.
Provide one-to-one supervision of the client during meal times and after meals (initially for 90 minutes, then decrease gradually). Do not allow the client to use the bathroom until at least 30 minutes after each meal.	The client may spill, hide, or discard food. The client may use the bathroom to vomit or dispose of concealed foods.
Provide a pleasant, relaxing environment for eating, and minimize distractions. Encourage the use of relaxation techniques, rest, and quiet before and after meals.	The client may have significant anxiety and guilt about eating, making meal time very stressful.
Encourage the client to seek out a staff member to talk about feelings of anxiety or guilt after eating or if the client has the urge to vomit.	Talking with a staff member promotes a focus on emotional issues rather than on food.
Allow the client increasing choices regarding food, meal time, and so forth.	The client needs to develop independence in eating habits.
Grant and restrict privileges based on weight gain (or loss) as a means of limit setting with the client. Do not focus on eating, meal times, calorie counts, or	Decreasing direct attention given to food and eating encourages the client to focus on emotional issues instead.

Nursing Interventions	Rationale
physical activity. If weight loss occurs, decrease privileges and talk with the client to examine the circumstances and explore the feelings involved.	
Monitor the client's vital signs, electrolytes, acid–base balance, liver enzymes, albumin, and other medical measures as indicated and ordered by the physician.	The client's physical health is a priority. Information regarding the client's clinical state is necessary to plan effective nursing care.
Monitor the client's intake and output. The intake and output record should be kept at the nursing station (not at the client's bedside or room) and should be completed by the nursing staff (not the client). Observations of intake and output should be made in as unobtrusive and matter-of-fact a manner as possible.	The client may provide inaccurate information on intake or output records. It is important to minimize direct attention given for eating and to remove emotional issues from food and eating.
Weigh the client daily, after the client has voided and before the morning meal, with the client wearing only his or her hospital gown. Measure weight in a matter-of-fact manner; do not approve or disapprove of weight gain or loss.	Consistency is necessary for accurate comparison of weight over time. The client may retain urine or conceal weights on his or her body to increase weight measurement. The client's weight gain or loss is not for your benefit or approval and is a measure of health, not of success or failure. A matter-of-fact attitude will help separate emotional issues, control, and approval or disapproval of the client from the client's eating (or noneating) behaviors.
Monitor the client's elimination patterns. The client's diet should include sufficient fiber and adequate amounts of fluids.	The client may be constipated or have less frequent stools. Bulk and fluid promote adequate elimination.
Discourage the client's use of enemas, laxatives, or suppositories.	The client may abuse laxative preparations as a means of controlling weight.
Observe and record the client's physical activity; be aware that this may be covert (eg, jogging in the shower, doing calisthenic exercises in bed).	The client may exercise to excess to control weight.
You may need to limit the client's exercise or structure activities into the client's treatment plan. Do not forbid all physical exercise unless the client is critically ill and exercise would be truly harmful or unsafe.	Restricting physical activity too severely may greatly increase the client's anxiety. (See Care Plan 45: Obsessive Thoughts or Compulsive Behavior.) Also, moderate exercise is a valuable long-term health behavior and should not be discouraged.
Provide skin care, especially over bony prominences.	The client is at risk for skin breakdown due to his or her nutritional state and lack of muscle and subcutaneous tissue.
Encourage the client to use a shower for bathing.	Sitting in a bathtub may be quite uncomfortable for the client due to bony prominences and lack of muscle or subcutaneous tissue.

(continued)
Implementation

Nursing Interventions	Rationale
Provide warm bedding. Be aware of room air temperatures.	The client is especially apt to feel cold because of decreased fat and subcutaneous tissue.
Provide or encourage dental hygiene. Referral to a dentist may be appropriate.	The client's teeth or gums may be in poor condition due to the effects of vomiting (decreased tooth enamel from contact with gastric fluids) and malnutrition.
Gradually decrease limits on meals and snacks, and allow the client more control over his or her food intake, choice of foods, preparation, and so forth.	The client needs to develop independent eating habits.
Give positive feedback for healthy eating behaviors.	Positive support tends to reinforce desired behaviors.
Be aware of your role in modeling healthy behavior.	You are a role model for the client.
Assess the client's knowledge of weight, nutrition, and so forth. Client teaching may be indicated; this should be done in factual and unemotional terms and should be limited in frequency and duration. Refer the client to a dietitian for detailed instruction if appropriate.	The client may have false ideas about food, weight, and nutrition. The client needs to decrease his or her emotional investment in food or eating. Areas outside the nursing area of expertise are best referred to other health professionals.
Do not engage in nonteaching interactions with the client on topics of food and eating.	This allows you to focus on emotional issues with the client and limits focusing on food and eating.
Discharge should not occur until the client has reached a healthy weight, as agreed in the treatment plan. This limit should be maintained without bargaining after the goal has been set (although the client may have initial input into the goal).	The client's physical health is a priority. Bargaining may undermine the limit. Allowing the client's input in the treatment plan can encourage cooperation.

Nursing Diagnosis	*Ineffective Individual Coping (5.1.1.1)* *Impairment of adaptive behaviors and problem-solving abilities of a person in meeting life's demands and roles.*

Assessment Data

Defining Characteristics	• Denial of illness • Inability to ask for help • Inability to problem solve • Inability to meet basic needs • Inability to meet role expectations • Feelings of helplessness or powerlessness • Depressive behavior • Anxiety • Guilt

✳ *(continued)*
Assessment Data

Defining Characteristics	• Anger
	• Suicidal ideas or feelings
	• Manipulative behavior
	• Regressive behavior
	• Hyperactivity
	• Sleep disturbances, such as early awakening
	• Social isolation
	• Decreased sexual interest
	• Rumination
Related Factors	• Refusal to eat
	• Denial or loss of appetite
	• Dread of certain foods
	• Disgust at the thought of eating
	• Preoccupation with food
	• Hiding or hoarding food
	• Preoccupation with losing weight
	• Unceasing pursuit of thinness
	• Intense fear of becoming obese
	• Family problems
	• Low self-esteem
	• Problems with sense of identity
	• Delusions
	• Body image distortions

✳
Expected Outcomes

Initial	*The client will:*
	• Be free of self-inflicted injury
	• Demonstrate decreased manipulative, depressive, or regressive behavior and suicidal ideas and feelings
	• Demonstrate increased feelings of self-worth
	• Demonstrate beginning trust relationships with others
	• Verbalize recognition of perceptual distortions (eg, distorted body image)
	• Participate in treatment program
	• Identify non–food-related coping mechanisms
	• Interact with others in non–food-related ways
	• Demonstrate increased social skills
	• Demonstrate more effective interpersonal relationships with family or significant others
	• Demonstrate change in attitudes about food and eating
Discharge	*The client will:*
	• Demonstrate non–food-related coping mechanisms
	• Verbalize a realistic perception of body image
	• Demonstrate decreased associations between food and emotions

✸ *(continued)*
Expected Outcomes

Discharge

- Demonstrate increased independence and age-appropriate behaviors
- Verbalize knowledge of illness and medications, if any
- Verbalize plans for continuing therapy after discharge, if appropriate

✸
Therapeutic Aims

- Protect the client from self-inflicted injury.
- Build a trust relationship.
- Avoid conflict with the client.
- Decrease withdrawn or depressive behavior.
- Prevent or decrease manipulative behavior.
- Promote self-esteem, social skills, and maturity.
- Decrease regressive behavior.
- Decrease the client's association between food and stress.
- Help the client develop non–food-related coping mechanisms.
- Promote improvement of the client's home environment and the client's ability to function in his or her family without anorexic behaviors.
- Prepare the client for discharge and successful reintegration into his or her home environment.

✸
Implementation

Nursing Interventions	Rationale
See Care Plan 24: Suicidal Behavior.	
Be aware of your own feelings about the client and his or her behaviors. Express your feelings to other staff members.	You may have strong feelings of helplessness, frustration, and anger in working with this client. Working through your own feelings will decrease the possibility of acting them out in your interactions with the client.
Be nonjudgmental in your interactions with the client. Do not express approval or disapproval or be punitive to the client.	Issues of control, approval, and guilt often are problems with the client. Nonjudgmental nursing care decreases the possibility of power struggles.
See Care Plan 1: Building a Trust Relationship, Care Plan 23: Depressive Behavior, and Care Plan 49: Withdrawn Behavior.	
Maintain consistency of treatment. One staff member per shift should be identified to have the final word on all decisions (although other staff members and the client may have input).	Consistency minimizes the possibility of manipulation of staff members by the client.
Supervise or remain aware of the client's interactions with other clients and with visitors.	Other clients or visitors, especially family members, may reinforce manipulative behavior or provide secondary gain for the client's not eating.
See Care Plan 36: Passive–Aggressive or Manipulative Behavior.	

✳ *(continued)*
Implementation

Nursing Interventions	Rationale
Do not restrict the client to his or her room as a restriction of privileges.	Social isolation may be something the client desires or may be considered part of the client's disorder.
Remember the client's age, and relate to the client accordingly. Expect age-appropriate behavior from the client.	The client may appear to be younger than his or her actual age. The client may want to be dependent and to be treated like a child and may fear or want to avoid maturity, responsibility, and independence.
Expect healthy behavior from the client.	There is a danger in labeling a client with an illness: You may then expect behaviors characteristic of the disorder and inadvertently reinforce those behaviors.
Encourage the client to do schoolwork while in the hospital if the client is missing school due to hospitalization.	Schoolwork is a normal part of an adolescent's usual routine. The client may receive secondary gain from not being expected to do schoolwork or by falling behind his or her age group in school.
Give the client positive support and honest praise for accomplishments. Focus attention on the client's positive traits and strengths (not on feelings of inadequacy).	Positive support tends to provide reinforcement for desired behaviors.
Do not flatter or be otherwise dishonest in interactions with or feedback to the client.	The client will not benefit from dishonest praise or flattery. Honest, positive feedback can help build self-esteem.
Foster successful experiences for the client: Arrange for the client to help other clients in specific ways; suggest activities to the client that are within his or her realm of ability. Begin by offering the client small tasks and activities that are easily accomplished, and then increase complexity as appropriate.	Any activity that the client is able to complete provides an opportunity for positive feedback.
Use group therapy and role playing with the client.	The client can share feelings and try out new behaviors in a supportive, nonthreatening environment.
Remain aware of your own behavior with the client. (Be consistent, truthful, nonjudgmental.)	Staff members are the client's role models for appropriate behavior and self-control.
Make referrals for recreational and occupational therapy as appropriate.	The client may need to learn non–food-related ways to relax, spend leisure time, and so forth.
Allow the client food only at specified snack and meal times. Do not talk with the client about emotional issues at these times. Encourage the client to ventilate his or her feelings at other times in ways not associated with food.	It is important for the client to separate emotional issues from food and eating.
Withdraw your attention if the client is ruminating about food or engaging in rituals with food or eating. See Care Plan 45: Obsessive Thoughts or Compulsive Behavior.	Minimizing attention given to these behaviors may help decrease them.

❊ *(continued)*
Implementation

Nursing Interventions	Rationale
Observe and record the client's perceptions of and responses to stress. Encourage the client to approach the staff at stressful times.	The client may be unaware of his or her responses to stress and may need to learn to identify stressful situations.
Talk with the client to identify others in his or her home environment with whom the client can talk and who can be supportive of the client. Identify non–food-related activities that may decrease stress or anxiety (eg, hobbies, writing, drawing).	The client needs to learn new skills to deal with stress.
As tolerated, encourage the client to express his or her feelings regarding achievement, family issues, independence, social skills, sexuality, and control.	These issues often are problem areas for anorexic clients.
See Care Plan 43: Anxious Behavior.	
Assess the client's home environment: Interview the client's family, make a home visit if possible, or observe the family's behavior at meal time. Encourage the family's participation in family therapy if indicated.	Research indicates that family dynamics may be involved in the development and progression of anorexia nervosa and that family therapy can be successful in eliminating the disorder (Doyen, 1982).
Encourage the client to ventilate his or her feelings about family members, family dynamics, family roles, and so forth.	Ventilation of feelings can help the client identify, accept, and work through his or her feelings, even if these are painful or uncomfortable for the client.
Send the client home for a specified time, then evaluate the success of this trial period with the client in the hospital prior to discharge. Observe and record the client's feelings, mood, and activities before and after time at home.	Hospitalization may decrease pressure for the client by removing the client from home and by interrupting family dynamics. Returning home may increase the client's stress and result in weight loss or other anorexic behaviors.
Involve the client's family or significant others with the client in teaching, treatment, and discharge and follow-up plans. Teaching should include dynamics of illness, nutrition, and medication use, if any.	Family dynamics may play a significant role in anorexia nervosa.
Arrange for follow-up therapy for the client and the family. Encourage contact with follow-up therapist before discharge.	Follow-up and long-term therapy can be effective in preventing future weight loss.
Refer the client and his or her family to local support groups or to national groups by mail (eg, the National Anorexic Aid Society for Anorexia Nervosa and Associated Disorders).	These groups can offer support, education, and resources to clients and their families.
See Care Plan 2: Discharge Planning.	

Bulimia Nervosa and Excessive Eating

Bulimia nervosa, also known as *bulimia* or *buliminarexia,* is an eating disorder characterized by an excessive intake of food, although not all clients who eat excessively have this disorder. Excessive eating behavior in bulimia involves compulsive eating or food *binges,* during which the client rapidly consumes very large amounts of food at one time; these episodes may occur from two or three times a week to several times a day. Binges may be terminated or followed by *purge behaviors,* which include self-induced vomiting or the excessive use of laxatives or diuretics (Hofland and Dardis, 1992). Clients with bulimia also may manifest other weight loss behaviors, such as prolonged fasting, excessive exercise, or misuse of diet pills.

Binge eating behavior may occur without purge behaviors; this is sometimes called *compulsive eating.* Excessive eating behaviors may be seen as a continuum of eating disordered behaviors involving excessive or compulsive eating with or without binge or purge behaviors. These disorders involve eating as a way of dealing with feelings and interpersonal issues. Not all people who are overweight have this type of disorder. Clients who eat excessively and compulsively can reach weights that are considered in the morbid obesity range, that is, more than 100 pounds over normal body weight; as a result, their health may be severely compromised. However, bulimic clients, especially those who use purging and fasting as weight control measures, may be at, near, or under their ideal body weight. Clients with bulimia often experience a distortion of body image (perceiving themselves as fat or too large even when thin), body image dissatisfaction, and an overpowering drive to be thin (Waller, Newton, Hardy, and Svetlik, 1990). Bulimic clients may be severely malnourished, and often experience medical complications, such as fluid and electrolyte imbalances, which can be severe and potentially life-threatening.

Bulimic clients usually are women, and the onset of bulimic behavior usually occurs in late adolescence or the early 20s; prevalence estimates of bulimia vary from 1% of adolescent and young adult females (Marshall, 1992) to as much as 79% in some groups (Hofland and Dardis, 1992). These clients often present with or have histories or family histories of substance abuse, impulsive behavior (including shoplifting and promiscuity), affective disorders (including major depression, self-mutilation, or suicidal behavior), anxiety disorders, or personality disorders (Mitchell, Specker, and de Zwaan, 1991; Palmer 1990). Many bulimics report a history of dieting behavior and report that binge episodes often are followed by feelings of depression, guilt, self-deprecation, panic, feeling out of control, shame, humiliation, worry, or anxiety (Marshall, 1992). In addition bulimic clients have been described as being dissatisfied with or impaired in social relationships and having high levels of depression and anxiety and low self-esteem (Agras, 1991).

Treatment of clients with bulimia often is long term and can involve the use of pharmacologic agents and psychotherapy. Antidepressant medications have been effective in bulimic clients; other drugs are being investigated for use in bulimia (Kennedy and Goldbloom, 1991; Walsh, 1991). Research indicates that both cognitive–behavioral and interpersonal psychotherapeutic methods can be successful in treating bulimia (Agras, 1991). Periods of hospitalization, if they occur, are relatively short and may occur only during medical or psychiatric crises. These clients may be seen initially on a medical unit due to physical complications from binge–purge behaviors, malnutrition, and so forth. It is important to identify eating disordered clients, refer them for therapy, and encourage them to follow through with treatment for the eating disorder.

Nursing Diagnoses Addressed in this Care Plan

Altered Nutrition: Less than Body Requirements
Altered Nutrition: More than Body Requirements
Ineffective Individual Coping

Related Nursing Diagnoses

Ineffective Denial
Noncompliance with Treatment Plan
Self-Esteem Disturbance
Sensory/Perceptual Alterations
Anxiety
Ineffective Family Coping (disabling or compromised)

Nursing Diagnosis

Altered Nutrition: More than/Less than Body Requirements (1.1.2.1/1.1.2.2)

The state in which an individual is experiencing an intake of nutrients which exceeds metabolic needs or is insufficient to meet metabolic needs.

Assessment Data

Defining Characteristics

- Weight gain or loss
- Body weight at least 20% over or under ideal body weight
- Overuse of laxatives, diet pills, or diuretics
- Sedentary activity level
- Dysfunctional eating patterns
- Binge eating
- Compulsive eating
- Diuretic use
- Laxative use

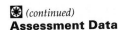 *(continued)*
Assessment Data

Related Factors	• Preoccupation with weight, food, or diets
	• Fatigue or lethargy
	• Inadequate nutritional intake
	• Excessive caloric intake
	• Secrecy regarding eating habits or amounts eaten
	• Recurrent vomiting after eating
	• Physical signs and symptoms: skin changes on dorsal surface of hand (ulceration or scarring) or finger calluses (from manually stimulating vomiting), hypertrophy of salivary or parotid glands, erosion of dental enamel (from acidity of emesis), ulcerations around mouth and cheeks (from emesis splashback).
	• Physical problems or changes (may be life-threatening): fluid and electrolyte imbalances, including dehydration and volume depletion, hypokalemia, hyponatremia, hypomagnesia, and hypocalcemia; cardiac problems, including electrocardiogram disturbances, heart failure, and myopathy; metabolic alkalosis or acidosis; seizures; hypotension; elevated aldosterone level; edema of hands and feet; fatigue; muscle weakness, soreness, or cramps; headache; nausea; laxative dependence; gastrointestinal problems (from vomiting and laxative misuse), including constipation, colitis, malabsorption disorders, delayed gastric emptying, gastric bleeding, ulcers, or rupture; sore throat; emetine toxicity (from ipecac misuse); elevated serum amylase; esophagitis, esophageal erosions, bleeding, stricture, or perforation; pancreatitis; hypoglycemia; disturbance in hormone levels; irregular menses.

Expected Outcomes

Initial	*The client will:*
	• Interrupt binge (binge–purge) eating patterns
	• Establish regular (adequate, not excessive) nutritional eating patterns
	• Maintain normal bowel elimination without laxatives
	• Be free of use of diuretics, laxatives, or diet pills
	• Evidence improvement in physical status related to complications of bulimia or excessive eating
Discharge	*The client will:*
	• Eliminate binge (binge–purge) eating patterns
	• Continue to evidence improvement in physical status related to complications of bulimia or excessive eating
	• Maintain regular (adequate, not excessive) nutritional eating patterns
	• Verbalize acceptance of stable body weight within 20% of ideal body weight

Therapeutic Aims

• Promote adequate nutritional intake and retention of food.
• Promote the client's sense of control.
• Help the client establish normal elimination patterns.
• Promote adequate dental care.

✳ Implementation

Nursing Interventions	Rationale
Help the client determine a daily meal plan that is appropriate for him or her, includes all food groups, and so forth. Consultation with a dietitian is helpful.	Though the client has been very preoccupied with food, he or she may lack knowledge about the type and amounts of food that constitute a healthful diet. The meal plan provides a structure for the client's eating behavior.
Initially, allow the client to avoid some "fattening" foods (foods the client fears or sees as bad), as long as his or her diet is nutritionally sound.	The client can exercise some control if allowed to make some decisions. Initially, his or her anxiety may be minimized by allowing the client to avoid certain foods.
Gradually include foods that the client has avoided as forbidden or fattening or has come to fear (eg, carbohydrates).	Including foods that the client has avoided may help the client learn that these foods are not harmful. Gradual introduction of fearsome foods will help minimize the client's anxiety.
Spend time with the client after meals. Avoid letting the client go to the bathroom unaccompanied or to an isolated area where secretive vomiting would be likely to occur.	Your presence is a deterrent to vomiting, because that behavior usually is secretive. Your presence is supportive because the client may feel guilty and anxious about having eaten.
When the client feels the urge to binge, go on a walk with the client or engage in other physical or distracting activities. Encourage the client to use physical activities independently, because he or she is more able to deal with these urges. However, discourage the client from using excessive exercise as a weight control measure.	Physical activity can provide a release for feelings that promote binge behavior. It also is a way to postpone eating until meal time.
Have the client measure and record weight daily. Avoid letting the client weigh more than once a day or skip daily weight measures.	The client may have avoided weight measurement because he or she is convinced of being overweight. Clients also tend to binge or purge based on feeling fat rather than on actual weight.
Discourage the client's use of diuretics, diet pills, or laxatives. Ask the client to relinquish these items. You may need to search the client's belongings, with the client's permission.	Continued use of diuretics, diet pills, or laxatives reinforces bulimic behavior and can have severe medical consequences.
Be alert to the possibility of the client asking friends or family to smuggle food, laxatives, or other drugs to him or her.	The client may feel panicky when binge foods, laxatives, or other drugs are not available—the client may feel out of control. The client's significant others can be supportive of the client's health by not reinforcing bulimic behaviors.
Be nonjudgmental and matter-of-fact in your approach to the client and his or her behavior.	This approach will not reinforce the client's already excessive feelings of guilt and shame.
Monitor the client's laboratory values for electrolyte imbalance.	Persistent vomiting, diuretic use, or use of laxatives can result in hypokalemia, hyponatremia, dehydration, and metabolic alkalosis or acidosis.

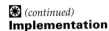 *(continued)*
Implementation

Nursing Interventions	Rationale
Discontinue the availability of laxatives. The client's diet should have adequate fiber to promote normal elimination.	Laxative dependence must be eliminated.
Encourage the client to drink fluids, especially water.	Adequate fluid intake promotes normal elimination.
Encourage the client to be physically active (though not to excess).	Physical activity promotes normal elimination.
If the client remains constipated, temporary use of glycerin suppositories will stimulate evacuation.	Judicious use of glycerin suppositories will not foster dependence as do laxatives.
Refer the client to a dentist, or encourage the client to seek dental care.	Due to frequent vomiting, erosion of tooth enamel, tooth sensitivity, poor dental hygiene, and dental caries are common.

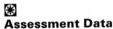

Nursing Diagnosis

Ineffective Individual Coping (5.1.1.1)
Impairment of adaptive behaviors and problem-solving abilities of a person in meeting life's demands and roles.

Assessment Data

Defining Characteristics

- Inability to meet basic needs
- Inability to ask for help
- Inability to problem-solve
- Inability to change behaviors
- Self-destructive behavior
- Suicidal thoughts or behavior
- Inability to delay gratification
- Poor impulse control
- Stealing or shoplifting behavior
- Desire for perfection
- Intolerance of self-weaknesses
- Feelings of worthlessness
- Feelings of inadequacy or guilt
- Unsatisfactory interpersonal relationships
- Self-deprecatory verbalization
- Denial of feelings, illness, or problems
- Anxiety
- Sleep disturbances

❋ *(continued)*
Assessment Data

Related Factors	
	• Low self-esteem
	• Excessive need to control
	• Feelings of being out of control
	• Preoccupation with weight, food, or diets
	• Distortions of body image
	• Overuse of laxatives, diet pills, or diuretics
	• Fatigue or lethargy
	• Secrecy regarding eating habits or amounts eaten
	• Bulimia nervosa
	• Fear of being fat
	• Recurrent vomiting
	• Binge eating
	• Compulsive eating
	• Substance use
	• Affective disorders, especially depression
	• Family history of substance abuse or affective disorders

❋
Expected Outcomes

Initial

The client will:

• Be free of self-inflicted harm
• Identify non–food-related methods of dealing with stress or crises
• Verbalize feelings of guilt, anxiety, anger, or an excessive need for control

Discharge

The client will:

• Demonstrate more satisfying interpersonal relationships
• Follow through with discharge planning, including support groups or therapy as indicated
• Verbalize more realistic body image
• Demonstrate alternative methods of dealing with stress or crises
• Verbalize increased self-esteem and self-confidence
• Eliminate shoplifting or stealing behaviors
• Express feelings in non–food-related ways
• Verbalize understanding of disease process and safe use of medications if any

❋
Therapeutic Aims

• Provide a safe environment.
• Help the client develop insight into his or her behavior and feelings.
• Promote the client's ability to express feelings.
• Promote knowledge regarding the eating disorder and associated behaviors, medications, and self-care.
• Promote the client's self-esteem and acceptance of himself or herself.
• Help the client develop realistic body image perceptions.
• Promote the client's ability to function in his or her family or relationships without dysfunctional eating behaviors.
• Help the client prepare for discharge and possible follow-up therapy.

Implementation

Nursing Interventions	Rationale
Set limits with the client about eating habits. Food will be eaten in a dining room setting, at a table, only at conventional meal times.	These limits will discourage previous binge behavior, which involves sneaking and gulping food, hiding food, and so forth. You will help the client return to normal eating patterns. Eating three meals a day will prevent starvation and subsequent overeating in the evening.
Encourage the client to eat with other clients, when tolerated.	Eating with other people will discourage secrecy about eating, though initially the client's anxiety may be too high to join others at meal time.
Encourage the client to express feelings, such as anxiety and guilt about having eaten.	Verbal expression of feelings can help decrease the client's anxiety and the urge to engage in purging behaviors.
Ask the client directly about thoughts of suicide or self-harm.	The client's safety is a priority. It is important to remember that you will not give the client ideas about suicide by addressing the issue directly.
See Care Plan 24: Suicidal Behavior.	
Encourage the client to keep a diary in which to write types and amounts of foods eaten and to identify feelings that occur before, during, and after eating, especially related to urges to engage in binge or purge behavior.	A diary can help the client examine his or her food intake and the feelings he or she experiences. Gradually, he or she may be able to see relationships among these feelings and behaviors. Initially, the client may be able to write these feelings and behaviors more easily than talking about them.
Encourage the client to describe and discuss feelings verbally. Begin to separate dealing with feelings from eating or purging behaviors. Maintain a nonjudgmental approach.	You can help the client begin to express feelings in a nonthreatening environment. Being nonjudgmental gives the client permission to openly discuss feelings that may be negative or unacceptable to him or her without fear of rejection or reprisal.
Discuss the types of foods that are soothing to the client and that relieve anxiety.	You may be able to help the client see how he or she has used food to deal with feelings or to comfort himself or herself.
Help the client explore ways of relieving anxiety and expressing feelings, especially anger, frustration, and anxiety, that are not associated with eating. Help the client identify ways to experience pleasure that are not related to food or eating.	It is important to help the client separate emotional issues from food and eating behaviors.
Give positive feedback for the client's efforts.	The client may have become accustomed to judging himself or herself on accomplishments (often food related), with no regard for feelings. Your sincere praise can promote the client's attempts to deal openly and honestly with anxiety, anger, and other feelings.

✳ *(continued)*
Implementation

Nursing Interventions	Rationale
Teach the client and his or her significant others about bulimic behaviors, physical complications, nutrition, food, and so forth. Refer the client to a dietitian for further instruction if indicated.	The client and his or her significant others may have little actual knowledge of the illness and of food, nutrition, and so forth. Factual information can be useful in dispelling incorrect beliefs and in separating food issues from emotional issues.
Teach the client and his or her significant others about the purpose, action, timing, and possible adverse effects of medications, if any.	Antidepressant and other medications are sometimes prescribed for bulimia. The client needs to be aware of the effects of the medication(s) and their safe use. Remember, some antidepressant medications may take 2 to 3 weeks to achieve a therapeutic effect.
Teach the client about the use of the problem-solving process.	Successful use of the problem-solving process can help increase the client's self-esteem and confidence.
Explore with the client his or her personal strengths. Making a written list is sometimes helpful.	You can help the client discover his or her strengths. It will not be useful, however, for you to list the client's strengths—he or she needs to identify them but may benefit from your supportive expectation that he or she will do so.
Discuss with the client the idea of accepting a less than "ideal" body weight.	The client's previous expectations of an ideal weight may have been unrealistic, and even unhealthy.
Encourage the client to incorporate fattening (or "bad") foods into the diet as he or she tolerates.	This will enhance the client's sense of control of overeating.
Encourage the client to develop these skills and use them in his or her daily life. Refer the client to assertiveness training books or classes if indicated.	Many bulimic clients are passive and nonassertive in interpersonal relationships. Assertiveness training may foster a sense of increased control, confidence, and healthy relationship dynamics.
Encourage the client to express his or her feelings about family members and significant others, their roles and relationships.	Expression of feelings can help the client to identify, accept, and work through his or her feelings in a direct manner.
Refer the client to long-term therapy if indicated. Encourage the client to follow through with therapy on an outpatient basis. Use of contracting with the client may be helpful to promote follow through.	Treatment for eating disorders often is long term. The client may be more likely to engage in ongoing therapy if he or she has contracted to do this.
Ongoing therapy may need to include family members or significant others to sustain and continue the client's non–food-related coping skills.	Dysfunctional relationships with family members or significant others are thought to be a primary issue with clients experiencing eating disorders.
Refer the client and his or her family and significant others to local or national support groups for people with eating disorders (for example, Anorexia Nervosa and Associated Disorders, Overeaters Anonymous).	These groups can offer support, education, and resources to clients and their families or significant others.

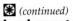 *(continued)*
Implementation

Nursing Interventions	Rationale
Refer the client to a chemical dependence treatment program or chemical dependence support group (for example, Alcoholics Anonymous), if appropriate. (See Care Plan 33: Chemical Dependence Treatment Program.)	Substance use is common among clients with bulimia.
See Care Plan 2: Discharge Planning.	

Section Ten

Chemical Dependence

Abuse of chemical substances may be chronic or acute, and may include the use or abuse of alcohol, licit (prescription or over-the-counter) drugs, and illicit drugs. The first two care plans in this section are concerned with acute or short-term treatment plans for the client who is withdrawing from alcohol or another chemical substance. Chemical dependence involves certain physiologic problems, often specific to the kind of substance used by the client, and emotional problems. It also may involve social, economic, vocational, and legal difficulties. Care Plan 33 describes a possible program that can be used in the long-term treatment of a client whose primary problem is substance abuse. Clients who have a dual diagnosis—a major psychiatric illness and chemical dependence—have special needs that are not necessarily met by traditional treatment for one or the other of their major problems. Considerations and care related to these clients are addressed in Care Plan 34. Finally, adult children of alcoholics may be encountered as clients or significant others in a number of situations in nursing. Care Plan 35 describes their characteristics and offers suggestions for nursing care planning.

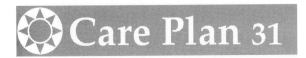

Alcohol Detoxification

Alcohol is a drug that causes central nervous system (CNS) depression. With chronic use and abuse the CNS is chronically depressed. An abrupt cessation of drinking causes a rebound hyperactivity of the CNS. This produces a variety of withdrawal phenomena. The particular phenomena are peculiar to each client, the client's pattern of use, and the chronicity of excessive alcohol intake. The most common withdrawal phenomena can be summarized as follows:

Tremors are characterized by irritability, rapid pulse, elevated blood pressure, diaphoresis, sleep disturbances, and coarse tremors. Tremors vary from shaky hands to involvement of the entire body.

Alcoholic hallucinosis are sensory experiences characterized by misperception and misinterpretation of real stimuli in the environment (not to be confused with hallucinations), sleep disturbances, or nightmares. The client remains oriented to person, place, and time.

Seizures are categorized as grand mal, or major motor seizures, though they are transitory in nature. Medical treatment is required.

Auditory hallucinations are true hallucinations but are caused by a cessation of alcohol intake rather than a psychiatric disorder, such as schizophrenia. The client hears voices, which usually are threatening or ridiculing. These "voices" may sound like someone the client knows.

Delirium Tremens (DTs) is the most serious phase of alcohol withdrawal. Twenty percent of all people who develop DTs die, even with medical treatment. DTs begin with tremors, rapid pulse, fever, and elevated blood pressure. Rather than improving in a few days, the client's condition worsens with time. The client becomes confused, is delusional, and has auditory, visual, and tactile hallucinations (frequently of bugs, snakes, or rodents). The client feels pursued and fearful. DTs may last from 2 to 7 days and may involve physical complications, such as pneumonia and cardiac or renal failure.

Nursing Diagnoses Addressed in this Care Plan

High Risk for Injury
Altered Health Maintenance

Related Nursing Diagnoses

Sleep Pattern Disturbance
Self-Care Deficit
High Risk for Violence: Self-Directed or Directed at Others
Sensory/Perceptual Alterations
Altered Nutrition: Less than Body Requirements
Fluid Volume Excess

Nursing Diagnosis

High Risk for Injury (1.6.1)
A state in which the individual is at risk of injury as a result of environmental conditions interacting with the individual's adaptive and defensive resources.

Risk Factors

- Confusion
- Disorientation
- Feelings of fear, dread
- Belligerent, uncooperative behavior
- Seizures
- Hallucinosis
- Delirium tremens
- Suicidal behavior
- Inability to distinguish potential harm
- Threatening or aggressive behavior
- Environmental misperceptions

Expected Outcomes

Initial

The client will:

- Be safe and free of injury
- Respond to reality orientation
- Demonstrate decreased aggressive or threatening behavior

Discharge

The client will:

- Abstain from alcohol and other drugs
- Verbalize risks related to alcohol intake

Therapeutic Aims

- Provide a safe environment.
- Protect the client from injury.
- Increase reality contact.
- Provide emotional support.

Implementation

Nursing Interventions	Rationale
Place the client in a room near the nurses' station or where the staff can observe the client closely.	The client's safety is a priority.
Institute seizure precautions according to hospital policy (padded tongue blade in room, padded side rails, side rails up, airway at bedside, and so forth).	Seizures can occur during withdrawal. Precautions can minimize chances of injury.
Provide only an electric shaver.	The client may be too shaky to use a razor with blades.
Monitor the client's sleep pattern; he or she may need to be restrained at night if confused or if he or she wanders or attempts to climb out of bed.	The client's physical safety is a priority.
Reorient the client to person, time, place, and situation as needed.	You provide reality orientation by describing situations, stating the date, time, and so forth.
Talk to the client in simple, direct, concrete language. Do not try to discuss the client's feelings, plans for treatment, or changes in life-style when the client is intoxicated or in withdrawal.	The client can respond to simple, direct statements from you. His or her ability to deal with complex or abstract ideas is limited by his or her physical condition. Attempts to discuss emotional issues will be frustrating to you and the client.
Reassure the client that the bugs, snakes, and so on are not really there.	You provide reality orientation for the client.
Tell the client that you know these sights appear real to him or her, and empathize with the fear that the client is experiencing.	Let the client know you believe what he or she is experiencing and feeling, but leave no doubt about it not being real.
Do not moralize or chastise the client for his or her alcoholism. Maintain a nonjudgmental attitude.	Remember that alcoholism is an illness and is out of the client's control at this time. Moralizing belittles the client.

Nursing Diagnosis	*Altered Health Maintenance (6.4.2)*
	Inability to identify, manage, or seek out help to maintain health.

Assessment Data

Defining Characteristics	• Physical symptoms (impaired nutrition, fluid and electrolyte imbalance, gastrointestinal disturbances, liver impairment)
	• Physical exhaustion
	• Sleep disturbances
	• Dependence on alcohol

✳ (continued)
Assessment Data

Related Factors	• Ineffective coping strategies
	• Failure to manage stress
	• Disruptions in major life areas: family, work, social, or legal

✳
Expected Outcomes

Initial	*The client will:*
	• Establish nutritious eating patterns
	• Establish physiologic homeostasis
	• Establish a balance of rest, sleep, and activity
	• Maintain personal hygiene and grooming
Discharge	*The client will:*
	• Maintain physiologic stability
	• Agree to participate in a treatment program
	• Identify needed health resources
	• Follow through with discharge plans regarding physical health, counseling, and legal problems, as indicated
Therapeutic Aims	• Promote homeostasis
	• Provide emotional support

✳
Implementation

Nursing Interventions	Rationale
Monitor the client's vital signs, especially pulse and blood pressure. Also observe the client for physical symptoms and changes. Alert the physician to any symptoms or changes observed.	The client's vital signs are the most reliable data to determine the client's need for medication.
Complete the physical assessment of the client; ask what and how much the client usually drinks, as well as the time and amount of his or her last drink of alcohol.	This information can help you anticipate the onset and severity of withdrawal symptoms.
Offer fluids frequently, especially juices and malts. Serve only decaffeinated coffee. Intravenous therapy may be indicated in severe withdrawal.	Caffeine will increase tremors. Malts and juices offer nutrients and fluids to the client.
Monitor the client's fluid and electrolyte balance.	Clients with alcohol abuse problems are at high risk for fluid and electrolyte imbalances.
Provide food or nourishing fluids as soon as the client can tolerate eating; have something available at night. (Bland food usually is tolerated best at first.)	Many clients who use alcohol heavily experience gastritis, anorexia, and so forth. Therefore, bland foods are tolerated most easily. It is important to reestablish nutritional intake as soon as the client tolerates food.

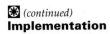 *(continued)*
Implementation

Nursing Interventions	Rationale
Administer medication to minimize the progression of withdrawal or complications and to facilitate sleep.	The client will be fatigued and needs rest. Also, he or she should be as comfortable as possible.
Encourage the client to bathe, wash his or her hair, and wear clean clothes.	Personal cleanliness will enhance the client's sense of well-being.
Assist the client as necessary; it may be necessary to provide complete physical care, depending on the severity of the client's withdrawal.	The level of client independence is determined by the severity of withdrawal symptoms. The client's needs should be met with the greatest degree of independence he or she can attain.
Teach the client that alcoholism is a disease that requires long-term treatment and follow-up. Refer the client to a chemical dependence treatment program.	Detoxification deals only with the client's physical withdrawal from alcohol but does not address the primary disease of alcoholism.
Refer the client's family or significant others to Alanon, Alateen, or Adult Children of Alcoholics, as indicated.	Alcoholism is an illness that affects all family members and significant others.

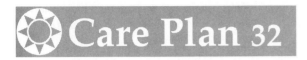

Drug Withdrawal

Two characteristics of physiologic addiction to drugs are *tolerance* (the need to increase the dose to achieve the same effect) and *withdrawal*. Withdrawal refers to the fact that physiologic symptoms will occur when drug ingestion ceases. Withdrawal symptoms occur at some time after the last dose of the drug and are specific to the type of drug taken. These symptoms can occur when drug ingestion is curtailed or eliminated, even when there is no demonstrable physiologic tolerance. In this situation the client may express a "need" (ie, psychologic dependence or reliance) for additional amounts of the substance, and this can lead to increased anxiety or agitation.

Withdrawal signs and symptoms for the major categories of drugs are as follows:

Opiates: morphine, heroin, Dilaudid (hydromorphone), codeine, Demerol (meperidine). Initially (8 to 12 hours after the last time the drug was taken): perspiration, yawning, lacrimation, rhinorrhea, and sneezing. These are followed by dilated pupils, anorexia, restlessness, insomnia, nausea, vomiting, chills, and abdominal cramps, all of which may persist for 72 hours after the last dose. These symptoms then subside during the next 4 to 7 days.

Central nervous system depressants: barbiturates, sedatives, and nonbarbiturate hypnotics (eg, Quaalude). Initially (10 to 16 hours after the last drug was taken): restlessness, anxiety, weakness, irritability, nausea, vomiting, tremors, and hyperreflexia. Two to three days after the last time the drug was taken: delirium, fever, and seizures. Without medical treatment, death may occur. *Note:* Withdrawal from barbiturates is a life-threatening situation in which seizures can be followed by coma and death.

Tranquilizers: Librium (chlordiazepoxide), Valium (diazepam), Tranxene, Equanil, Ativan (lorazepam), Serax, Xanax. Initially (6 to 10 hours after the last dose was taken): restlessness, irritability, insomnia, perspiration. These are followed by increasing agitation, nausea, vomiting, environmental misperceptions, and possibly hostile or aggressive behavior.

Stimulants: amphetamines, cocaine, crack, PCP. General symptoms: excessive sleeping, lassitude, headache, depression. Specifically, amphetamines may produce a "crash"—the client is paranoid, feels persecuted, and may act out physically 10 to 12 hours after the last drug was taken.

Note: Violent, aggressive behavior is common while people are under the influence of PCP. Sudden death has been documented by people using PCP, crack, or cocaine, even with first-time use.

Clients with drug use or abuse problems may have poor general health, especially in the area of nutrition. These clients are at increased risk for infections, hepatitis, gastrointestinal disturbances, and so forth. Clients who abuse prescription drugs have the same problems and difficulties as clients who abuse illicit drugs. Clients who use illicit drugs have the additional problem of unknowingly taking larger amounts than intended, or ingesting additional substances of which they are unaware. Adult females and adolescents of both sexes often develop drug tolerance and experience complications from drug use more rapidly than adult males. Clients who are intravenous drug users are at increased risk for human immunodeficiency virus (HIV) infection and acquired immunodeficiency syndrome (AIDS). It is especially important to educate these clients about HIV transmission related to needle sharing and sexual activity. (See Basic Concepts: HIV Disease and AIDS.)

Do not ask or even listen if the client attempts to reveal the names or locations of illicit drug sources to you. You do not need this information to work with the client. If you inadvertently gain knowledge of this nature, it is treated as confidential and not used for legal action.

Nursing Diagnoses Addressed in this Care Plan

High Risk for Injury
Altered Health Maintenance

Related Nursing Diagnoses

High Risk for Violence: Self-Directed or Directed at Others
Sleep Pattern Disturbance
Noncompliance
Sensory/Perceptual Alterations
High Risk for Infection
Fluid Volume Deficit
Altered Nutrition: Less than Body Requirements

Nursing Diagnosis

Risk Factors

High Risk for Injury (1.6.1)

The state in which the individual is at risk of injury as a result of environmental conditions interacting with the individual's adaptive and defensive resources.

- Fearfulness
- Mood alteration, drastic mood swings
- Confusion
- Disorientation
- Seizures
- Hallucinations
- Delusions

❋ *(continued)*
Risk Factors

- Physical pain or discomfort
- Uncooperative, hostile behavior
- Disturbances of concentration, attention span, or ability to follow directions

❋
Expected Outcomes

Initial

The client will:

- Be safe and free of injury
- Demonstrate decreased aggressive or hostile behavior
- Respond to reality orientation
- Verbally express feelings of fear or anxiety

Discharge

The client will:

- Abstain from the use of chemicals
- Verbalize risks related to drug ingestion

❋
Therapeutic Aims

- Prevent injury.
- Provide emotional support.
- Provide a safe environment.

❋
Implementation

Nursing Interventions	Rationale
Place the client in a room near the nurses' station or where the staff can observe the client closely.	The client's safety is a priority.
It may be necessary to assign a staff member to remain with the client at all times.	One-to-one supervision may be required to ensure the client's safety.
Institute seizure precautions as needed, according to hospital policy (padded tongue blade in room, padded side rails, airway at bedside).	You should be prepared for the possibility of withdrawal seizures.
Restraints may be necessary to keep the client from harming himself or herself.	If the client cannot be protected from injury in any other manner, restraints may become necessary. Restraints are not to be used punitively.
Do not moralize or chastise the client for his or her substance use. Maintain a nonjudgmental attitude.	Remember that substance use and abuse is an illness and out of the client's control at this time. Moralizing belittles the client.
Talk with the client using simple, concrete language. Do not attempt to discuss the client's feelings, plans for treatment, or possible changes in the client's lifestyle while the client is drug influenced or in acute or severe withdrawal.	The client's ability to process abstractions is impaired during withdrawal. You and the client will be frustrated if you attempt to address interpersonal or complex issues at this point.
Reorient the client to person, time, place, and situation as indicated when the client is confused or disoriented.	Presentation of concrete facts facilitates the client's reality contact.

❀ *(continued)*
Implementation

Nursing Interventions	Rationale
Decrease environmental stimuli (bright lights, television, visitors) when the client is restless, irritable, or tremulous. Avoid lengthy interactions; keep your voice soft; speak clearly.	Your presence and soft tones can be calming to the client. He or she is not able to deal with excessive stimuli.

Nursing Diagnosis

Altered Health Maintenance (6.4.2)
Inability to identify, manage, or seek help to maintain health.

Assessment Data

Defining Characteristics

- Dependence on drugs
- Physical discomfort
- Physical symptoms (impaired nutrition, fluid and electrolyte imbalance)
- Sleep disturbances
- Low self-esteem
- Feelings of apathy

Related Factors

- Ineffective coping strategies
- Failure to manage stress
- Disruptions in major life areas: work, family, social
- Financial difficulties or legal involvement (depending on type, amount, and cost of drug used)

❀ Expected Outcomes

Initial

The client will:

- Establish nutritious eating patterns
- Establish a balance of rest, sleep, and activity
- Establish physiologic homeostasis

Discharge

The client will:

- Verbalize knowledge of prevention of HIV transmission
- Agree to participate in a treatment program
- Follow through with discharge plans regarding employment, legal involvement, family problems, and financial difficulties

❀ Therapeutic Aims

- Promote adequate rest, nutrition, hydration, and hygiene.
- Minimize physical discomfort.
- Facilitate referral to a treatment program.

Implementation

Nursing Interventions	Rationale
Obtain the client's history, including the kind, amount, route, and time of last drug use. Consult the client's family or significant others to obtain or validate the client's information if necessary. *Note:* The client may report an inaccurate estimate of drug use (either minimized or exaggerated).	Baseline data can help you anticipate the onset, type, and severity of physical withdrawal symptoms.
Be aware of PRN medication orders to decrease physical symptoms. Do not allow the client to be needlessly uncomfortable, but do not use medications too liberally. *Note:* The client is already experiencing drug effects.	Judicious use of PRN medications can decrease the client's discomfort yet not jeopardize his or her health during withdrawal.
You may need to obtain drug or urine specimens (or both) for drug screening on admission, per the physician's orders and client's consent. Stress that this information is needed to help treat the client and that information obtained by the nurse or the medical staff is not for legal or prosecution purposes. (*Note:* Clients involved in vehicular accidents or charged with criminal activity may be an exception in some states.)	Drug screens can positively identify substances the client has ingested. In the case of illegal drugs, often other substances are included of which the client has no knowledge. The client and his or her family must be reassured that treatment is separate from legal issues. However, depending on the client's legal situation and state laws, information from laboratory tests may need to be surrendered to authorities.
Remain nonjudgmental in your approach to the client and his or her significant others.	Your nonjudgmental approach can convey acceptance of the client as a person, which is separate from any drug-taking behavior.
Monitor the client's intake and output and any pertinent laboratory values, such as electrolytes.	The client in withdrawal is at risk for fluid and electrolyte imbalances.
Encourage oral fluids, especially juice, fortified malts, or milk. If the client is vomiting, intravenous therapy may be necessary.	Milk, juice, and malts provide a maximum of nutrients in a small volume. Fluids usually are tolerated best by the client initially.
Talk with the client quietly in short, simple terms. Do not chatter or make social conversation.	Excessive talking on your part may be irritating to the client in withdrawal.
Be comfortable with silence. You may touch or hold the client's hand if these actions comfort or reassure the client.	Your physical presence conveys your acceptance of the client.
Encourage the client to bathe, wash his or her hair, and wear clean clothes.	Personal cleanliness will enhance the client's sense of well-being.
Assist the client as necessary; it may be necessary to provide complete physical care depending on the severity of the withdrawal symptoms.	You should attend to the client's hygiene only when he or she cannot do so independently.
Teach the client that chemical dependence is an illness and requires long-term treatment and follow-up. Refer the client to a chemical dependence treatment program.	A drug withdrawal program deals only with the client's physical dependence to the drug(s). Further therapy is needed to address the primary problem of chemical dependence.

(continued)
Implementation

Nursing Interventions	Rationale
Refer the client's family or significant others to Alanon, Alateen, or Adult Children of Alcoholics as indicated.	Family and significant others are affected by the client's substance use and also need help with their own issues.
Teach the client about the prevention of HIV transmission.	Clients who use intravenous drugs are at increased risk for HIV transmission by sharing needles and by sexual activity, especially when judgment is impaired.
If the client is HIV positive, refer him or her for medical treatment and counseling related to HIV disease.	Clients who are HIV positive face the risk of AIDS as well as the loss of friends, family, housing, insurance, employment, and so forth. Clients may be unaware of available medical treatment and supportive resources.

Chemical Dependence Treatment Program

Chemical dependence or *addiction* generally is viewed as an illness by health care professionals today, though that is not true of all health professionals or the general public. Various theories about the cause and development of chemical dependence include heredity, genetic predisposition, body chemistry imbalances, maladaptive response to stress, and personality traits or disorders. Chemical dependence is not a moral weakness nor is it caused by a lack of will power.

Clients with chemical dependence exhibit "symptoms and maladaptive behavior changes associated with more or less regular use of psychoactive substances that affect the central nervous system" (DSM-III-R, 1987). This use and resultant behaviors continue in spite of negative consequences, such as impaired performance at work, legal difficulties, family or marital discord, or threats to the client's physical health. In addition, the client may have tried to decrease the chemical use unsuccessfully, may use more of the chemical than he or she intends, may experience withdrawal symptoms, and may spend a great deal of time obtaining, consuming, or recovering from the effects of the chemical (DSM-III-R, 1987).

Detoxification must occur before the client can become successfully involved in treatment. It is important to involve the client's significant others in the treatment (whenever possible) to work toward resolving the problems and feelings surrounding the client's chemical use and to facilitate recovery for the client and affected family members. (See Care Plan 35: Adult Children of Alcoholics.)

The multiple abuse of alcohol and tranquilizers or other drugs is common. For recovery to be effective the client must avoid simply transferring his or her use from one chemical to another. For example, if a client quits using alcohol, he or she must not rely on tranquilizers or "nerve pills" to deal with stress or other daily life situations.

It can be common for clients with chemical dependency also to be diagnosed as having a personality disorder. Although this may be a factor in their treatment, it usually does not preclude success in such a program. However, if the client has a major psychiatric disorder, such as bipolar affective disorder or schizophrenia, there may need to be significant alterations in his or her chemical dependence treatment. (See Care Plan 34: Dual Diagnosis.)

Clients who have used intravenous drugs are at increased risk for human immunodeficiency virus (HIV) infection, acquired immunodeficiency syndrome (AIDS), and AIDS-related complex (ARC) from sharing infected needles or from unprotected sexual behavior, particularly when judgment is impaired under the influence of alcohol or drugs. (See Basic Concepts: HIV Disease and AIDS.)

Nursing Diagnoses Addressed in this Care Plan

Ineffective Denial
Ineffective Individual Coping

Related Nursing Diagnoses

Altered role performance
Noncompliance
Impaired Social Interaction
Ineffective Family Coping: Disabling

Nursing Diagnosis	*Ineffective Denial (5.1.1.1.3)*

The state of a conscious or unconscious attempt to disavow the knowledge or meaning of an event to reduce anxiety or fear to the detriment of health.

Assessment Data

Defining Characteristics	• Denial of the illness
	• Minimization of chemical or substance use
	• Blaming others for problems
	• Reluctance to discuss self or problems
	• Lack of insight
	• Failure to accept responsibility for behavior
	• Views self as different from others

Related Factors	• Rationalization of problems
	• Intellectualization
	• Martial or family problems
	• Financial problems
	• Difficulties with employment—fired, unemployed, threat of job loss

Expected Outcomes

Initial	*The client will:*

• Participate in treatment program
• Identify negative effects of his or her behavior on others
• Abstain from drug and alcohol use
• Verbalize acceptance of responsibility for own behavior
• Express acceptance of chemical dependence as an illness

Discharge	*The client will:*

• Maintain abstinence from chemical substances
• Demonstrate acceptance of responsibility for own behavior
• Verbalize knowledge of illness, treatment plan, and prevention of HIV transmission
• Follow through with discharge plans regarding employment, support groups, and so forth

Therapeutic Aims

- Provide information and education about chemical dependence.
- Promote realistic self-evaluation about chemical use, behaviors, and self-responsibility.

Implementation

Nursing Interventions	Rationale
Avoid the client's attempts to focus only on external problems (such as marital, financial, or employment problems) without relating them to the problem of chemical use.	The problem of chemical use must be dealt with first because it affects all other areas.
Provide the client and his or her family or significant others with factual information about chemical use. Do this in a matter-of-fact, rather than argumentative, manner. Dispel common myths such as "I'm not an alcoholic if I only drink beer or only drink on weekends," "I can learn to just use drugs socially," and so forth.	Most clients lack factual knowledge about chemical use as an illness. If the client can engage you in semantic arguments, the client can keep the focus off himself or herself and personal problems.
Encourage the client to identify behaviors that have caused family difficulties and other problems in his or her life.	It is important for the client to see the relationship between his or her problems and behavior.
Do not allow the client to rationalize or explain away difficulties or to blame problems on others or on circumstances beyond the client's control.	Rationalizing and blaming others gives the client an excuse to continue his or her behavior.
Consistently redirect the client's focus to his or her own problems and to what he or she can do about them.	You can facilitate the client's acceptance of responsibility for his or her own behavior.
Encourage all other clients in the program to provide feedback for each other.	Peer feedback usually is valued by the client, because it is coming from others with similar problems.
Positively reinforce the client when he or she identifies and expresses feelings or shows any insight into his or her behaviors and consequences.	You convey acceptance of the client's attempts to express feelings and to accept responsibility for his or her own behavior.

Nursing Diagnosis

Ineffective Individual Coping (5.1.1.1)
Impairment of adaptive behaviors and problem-solving abilities of a person in meeting life's demands and roles.

Assessment Data

Defining Characteristics
- Isolative behavior
- Low self-esteem
- Lack of impulse control

❊ *(continued)*
Assessment Data

Defining Characteristics	• Superficial relationships
	• Inability to form and maintain intimate personal relationships
	• Lack of effective problem-solving skills
	• Avoidance of problems or difficult situations
	• Ineffective coping skills
Related Factors	• Physical symptoms or problems
	• Sleep disturbances
	• Personality disorder
	• Impaired nutrition or eating disorder
	• Dependence on alcohol or other drugs

❊
Expected Outcomes

Initial	*The client will:*
	• Express feelings directly and openly
	• Engage in realistic self-evaluation
	• Verbalize process for problem solving
	• Practice nonchemical alternatives to dealing with stress or difficult situations
Discharge	*The client will:*
	• Develop a healthful daily routine regarding eating, sleeping, and so forth
	• Verbalize increased self-esteem, based on accurate information
	• Demonstrate effective communication with others
	• Demonstrate alternative (nonchemical) methods of dealing with feelings, problems, and situations

❊
Therapeutic Aims

• Promote development of alternative coping strategies.
• Direct client's focus to the "here-and-now."
• Facilitate development of discharge plans, including community follow-up and support system.

❊
Implementation

Nursing Interventions	Rationale
Encourage the client to explore alternative ways of dealing with stress and difficult situations.	The client may have minimal or no experience dealing with life stress without chemicals. The client may be learning for the first time how to cope, problem solve, and so forth.
Help the client develop skills in defining problems, planning problem-solving approaches, implementing solutions, and evaluating the process.	You can provide knowledge and practice of the problem-solving process in a nonthreatening environment.
Help the client identify and express his or her feelings in acceptable ways, and give positive reinforcement for doing so.	You are a sounding board for the client. Your feedback encourages the client to continue to express feelings.

❄ *(continued)*
Implementation

Nursing Interventions	Rationale
Involve the client in a group of his or her peers to provide confrontation, positive feedback, and the sharing of feelings.	Groups of peers in substance abuse treatment programs are a primary mode of treatment. Peers usually are honest and supportive yet unafraid of confrontation. The clients' common experiences validate the feedback.
Focus the client's attention on the "here-and-now" situation—what can the client do now to redirect his or her behavior and life?	The client cannot change what has happened. Once the client acknowledges responsibility for his or her past behavior, it is not helpful or healthy to ruminate about the past and feel guilty.
Avoid discussion of unanswerable questions, such as why the client uses chemicals.	Asking why is frustrating as well as fruitless; there is no answer.
Guide the client to the conclusion that sobriety is a choice he or she can make.	Sobriety, including abstinence from all chemicals, is associated with greater success in recovery.
Help the client view life and the quest for sobriety in feasible terms. The client may be overwhelmed by thoughts such as "How can I avoid using chemicals for the rest of my life?" A much more attainable goal is posed by "What can I do today to stay sober?" The client needs to believe he or she can succeed to do so.	The client can deal more easily with shorter periods of time. Dealing with "forever" is abstract and very difficult. The client needs to talk in terms of today, which is more manageable.
Refer the client to a chaplain or spiritual advisor of his or her choice, if indicated.	The client may be overwhelmed with guilt or despair. Spiritual resources may help the client maintain sobriety and find social support.
Teach the client and his or her significant others about prevention of HIV transmission, and refer them for HIV testing and counseling if appropriate.	Clients who use chemicals are at increased risk for HIV transmission by sharing needles and by sexual activity, especially when judgment is impaired by chemical use.
Refer the client to vocational rehabilitation, social services, or other resources as indicated.	The client may need a variety of services, depending on his or her situation.
Refer the client and his or her family or significant others to Alcoholics Anonymous, Alanon, Alateen, Adult Children of Alcoholics, or other support groups as indicated for continued support following discharge.	Many clients (and families or significant others) benefit from continued support for sobriety after discharge. Note: Many groups are modeled on the basic 12-step program, including gay, lesbian, and non-Christian groups.
Refer the client for treatment for other problems as indicated.	Chemical dependency often is associated with post-traumatic behavior, eating disorders, abusive relationships, and so forth.

Dual Diagnosis

Chemical dependence is a complicating factor with many clients who are chronically mentally ill. It is hypothesized that these clients use chemicals in an attempt to self-*medicate* (alleviate symptoms of illness), to fit in with peers, and to reduce social tension and anxiety or that chemical dependence exists as a primary illness. In a study by Perkins, Simpson, and Tsuang (1986) clients who abused drugs were categorized into three groups: (1) those with no psychotic symptoms, (2) those with acute psychotic symptoms (less than 6 months), and (3) those with chronic psychotic symptoms (longer than 6 months, meeting DSM-III-R criteria for major mental illness). The pattern of drug use was essentially the same for all three groups. Among the clients with acute or no psychotic symptoms, there were no significant differences in occupational status or residential outcome. However, clients with psychotic symptoms persisting for more than 6 months rated significantly lower in both areas. In addition, this group had a positive family history for schizophrenia and major affective disorders. This led the researchers to expect an overall difficult course and poor prognosis for this category of clients, who are described as having *dual diagnoses:* major mental illness and chemical dependence. (*Note:* Some literature defines dual diagnosis as mental illness and mental retardation. These clients are not included in this discussion.)

Alcoholism and bipolar affective disorder tend to be familial. It is common for clients with bipolar affective disorder to describe efforts to use drugs or alcohol to self-medicate attempting to level high and low mood swings. The result of these clients' chemical use, however, is an exacerbation (not relief) of symptoms. This also is true for clients with a diagnosis of schizophrenia.

Traditional methods of treatment for major psychiatric illness or primary chemical dependence treatment programs generally are reported to have little lasting success in treating clients who are dually diagnosed (Fariello and Scheidt, 1989). For clients with schizophrenia, cognitive impairment and decreased ability to process abstract concepts are major barriers to successful participation in chemical dependency treatment programs. Likewise, treatment designed to manage psychotic symptoms is less successful when the client drinks alcohol or uses chemical substances, which tend to exacerbate symptoms. Some clients with bipolar affective disorder have difficulty in some chemical dependence treatment programs with reconciling the concept of being drug-free with their instructions to remain compliant with Lithium or other chemotherapy regimens. In addition, the impulsiveness associated with bipolar affective disorder interferes with the ability to remain alcohol or drug free.

It would seem that an approach that considers both problems simultaneously, as opposed to either type of treatment alone, might be more successful for the dually diagnosed client. It also may be necessary to modify the treatment goals for the individual. For example, the goal for a client to achieve 1 or more years of sobriety and experience the social reward of that accomplishment is not realistic for the client who also is schizophrenic.

Little literature exists on the topic of dual diagnosis. The articles that have been written suggest that dually diagnosed clients are a difficult challenge and involve an area that needs further research to produce more effective methods of treatment.

NOTE: The care plan is based on community treatment because, although clients may be readily stabilized in the hospital setting, their treatment presents a greater challenge following discharge.

Nursing Diagnoses Addressed in this Care Plan

Noncompliance
Ineffective Individual Coping

Related Nursing Diagnoses

Altered Health Maintenance
Altered Thought Processes
Sensory/Perceptual Alterations
Diversional Activity Deficit
Impaired Home Maintenance Management
Self-Esteem Disturbance
Impaired Social Interaction

Nursing Diagnosis	*Noncompliance (5.2.1.1)*
	A person's informed decision not to adhere to a therapeutic recommendation.

Assessment Data

Defining Characteristics	• Frequent ingestion of alcohol or drugs
	• Neuroleptic blood levels outside therapeutic range
	• Exacerbation of symptoms
	• Failure to keep appointments or follow through on referrals
Related Factors	• Poor impulse control
	• History of self-medication
	• Nontherapeutic home environment
	• Incongruence between therapeutic regimen and personal values or desires
	• Knowledge or skill deficit

❀ Expected Outcomes

Initial	*The client will:*

- Establish a regular chemotherapy regimen
- Verbalize the need for medication compliance
- Identify difficulties associated with alcohol or chemical use

Discharge	*The client will:*

- Report instances of alcohol or drug use accurately
- Report medication compliance accurately
- Experience diminished or absent psychiatric symptoms

❀ Therapeutic Aims

- Provide knowledge about medication, alcohol or drugs, and associated risks.
- Promote accurate reporting of symptoms and compliance.

❀ Implementation

Nursing Interventions	Rationale
Discuss patterns of drug and alcohol use in a non-judgmental manner.	Asking the client about his or her chemical use in a nonpunitive manner increases your chance of obtaining accurate information.
Indicate that your need to know is based on the need for accurate data to assess the client, not for criticism.	This conveys genuine concern for the client, which enhances trust.
Assist the client to draw correlations between increased chemical use and increased psychiatric symptoms.	The effect of increased symptoms caused by alcohol use may not be apparent to the client.
Inform the client of drug interactions between medications and other substances.	Factual information is a sound basis for future problem solving.
Encourage the client to ask questions if he or she is uncertain about taking medications when drinking and so forth.	Safety is a priority. The client who has been using drugs or alcohol is at a greater risk for an overdose.
If the client is having symptoms such as not sleeping, encourage him or her to report that information to a health professional for assistance before instituting self-medication or using drugs or alcohol to alleviate the symptoms.	A change in medication or dosage may resolve the client's difficulties without placing him or her at risk.
Give positive feedback for honest reporting.	If the client perceives a greater reward for honesty than for strict adherence, he or she is more likely to report honestly.

Nursing Diagnosis

Ineffective Individual Coping (5.1.1.1)

Impairment of adaptive behaviors and problem-solving abilities of a person in meeting life's demands and roles.

Assessment Data

Defining Characteristics	• Poor impulse control • Low self-esteem • Lack of social skills • Dissatisfaction with life circumstances • Lack of purposeful daily activity
Related Factors	• Inadequate or ineffective support system • Major psychiatric illness • Lack of future plans or orientation

Expected Outcomes

Initial	*The client will:* • Take only prescribed medication • Interact appropriately with staff and other clients • Express feelings openly • Develop plans to manage unstructured time
Discharge	*The client will:* • Demonstrate appropriate social skills • Identify social activities in drug- and alcohol-free environments • Verbalize increased feelings of self-worth • Maintain contact or relationship with a professional in the community • Identify a community support group that meets the needs of dually diagnosed clients

Therapeutic Aims

• Promote self-esteem and a sense of personal control.
• Facilitate development of social and recreational skills.
• Promote realistic goal-setting.

Implementation

Nursing Interventions	Rationale
Encourage open expression of feelings.	Verbalizing feelings is an initial step toward dealing constructively with those feelings.
Validate the client's frustration or anger in dealing with dual problems.	Expressing feelings outwardly, especially negative ones, may relieve some of the client's stress and anxiety.
Consider alcohol or chemical use as a factor that influences the client's ability to live in the commu-	For the dually diagnosed client, chemical use is not necessarily the major problem he or she experiences,

✳ *(continued)*
Implementation

Nursing Interventions	Rationale
nity, as you would other factors, such as taking medications, keeping appointments, adequate eating and sleeping patterns, and so forth.	only one of several problems. Overemphasis on any single factor, even chemical use, is not a guarantee of success.
Maintain frequent contact with the client, even if it is only brief telephone calls.	Frequent contact decreases the length of time the client feels "stranded" or left alone to deal with problems.
Give positive feedback for abstinence on a day-by-day basis.	Positive feedback reinforces abstinent behavior.
If drinking or substance use occurs, discuss the events that led to the incident with the client in a nonjudgmental manner.	The client may be able to see the relatedness of the events or a pattern of behavior while discussing the situation.
Discuss ways to avoid similar circumstances in the future.	Anticipatory planning may prepare the client to avoid similar circumstances in the future.
Assess the amount of unstructured time with which the client must cope.	The client is more likely to experience frustration or dissatisfaction, which can lead to substance use, when he or she has excessive amounts of unstructured time.
Assist the client to plan weekly, or even daily, schedules of purposeful activities: errands, appointments, taking walks, and so forth.	Scheduled events provide the client with something to anticipate or look forward to doing.
Writing the schedule on a calendar may be beneficial.	Visualization of the schedule provides a concrete reference for the client.
Recording a journal of activities, feelings, and thoughts may be helpful to the client.	A journal can provide a focus for the client and can yield information that is useful in future planning. The client also may record information that would otherwise be forgotten or overlooked.
Teach the client social skills. Describe and demonstrate specific skills, such as eye contact, attentive listening, nodding, and so forth. Discuss the kind of topics that are appropriate for social conversation, such as the weather, news, local events, and so forth.	The client may have little or no knowledge of social interaction skills. Modeling the skills provides a conceret example of the desired skills.
Give positive support to the client for appropriate use of social skills.	Positive feedback will encourage the client to continue socialization attempts and enhance his or her self-esteem.
Refer the client to volunteer or vocational services if indicated.	Purposeful activity makes better use of the client's unstructured time, and can enhance the client's feelings of worth and self-esteem.
Refer the client to community support services that address mental health and chemical dependence-related needs.	Problems for clients who are dually diagnosed are complicated and long term, requiring ongoing and extended assistance.

Adult Children of Alcoholics

The term *adult child of an alcoholic* (ACA) refers to a person who "has been raised in a family where one or both parents were addicted to alcohol and who has been subjected to the many dysfunctional aspects associated with parental alcoholism" (Ackerman, 1987). The significance of being an ACA, or *adult child*, has gained attention in only the last 15 years, even though alcoholism as a family illness has been recognized for much longer.

The National Association for Children of Alcoholics (NACoA) was founded in 1983 to support and serve as a resource for children of alcoholics and for those in a position to help them—therapists, educators, physicians, nurses, social workers, and so forth. The NACoA cites the following information in describing the magnitude of this problem:

An estimated 28 million Americans have at least one alcoholic parent.
Children of alcoholics are at the highest risk of developing alcoholism and are prone to learning disabilities, eating disorders, stress-related medical problems, and compulsive achieving.
Alcohol is a significant factor in up to 90% of child abuse cases.
One of three families reports alcohol abuse by a family member.
More than one half of all alcoholics have an alcoholic parent.

In addition to being in high-risk categories for alcoholism and eating disorders, children of alcoholics often develop an inability to trust, an extreme need to control, an excessive sense of responsibility, and denial of feelings; these problems persist through adulthood. ACAs also are more likely than the general population to marry individuals who develop alcoholism, thus perpetuating the problems. Some authors also propose that behaviors related to ACAs exist for many people raised in homes in which one or both parents were "emotionally unavailable" for any reason, with or without alcohol use.

Self-help support groups, therapy groups, and a wide variety of popular books were developed in the 1980s to deal with the problems of adult children. In the 1990s the concept has broadened to *codependence*, including many of the problems and behaviors previously identified in adult children. The concept of codependence, however, is not as tightly coupled with parental or spousal alcoholism. Although clients are unlikely to be hospitalized solely for being codependent or an adult child, the nurse may find that many clients have similar issues as complicating factors in their lives.

Nursing Diagnoses Addressed in this Care Plan

Ineffective Individual Coping
Chronic Low Self-Esteem

Related Nursing Diagnoses

Powerlessness
Post-Trauma Response
Altered Role Performance
Ineffective Family Coping: Disabling

Nursing Diagnosis

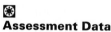

Ineffective Individual Coping (5.1.1.1)

Impairment of adaptive behaviors and problem-solving abilities of a person in meeting life's demands and roles.

Assessment Data

Defining Characteristics	• Inability to trust
	• Excessive need or desire for control, either overtly or covertly expressed
	• Very responsible or very irresponsible behavior
	• Difficulty with authority
	• Impulsive behavior
	• Lack of effective assertiveness skills
	• Intolerance of changes
	• Difficulty setting and keeping limits
	• Conflict avoidance behaviors

Related Factors	• Addictive behavior (eg, to excitement or chaos in daily life or relationships)
	• Eating disorders
	• History of abuse
	• Exaggerated negative response to alcohol or drug use by others
	• Chemical dependence

Expected Outcomes

Initial	*The client will:*
	• Discuss situations involving conflict
	• Demonstrate choices based on self-approval rather than seeking the approval of others
	• Participate in treatment programs for associated or other problems

Discharge	*The client will:*
	• Demonstrate appropriate use of assertiveness skills
	• Follow through with commitments
	• Demonstrate use of effective problem-solving skills
	• Verbalize plans for chemical dependence treatment, if indicated, or support groups after discharge

Therapeutic Aims

- Promote development of problem-solving and assertiveness skills.
- Facilitate development of coping skills.

Implementation

Nursing Interventions	Rationale
Teach the client a step-by-step approach to solving problems: identifying problems, exploring alternatives, evaluating consequences of alternatives, and making a decision.	The client may never have learned a process for solving problems or have seen rational problem-solving implemented.
Have the client make a list of actual situations that are difficult or threatening for him or her.	The client's emotional investment in learning to problem solve is enhanced by using actual, rather than hypothetical, situations.
Develop a list of approaches to these situations, followed by the client's feelings about each choice.	Learning to identify his or her own feelings and to couple feelings with choices can be a new experience for the client.
Assist the client to determine the pros and cons of each choice.	Practicing the problem-solving process will develop proficiency in its use.
Encourage the client to select a choice and make specific plans for implementation.	Adult children typically have difficulty following through. Specific plans will increase the likelihood that the client will do so.
Provide education about assertiveness skills (ie, passive, aggressive, and assertive responses).	The client may be unaware of the basis for assertiveness skills.
Teach the client about limit setting, and encourage the use of limit-setting skills and awareness in relationships.	ACAs often have little or no knowledge, experience, or skill in using limit setting.
Encourage the client to use "I" statements to express his or her needs or desires. Practice the client's use of these statements with him or her.	Using "I" statements encourages the client to focus on and accept responsibility for his or her own feelings and wishes.
Role play previously identified situations with the client, incorporating assertiveness skills.	Anticipatory practice helps the client be better prepared for actual implementation.
Encourage the client to begin implementation of an approach to deal with one of the identified situations, beginning with the least threatening situation.	The least threatening situation has the greatest chance of being a successful initial experience for the client.
Provide time to discuss the client's attempts, focusing on how he or she felt.	If the situation was successful, the client's feelings of self-worth increase. If he or she was unsuccessful, the client learns that one can survive making mistakes or having negative experiences.
Give positive feedback for attempts to use new skills, not just for successful resolution of the situation.	The client needs positive feedback for trying, not just for "winning."

(continued)
Implementation

Nursing Interventions	Rationale
If the client was unsuccessful in resolving the problem, help him or her to evaluate alternatives and make another attempt to solve the problem. Do not punish the client or withdraw your attention when the client is unsuccessful.	This will promote the client's ability to follow through, and he or she can have another opportunity for success, even following unsuccessful experiences. The client's early experiences of mistakes or lack of success may have been followed by punishment or withdrawal of parental attention.

Nursing Diagnosis
Assessment Data

Chronic Low Self-Esteem (7.1.2.1)
Long standing negative self evaluation or feelings about self or self capabilities.

Defining Characteristics

- Excessive need to control emotions
- Denial of feelings
- Difficulty expressing feelings
- Fear of emotional abandonment
- Chronic feelings of insecurity
- Reluctance to discuss personal issues
- Guilt feelings
- Harsh judgment of own behavior
- Consistent feelings of failure
- Impaired spontaneity or ability to have fun
- Reluctant to try new things

Related Factors

- Dysfunctional or unsatisfactory relationships (eg, the client may play the role of the victim or have difficulty with intimacy)
- Views self as "different" from other people
- Extreme loyalty to others, even when undeserved

Expected Outcomes

Initial

The client will:

- Verbalize recognition of alcoholism as an illness
- Verbally identify his or her feelings in a nonjudgmental manner
- Focus on self in the present rather than past experiences

Discharge

The client will:

- Verbalize realistic self-evaluation
- Demonstrate the ability to engage in spontaneous activities for the sake of having fun
- Express feelings to others without guilt
- Verbalize knowledge about alcoholism and related family problems

❂ Therapeutic Aims

- Facilitate expression of honest feelings.
- Focus on present.
- Promote self-esteem and personal growth.

❂ Implementation

Nursing Interventions	Rationale
Encourage the client to remember and discuss experiences of growing up, family interactions, and so forth.	Adult children have frequently kept the "family secrets," especially those related to alcoholism, and shared them with no one.
Provide education to the client and his or her family or significant others about alcoholism as a family illness.	Accurate information helps the client to recognize the parent's alcoholism as a source of many family problems and that the client was not responsible for the illness or the problems.
Encourage the client to identify characteristics of himself or herself and family members.	The client's sense of personal identity may be enmeshed with the entire family. The client may have difficulty seeing himself or herself as a separate person.
Encourage the client to verbalize all feelings, especially negative ones, such as anger, resentment, loss, and so forth, to staff members.	Adult children often have learned to "stuff" or deny feelings and are not skilled at identifying them.
Give positive feedback for honest expression of feelings.	Positive feedback increases the frequency of desired behavior.
Suggest appropriate ways of expressing feelings, such as talking and writing in a journal.	The client needs to identify the most comfortable and beneficial way of appropriately expressing feelings.
Assist the client to view himself or herself realistically in the present and to allow the past to become history.	Once the client has sorted through past feelings and experiences openly, he or she can put them in the past and "let go" of them. This can enhance opportunities for future growth.
Encourage the client to make a list of his or her strengths and areas he or she would like to change.	A written list gives the client a concrete focus, so he or she is not so likely to feel overwhelmed. The client may have the most difficulty identifying positive qualities.
Practice giving and receiving compliments with the client.	Receiving compliments may be a new experience for the client and can increase self-esteem. Giving compliments to others helps the client focus on communication skills.
Involve the client in small group discussions with others having similar issues, if possible.	Groups of adult children allow the clients to find that they are not alone in their feelings and that others share some of the same doubts, fears, and so forth.

(continued)
Implementation

Nursing Interventions	Rationale
Encourage the client to begin or continue using a journal to focus on present thoughts, feelings, and their relatedness.	Use of a journal can help increase the client's awareness of his or her feelings and behavior, promote insight, and help the client focus on self-approval, rather than seeking the approval of others.
With the client, review journal entries as a basis for identifying aspects of personal growth for the client.	The client is struggling with issues that often are many years old. Progress can be more easily identified if he or she has a means for recognizing steps in growth and positive change.
Assist the client to set small achievable daily or weekly goals.	Small goals seem possible to attain and will not discourage or overwhelm the client.
Provide the client with a reading list of resources related to ACAs.	The client will not be able to assimilate all the possible information in a short time. A reading list provides an ongoing resource for the client as he or she is ready for new information.
Refer the client to a support group for adult children.	The client is dealing with feelings and behaviors that have been accumulating for a lifetime. Resolving these issues and making personal changes also is a long process and is facilitated by the ongoing support of others in similar situations.
See Care Plan 53: Sexual, Emotional, or Physical Abuse.	Adult children frequently have issues involving some type of abuse.

Section Eleven

Personality Disorders

A *personality disorder* is evidenced by a client demonstrating maladaptive coping mechanisms (the usual ways in which he or she deals with others and the environment). Behaviors addressed in this section of the *Manual* are often related to personality disorders, but not all clients manifesting the behaviors found here have a personality disorder. A particular client may have problems primarily related to a specific behavior, such as manipulation, or a behavior such as manipulation may be manifested in a client whose primary problem is addressed elsewhere in this *Manual* (eg, psychosomatic problems or anorexia nervosa).

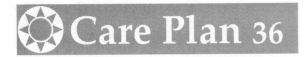

Passive–Aggressive or Manipulative Behavior

Passive–aggressive behavior is a type of indirect expression of feelings whereby a client does not express aggressive (angry, resentful) feelings verbally but denies these feelings and reveals them instead through behavior. This behavior may indicate a personality disorder that is characterized by the use of passive behavior to express hostility. This behavior includes obstructionism, pouting, procrastination, stubbornness, and intentional inefficiency. Psychological testing of a client displaying these behaviors may be appropriate to determine the presence of a personality disorder.

Manipulative behavior is characterized by the client's attempts to control his or her interactions and relationships with others often to satisfy some immediate desire or need or to avoid discomfort, change, or growth. Clients who manifest manipulative behavior may have little genuine motivation to change their ways of relating to others and of dealing with situations in general. In seeking treatment the client may be wanting merely to get out of a bind, crisis, or stressful situation. Involve the client in care planning if possible.

It is especially important to remember your professional role when working with clients who manifest passive–agressive or manipulative behavior. It is neither necessary nor particularly desirable for the client to like you personally. It is not your purpose to be a friend to the client, nor is it to the client's purpose to be a friend to you. Maintaining your professional role with the client will be a firm basis on which to establish a therapeutic relationship in the best interest of the client.

Nursing Diagnosis Addressed in this Care Plan

Ineffective Individual Coping

Related Nursing Diagnoses

Impaired Social Interaction
Self-Esteem Disturbance
Noncompliance
Ineffective Family Coping: Disabling

Nursing Diagnosis	*Ineffective Individual Coping (5.1.1.1)* *Impairment of adaptive behaviors and problem-solving abilities of a person in meeting life's demands and roles.*

Assessment Data

Defining Characteristics	• Lack of insight • Inability or refusal to express emotions directly (especially anger) • Refusal to participate in activities • Forgetfulness • Dishonesty • Anger or hostility • Superficial relationships with others • Somatic complaints • Seductive behavior or sexual acting out • Low self-esteem
Related Factors	• Denial of problems or feelings • Resistance to therapy • Preoccupation with other clients' problems ("playing therapist") or with staff members to avoid dealing with his or her own problems • Intellectualization or rationalization of problems • Dependency • Manipulation of staff or family • Attempting to gain special treatment or privileges

Expected Outcomes

Initial	*The client will:* • Verbalize self-responsibility for behavior • Express feelings directly, verbally and nonverbally • Participate in the treatment program, activities, and so forth • Communicate directly and honestly with staff and other clients about himself or herself • Verbalize fewer somatic complaints • Develop or increase feelings of self-worth • Demonstrate decreased manipulative, attention-seeking, or passive–aggressive behaviors
Discharge	*The client will:* • Demonstrate independence from the hospital environment and staff • Demonstrate increased responsibility for himself or herself • Verbalize knowledge of problem behavior, treatment plan, and other therapies • Express feelings, including anger, directly and in a nondestructive manner • Demonstrate increased feelings of self-worth • Demonstrate mature interactions with others • Demonstrate problem-solving skills when dealing with situations or others

❋ Therapeutic Aims

- Decrease manipulative, attention-seeking behavior.
- Promote direct and clear expression of feelings.
- Facilitate the client taking responsibility for self, problems, and behavior.
- Promote effective coping skills.

❋ Implementation

Nursing Interventions	Rationale
State the limits and the behavior you expect from the client. Do not debate, argue, rationalize, or bargain with the client.	Specific limits let the client know what is expected from him or her. Arguing, bargaining, justifying, and so forth interject doubt and undermine the limit.
Be consistent, not only with this particular client, but also with all other clients; that is, do not insist that this client follow a rule, while excusing another client from the same rule.	Consistency provides structure and reinforces limits. Making exceptions undermines limits and encourages manipulative behavior.
Enforce all unit and hospital policies or regulations. Without apologizing, point out reasons for not bending the rules.	Institutional regulations provide a therapeutic structure. Apologizing for regulations undermines this structure and encourages manipulative behavior.
Be direct and use confrontation with the client if necessary; however, be sure to examine your own feelings. Do not react to the client punitively or in anger.	You are a role model of appropriate behavior and self-control. There is no justification for punishing a client. Remember, the client is acceptable as a person regardless of his or her behaviors, which may or may not be acceptable.
Do not discuss yourself, other staff members, or other clients with this client.	Your relationship with the client is professional, and sharing personal information about yourself or others is inappropriate.
Set limits on the frequency and length of interactions with the client, particularly those with therapists significant to the client. Set definite and limited appointment times with therapists (like Thursday, 2:00 to 2:30 PM), and allow interactions only at those times.	Setting and maintaining limits can help decrease attention-seeking behaviors and reinforce appropriate behaviors.
Do not attempt to be popular, liked, or the "favorite staff member" of this client.	It is not necessary nor particularly desirable for the client to like you personally. A professional relationship is based on the client's therapeutic needs, not personal feelings.
Do not accept gifts from the client or encouarge a personal dependency relationship.	Maintaining your professional role is therapeutic for the client. Your acceptance of personal gifts from the client may foster manipulative behavior. (For example, the client may have expectations that you grant special favors.)
Withdraw your attention from the client if he or she begins saying that you are "the only staff member I can talk to . . . " or "the only one who understands"	It is important that the client establish and maintain trust relationships with a variety of people, staff, and other clients. If you are "the only one," the client may

✳ *(continued)*
Implementation

Nursing Interventions	Rationale
and so forth; confront the client with the idea that this is not a desirable situation. Emphasize the importance of the milieu in his or her therapy.	be too dependent or may be flattering you as a basis for manipulation.
Discuss the client's perceptions and feelings (eg, anger, hurt, feelings of being rejected or unworthy) about being denied special privileges. Encourage the client's expression of those feelings.	The client's ability to identify and express feelings is impaired. You can help the client, especially with emotions that may be uncomfortable for him or her. The client may not be used to accepting limits.
Discuss the client's problems in relation to being discharged and returning to his or her life at home, rather than in relation to unit dynamics or policies. Do, however, point out how the client's behavior on the unit reflects general behavior patterns in the client's life.	Focusing on unit activities may be a way for the client to avoid his or her real problems. Also, the goal is for the client to manage his or her behavior effectively in the community, not to be a "good patient."
Discuss the client's behavior with him or her in a nonjudgmental manner, using examples in a non-threatening way.	Providing nonjudgmental feedback can help the client to acknowledge problems and develop insight.
Help the client identify the results and the dynamics of his or her behavior and relationships. (You might say, "You seem to be . . . " or "What effect do you see . . . ?")	Reflection and feedback can be effective in increasing the client's insight.
Encourage the client to express feelings.	Appropriate expression of feelings is a healthy, adult behavior.
In your interactions with the client, emphasize expression of feelings rather than intellectualization.	The client may use intellectualization as a way of avoiding feelings and dealing with his or her emotions.
Be kind but firm with the client. Make it clear that limits and caring are not mutually exclusive, that you set and maintain limits because you care, that the client can feel hurt from someone who cares about him or her, that caring and discipline are not opposites.	The client is acceptable as a person regardless of his or her behaviors, which may or may not be acceptable. Because you care about the client's well-being, you set and maintain limits to encourage the client's growth and health.
Involve the client in care planning to assess his or her motivation and establish goals, but do not allow the client to dictate the terms of therapy or treatment (for example, what type of therapy, which therapists, length and frequency of interactions). Involve the client in the full treatment program.	Including the client in planning his or her care can encourage the client's sense of responsibility for his or her health. Allowing the client to dictate his or her care may encourage manipulation by the client.
Withdraw your attention when the client refuses to be involved in activities or other therapies or when the client's behavior is otherwise inappropriate.	It is important to minimize attention given to unacceptable behaviors. Withdrawing attention can be more effective than negative reinforcement in decreasing unacceptable behaviors.

✿ (continued)
Implementation

Nursing Interventions	Rationale
Give attention and support when the client exhibits appropriate behavior—attends activities, expresses feelings, and so forth.	Positive feedback provides reinforcement for the client's growth and can enhance self-esteem. It is essential that the client be supported in positive ways and not given attention only for unacceptable behaviors.
Teach the client a step-by-step approach to solving problems: identifying problems, exploring alternatives, evaluating consequences of alternatives, and making a decision.	The client may be unaware of a logical process for examining and resolving problems.
When the client voices a somatic complaint, treat the issue immediately; refer the client to a nurse or physician or treat according to his or her individual care plan. Then, tell the client that you will discuss other things (such as feelings). Do not engage in lengthy conversations about the client's physical complaints or physical condition.	Treating the somatic complaint in a matter-of-fact, consistent manner will minimize reinforcement of attention-seeking behavior. Emphasizing the client's feelings rather than physical complaints can help reinforce verbalization of feelings.
Observe and note patterns in somatic complaints. (Does the client have a headache when he or she is supposed to go to an activity or a stomachache when verbally confronted?)	The client may voice these complaints because he or she finds a situation stressful, or the client may use these complaints to avoid activities, and so forth.
Teach the client social skills. Describe and demonstrate specific skills, such as eye contact, attentive listening, nodding, and so forth. Discuss the types of topics that are appropriate for social conversation, such as the weather, news, local events, and so forth.	The client may have little or no knowledge of social interaction skills. Modeling provides a concrete example of the desired skills.
Set and maintain limits on seductive or sexual behavior that are inappropriate or unacceptable.	The client may use seductive behavior (that is familiar to him or her) to approach others, particularly if he or she lacks appropriate social skills. The use of sexual or seductive behavior also may be manipulative.
Teach the client and his or her family or significant others about prevention of human immunodeficiency virus (HIV) transmission.	Clients who act out sexually are at increased risk for HIV transmission.

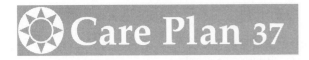

Dependency or Inadequacy

Clients who are very dependent or who lack adequate skills to deal effectively with daily life may be repeatedly admitted to a hospital with varying complaints or precipitating factors. They may report a complex group of problems related to inadequate coping with day-to-day life, resulting in a poor job history or legal problems from writing bad checks . These clients may survive adequately outside the hospital until faced with a change or crisis, which precipitates their admission to a hospital. They may be diagnosed as having personality disorders (passive–dependent, inadequate, passive–aggressive), depression, adjustment disorders, or other psychiatric problems, such as suicidal behavior.

Clients who are dependent may rely on a significant other in their lives for help in day-to-day living. The loss of this person could precipitate an admission to the hospital, and the client may then transfer his or her dependency needs to a hospital or to staff members.

Nursing Diagnoses Addressed in this Care Plan

Ineffective Individual Coping
Powerlessness

Related Nursing Diagnoses

Impaired Social Interaction
Social Isolation
Hopelessness
Self-Esteem Disturbance

Nursing Diagnosis	*Ineffective Individual Coping (5.1.1.1)*

Impairment of adaptive behaviors and problem-solving abilities of a person in meeting life's demands and roles.

Assessment Data

Defining Characteristics	• Inadequate skills for daily living or to meet changes and crises • Low frustration tolerance • Poor impulse control • Poor judgment • Anxiety • Anger or hostility (often covert)
Related Factors	• Manipulative behavior • Self-mutilating behavior • Depression • History of repeated hospital admissions • Physical symptoms • Drug or alcohol abuse • Suicidal threats or gestures

Expected Outcomes

Initial	*The client will:* • Be free of injury • Demonstrate decreased manipulative, attention-seeking behavior • Verbally express feelings, especially anger
Discharge	*The client will:* • Discuss relationship of physical complaints, legal difficulties, or substance use to ineffective coping • Verbalize adequate skills to deal with life changes or crises • Demonstrate adequate daily living skills

Therapeutic Aims

• Provide a safe environment.
• Decrease acting-out behaviors.
• Promote a healthy expression of feelings.
• Promote coping skills.

Implementation

Nursing Interventions	Rationale
Assess the client's immediate environment, possessions, and hospital room for potentially dangerous objects.	The client's safety is a priority.

✳ *(continued)*
Implementation

Nursing Interventions	Rationale
Provide adequate supervision while the client is involved in activities, with other clients or off the unit.	Self-destructive acting out is more likely to occur during unsupervised times.
Treat any self-mutilating act in a matter-of-fact manner. Give or obtain any physical treatment needed, then change the focus away from the act itself, and try to interact with the client about how he or she is feeling.	The more attention the client receives for these behaviors, the more likely the client is to repeat the behaviors.
Withdraw your attention from the client when acting-out behavior occurs; if the behavior is nondestructive, it may be ignored.	Decreased attention tends to decrease the behavior.
If intervention is required (eg, in the event of destructive behavior), take the client to a secluded, physically safe area without delay.	Immediate isolation minimizes the attention the client receives. The client is removed from the audience.
Encourage the client to express feelings verbally or in other ways that are nondestructive and acceptable to the client (eg, writing, drawing, or physical activity).	The client may need specific direction for the acceptable expression of feelings. He or she may never have learned to do so previously.
Give the client positive feedback when he or she is able to express anger verbally or in a nondestructive manner.	Positive feedback can give the client confidence and incentive to continue the positive behavior.
Teach the client needed social skills. Describe and demonstrate specific skills, such as eye contact, attentive listening, nodding, and so forth. Discuss the type of topics that are appropriate for casual social conversation, such as the weather, news, local events, and so forth.	The client may have little or no knowledge of social interaction skills. Modeling provides a concrete example of the desired skills.
Encourage the client to take direct action to meet personal needs. Do not help the client unless it is necessary. For example, allow the client to obtain a newspaper to check want ads and identify possible jobs or housing, to make appointments, and so forth on his or her own as much as possible.	The client needs to learn independent living skills. This cannot happen if he or she does not do things without assistance, even though it is uncomfortable initially.
Work with the client to help him or her anticipate future needs and situations prior to discharge ("What will you do if . . . ?"). It may help to write down specific strategies, people to contact, and so forth.	Because the client deals with change poorly (by history), any anticipatory plans can help diffuse the emotional charge of change in the client's life. This can help the client develop skills in anticipating and planning for events or changes.
Teach the client a step-by-step approach to solving problems; identifying problems, exploring alternatives, evaluating consequences of alternatives, and making a decision.	The client may be unaware of a logical process for examining and resolving problems.

Nursing Diagnosis

Powerlessness (7.3.2)

Perception that one's own action will not significantly effect an outcome; a perceived lack of control over a current situation or immediate happening.

Assessment Data

Defining Characteristics	• Dependency on others to meet needs • Feelings of inadequacy, dependency, worthlessness, failure, or hopelessness • Apathy • Doubt about role performance • Perceived lack of control
Related Factors	• Life-style of helpless behavior • Lack of satisfactory interpersonal relationships

Expected Outcomes

Initial	*The client will:* • Identify present skills and level of functioning • Verbalize feelings openly
Discharge	*The client will:* • Verbalize increased feelings of self-worth • Terminate staff–client relationships • Identify people and resources in the community for support

Therapeutic Aims

• Promote self-esteem and independence.
• Terminate staff–client relationships effectively.
• Promote supportive relationships in the community.

Implementation

Nursing Interventions	Rationale
Encourage the client to ventilate his or her feelings, including anger, hostility, worthlessness, or hopelessness. Give the client support for expressing feelings openly and honestly.	The client can learn to ventilate feelings in a safe situation with you. Positive support encourages the client to continue to do so.
Encourage the client to share his or her feelings with other clients, in small informal groups at first, progressing to larger, more formal groups.	Including others as soon as the client can tolerate it will minimize the client's dependence on one person or on hospital staff for communication.
Beginning with the initial interview, always work toward the goal of the client's discharge and independence from the hospital. Reinforce this concept with the client throughout the hospitalization.	With the dependent client it is essential to communicate the temporary nature of your relationship with him or her.

❄ *(continued)*
Implementation

Nursing Interventions	Rationale
Rotate staff members who work with the client to avoid the client's developing dependence on particular staff members. It is not desirable to be the "only one" the client can talk to.	The client must learn self-reliance and avoid dependence on one or two people.
Remember: Do not give the client the addresses or phone numbers of staff members. Do not allow the client to socialize with staff members or contact them personally after discharge.	It is essential to separate professional and social relationships.
Encourage the client to identify and build a support system in the community that is as independent from the hospital as possible. If the client cannot maintain such a level of independence at this time, continued therapy as an outpatient (individual or group therapy), support groups, or a hospital-sponsored social club may be indicated.	Use of an outside support system is a less dependent situation than hospitalization.
When necessary, work with other agencies in the community to meet the client's needs. However, do not undermine the client's progress by unnecessarily encouraging his or her dependence on more institutions. Also, these clients may have all but exhausted community resources in the past, so work in this area may need special attention.	If other assistance is needed to maintain the client in the community, it should be used. First, however, the client should do all he or she can independently.

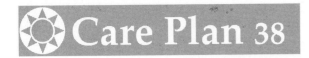 **Care Plan 38**

Antisocial Behavior

The client with antisocial behavior frequently is in conflict with society's social, moral, or legal norms. The history of the client's problems usually begins in grade school with truancy, poor grades, disruptive behavior in class, and fighting with other children.

The client with antisocial behavior may be charming, full of fun, and entertaining on a superficial, social level. He or she usually has the ability to succeed, is of average or above-average intelligence, and creates a good first impression. This client rarely sees himself or herself as having difficulties and usually does not seek help voluntarily, unless it is to avoid unpleasant consequences (he or she may consent to hospitalization to avoid jail, divorce, debts, and so forth). The client may return to jail or hospitals repeatedly. It may take several years to modify the pattern of behavior to meet long-term goals. Thus, clients with an antisocial personality disorder or who demonstrate antisocial behavior can be very frustrating for staff members within a hospital setting.

Nursing Diagnosis Addressed in this Care Plan

Ineffective Individual Coping

Related Nursing Diagnoses

High Risk for Violence: Self-Directed or Directed at Others
Impaired Social Interaction
Noncompliance

Nursing Diagnosis

Ineffective Individual Coping (5.1.1.1)
Impairment of adaptive behaviors and problem-solving abilities of a person in meeting life's demands and roles.

Assessment Data

Defining Characteristics	• Low frustration tolerance • Impulsive behavior • Inability to delay gratification • Poor judgment • Conflict with authority • Difficulty following rules and obeying laws • Lack of feelings of remorse • Socially unacceptable behavior • Dishonesty
Related Factors	• Ineffective interpersonal relationships • Manipulative behavior • Drug or alcohol use or abuse • Poor employment record • Failure to learn or change behavior based on past experience or punishment • Failure to accept or handle responsibility

Expected Outcomes

Initial	*The client will:* • Not harm self or others • Identify behaviors leading to hospitalization • Function within limits of therapeutic milieu
Discharge	*The client will:* • Demonstrate nondestructive ways to deal with stress and frustration • Identify ways to meet own needs that do not infringe on the rights of others • Achieve or maintain satisfactory work performance

Therapeutic Aims

• Decrease manipulative, dishonest, and socially unacceptable behavior.
• Improve impulse control.
• Promote compliance.

Implementation

Nursing Interventions	Rationale
Encourage the client to identify the actions that precipitated hospitalization (eg, debts, marital problems, law violation).	These clients frequently deny responsibility for consequences to their own actions.

✹ *(continued)*
Implementation

Nursing Interventions	Rationale
Give positive feedback for honesty. The client may try to act as though he or she is "sick" or "helpless" or use other techniques to avoid responsibility.	Honest identification of the consequences for the client's behavior is necessary for future behavior change.
Identify behaviors that are unacceptable for the client. These may be general (stealing others' possessions) or specific (embarrassing Ms. X by using profane language or telling lewd jokes).	You must supply limits when the client is unable or unwilling to do so. Limits must be clear, concrete, and not open to misinterpretation.
Develop specific consequences for the identified unacceptable behaviors (the client may not go to the gym that day, television-watching is revoked, and so forth). The consequence must involve something the client enjoys to be effective.	Unpleasant consequences may help decrease or eliminate unacceptable behaviors.
Avoid any discussion or debate about why the rules or requirements exist. State the requirement or rule in a matter-of-fact manner. The client may attempt to get special concessions or bend the rules "just this once" with numerous reasons, excuses, and justifications. Avoid arguing with the client.	Your refusal to be manipulated or charmed will help decrease manipulative behavior.
Inform the client of unacceptable behaviors and the resulting consequences in advance of their occurrence.	The client must be aware of expectations and consequences.
Avoid discussing another staff member's actions or statements with the client until the other staff member is present.	The client will attempt to focus attention on others to decrease attention to himself or herself.
Communicate and document in the client's care plan all behaviors and consequences in specific terms for all staff members. The client may attempt to gain favor with individual staff members or play one staff member against another. ("Last night the nurse told me I could do that.")	If all team members follow only the written plan, the client will not be able to manipulate changes in the plan.
Be consistent and firm with the care plan. Do not make independent changes in rules or consequences. Any change should be made by the staff as a group, and the new information should be conveyed to all staff members working with this client, including professionals in other disciplines. (Also, you may designate a primary staff person to be responsible for minor decisions and refer all questions to this person.)	Consistency is essential. If the client can find just one person to make independent changes, any plan will become ineffective.
Avoid trying to coax or convince the client to do the "right thing."	The client must decide to begin accepting personal responsibility for his or her own behavior and the consequences resulting from poor choices.

Implementation

Nursing Interventions	Rationale
Provide consequences immediately after the behavior in a matter-of-fact manner.	A consequence must closely follow the unacceptable behavior to be most effective. If you are angry, the client may take advantage of it. It is better to get out of the situation if possible and let someone else handle it. Do not react to the client in an angry or punitive manner.
Provide immediate positive feedback or reward for acceptable behavior.	Immediate positive feedback will help increase the frequency of the acceptable behavior. The client must receive attention for positive behaviors, not just unacceptable ones.
Require gradually longer periods of acceptable behavior to obtain the reward. Inform the client of changes in requirements and rewards as these decisions are made. For example, at first the client must demonstrate acceptable behavior for 2 hours to earn 1 hour of television time. Gradually, both the requirement and the reward are increased. The client could progress to 5 days of acceptable behavior and earn a 2-day weekend pass.	This gradual progression will help develop the client's ability to delay gratification. This is necessary if he or she is to function effectively in society.
Encourage the client to identify sources of frustration, how he or she dealt with it previously and the unpleasant consequences that resulted.	This activity should facilitate the client's ability to accept responsibility for his or her own behavior.
Explore alternative, socially and legally acceptable methods of dealing with identified frustrations.	The client has the opportunity to learn to make alternative choices.
Help the client try alternatives as situations arise. Give positive feedback when the client uses alternatives successfully.	The client can role play alternatives in a nonthreatening environment.
Include exploration and information on job seeking, work attendance, debt paying, court appearances, and so forth when working with the client in anticipation of discharge.	The client may have had little or no successful experience in these areas. Dealing with consequences and working are responsible behaviors. The client can benefit from assistance in these areas.

Borderline Personality Disorder

The client with a *borderline personality disorder* exhibits a multitude of difficulties in many different life areas and has many features similar to other personality disorders. A pervasive pattern of instability is the essential feature of this disorder (DSM-III-R, 1987) and encompasses self-image, interpersonal relationships, mood, and behavior. Frequently, these clients are described as socially contrary, generally pessimistic, demanding, and self-destructive. This disorder is more common in females and is evident by early adulthood.

Interpersonal relationships are characterized by alternating periods of clinging dependency and hostile rejection. The friend or significant other may be idolized at times and then devalued later for no apparent reason. Relationships are very intense, and the client usually will go to extremes to avoid feeling lonely, bored, or abandoned, which are frequent complaints.

Clients with a borderline personality disorder have a persistent identity disturbance, which involves sexual orientation, their value or belief system, future goals regarding career and family, self-image, and general uncertainty about major life issues.

Mood swings, from anger to anxiety to elation and so forth are common. These clients frequently are described as being on an "emotional roller coaster" (DuBrul, 1989). They display a sense of entitlement (feeling they deserve to have anything they want) and an insatiable need for special attention. When their desires are not fulfilled immediately, they can react with intensely expressed emotions, in the form of temper tantrums, rages, or aggressive or self-destructive behavior, such as suicidal threats or gestures, self-mutilating behavior, or excessive drinking episodes. These clients also are impulsive, unable to delay gratification or tolerate the frustrations or anxiety of daily life.

Under extreme stress the client with a borderline personality disorder can display psychotic symptoms of brief duration. Also it is common for these clients to seek hospitalization. In the milieu they can be frustrating for the treatment team because they engage in many "staff-splitting" behaviors (creating conflict or disharmony among staff members) and tend to influence other, more vulnerable clients to join their "war" against staff. Extended hospitalizations for these clients usually are discouraged, if possible, to prevent a continuing downward spiral in the client's level of functioning (Wester, 1991).

Some clients are not as severely impaired, and though they experience many dissatisfactions in major life areas, they are intermittently capable of moderate moods, employment, and the absence of outbursts. Participation in community support services frequently is helpful for these clients.

Nursing Diagnoses Addressed in this Care Plan

High Risk for Violence: Self-Directed or Directed at Others
Ineffective Individual Coping
Impaired Socialization

Related Nursing Diagnoses

Noncompliance
Self-Esteem Disturbance
Social Isolation

Nursing Diagnosis

High Risk for Violence: Self-Directed or Directed at Others (9.2.2)
A state in which an individual experiences behaviors that can be physically harmful to the self or others.

Risk Factors

- Impulsive behavior
- Displays of temper
- Inability to control anger
- Physically self-damaging acts
- Attention-seeking behavior
- Aggressive behavior
- Ineffective coping skills

Expected Outcomes

Initial

The client will:

- Be free of injury
- Not harm others or destroy property
- Respond to external limits

Discharge

The client will:

- Eliminate acting-out behaviors (temper tantrums, suicidal threats)
- Participate in a treatment program

Therapeutic Aims

- Provide a safe environment.
- Promote behavior containment within acceptable limits.

Implementation

Nursing Interventions	Rationale
In your initial assessment of the client, find out if he or she has any history of suicidal behavior or present suicidal ideation or plans.	The client's physical safety is always a priority. Absence of a suicidal history does not preclude risk; however, presence of a suicidal history increases the likelihood of suicidal risk.
You may wish to place the client in a room near the nursing station or where the client can be observed easily; avoid placing the client in a room near the exit, stairwell, and so forth.	The client is easier to observe and has less chance to leave the area undetected.
See Care Plan 24: Suicidal Behavior and Care Plan 52: Aggressive Behavior.	
Closely supervise the client's use of sharp or other potentially dangerous objects.	The client may use these items for self-destructive acts.
Be consistent with the client. Set and maintain limits regarding behavior, responsibilities, unit rules, and so forth.	Consistent limit setting is essential to decrease negative behaviors.
Withdraw your attention as much as possible if the client acts out.	Withdrawing your attention will tend to decrease acting out.
See Basic Concepts: Limit-setting.	

Nursing Diagnosis

Ineffective Individual Coping (5.1.1.1)
Impairment of adaptive behaviors and problem-solving abilities of a person in meeting life's roles and demands.

Assessment Data

Defining Characteristics

- Inconsistent behavior
- Uncertainty about identity (eg, role, self-image, career choices, loyalties)
- Poor impulse control
- Inability to delay gratification
- Inability to tolerate frustration, anxiety
- Dissatisfaction with life
- Mood swings
- Alcohol or drug use
- Frequent somatic complaints

Related Factors

- Noncompliance with or sabotage of treatment efforts
- Sense of entitlement
- History of frequent hospitalizations or therapy

❀ *(continued)*
Assessment Data

Related Factors	• Staff-splitting behavior
	• Manipulation of others for client's own needs
	• Aggressive, suicidal, or self-destructive behavior

❀
Expected Outcomes

Initial	*The client will:*
	• Verbalize or demonstrate resolution of the immediate crisis that precipitated hospitalization
	• Participate in treatment program
	• Ask for what he or she needs in an acceptable manner
	• Diminish efforts to manipulate staff or other clients
Discharge	*The client will:*
	• Demonstrate impulse control
	• Delay gratification of needs and requests without acting out
	• Eliminate the need for inpatient hospitalization
	• Verbalize plans for moderation of life-style

❀
Therapeutic Aims

• Promote participation in treatment program.
• Provide structure for daily activities routine.
• Decrease manipulative behavior.

❀
Implementation

Nursing Interventions	Rationale
Give the client support for direct communication and for fulfilling assigned tasks and personal responsibilities.	Positive support tends to increase positive behaviors.
It may be helpful in maintaining consistency to assign the responsibility for decisions regarding the client to one staff member.	If only one person makes final decisions, there is less opportunity for manipulation by the client.
Do not assume that physical complaints are not genuine or that the client is just manipulating or seeking attention.	The client may be physically ill. This must be validated or ruled out.
The medical staff should investigate each complaint within a certain time period or at a structured time. Then do not give attention for the client's continued conversation about physical complaints.	After the medical staff deals with physical problems, you are free to deal with the client's interpersonal issues. Physical symptoms must not be used by the client to avoid dealing with emotional problems.
Attempt to determine in your initial assessment of the client the extent of the client's substance use. Interview the client's significant others if necessary.	If substance use exists, it will need to be handled in an effective manner.

✷ *(continued)*
Implementation

Nursing Interventions	Rationale
When talking with the client concerning the above problems, focus on self-responsibility and active approaches that the client can take in his or her life. Avoid reinforcing the client's passivity, feelings of hopelessness, and so forth.	If the client is blaming others or the system for his or her problems, it is unlikely the client will accept responsibility for making changes.
Teach the client a step-by-step approach to solving problems: identifying problems, exploring alternatives, evaluating consequences of alternatives, and making a decision.	The client may be unaware of a logical process for solving problems.
In your initial assessment and in subsequent conversations, ask for the client's perceptions of his or her skills, level of functioning, and independence.	The client's perception of self is an essential component of baseline data.
Observe how the client functions in various situations: Can the client use the telephone or directory? How does the client interact with peers? with authority figures? How does the client function with regard to structured activities, unstructured time, and competitive situations?	You need to assess what the client can do and what skills he or she needs to develop.
Give the client feedback regarding your observations; involve the client in planning to work on deficient areas or to use and augment strengths. Together try to arrive at reasonable and realistic goals. Using written lists, priority schedules, and so forth may help structure the client's tasks.	Involving the client facilitates his or her acceptance of responsibility. Using schedules and lists helps achieve an independent life-style.
Work with professionals in other disciplines (vocational rehabilitation, education, psychology) for testing of the client and for help in specific situations (like job interview training).	Using other health professionals for areas beyond nursing's scope enhances the client's chance for success.
Encourage the client to express personal feelings or concerns, including identity questions, uncertainties, fears, and so on. Remain nonjudgmental in these discussions, and reassure the client that you will not ridicule him or her or take his or her concerns lightly.	A nonjudgmental attitude will help the client feel safe in sharing concerns with you. It is unlikely that the client has relationships with others that would allow discussing personal concerns without fear of rejection.
Encourage the client to identify any particular problem or life situation that precipitated hospitalization.	The client may have difficulty identifying his or her role in the situation that led to hospitalization.
Help the client obtain aid and use resources, such as social services or vocational rehabilitation as needed and appropriate.	The client may need these resources to live in the community but may be unaware of how to obtain the services.
You may need to work with professionals in other disciplines (eg, social work or law) as they work with the client on his or her legal problems. Take care to	Legal difficulties are beyond the scope of nursing. Your responsibility is appropriate referral.

✸ *(continued)*
Implementation

Nursing Interventions	Rationale
promote the client's autonomy and development to deal with problems independently. Do not reinforce the client's patterns of dependence on others.	
Help the client identify his or her strengths realistically, as well as successful coping behaviors that the client has used in the past. It may help to have the client make a written list. Encourage the client to try to use these coping behaviors in present and future situations.	The client's self-perception may be one of hopelessness or helplessness. The client needs your assistance to recognize strengths.
Throughout the client's hospitalization discuss discharge planning in a positive manner, beginning with the initial interview or assessment.	The client receives the message that he or she can be independent and that hospitalization is temporary.

✸

Nursing Diagnosis	*Impaired Socialization (3.1.1)*
	The state in which an individual participates in an insufficient or excessive quantity or ineffective quality of social exchange.

✸
Assessment Data

Defining Characteristics	• Intolerance of being alone • Chronic feelings of boredom or emptiness • Alternate clinging and avoidance behavior in relationships • Excessive dependency needs
Related Factors	• Manipulation of others for own needs • Sense of entitlement • Acting out or risky behavior • Lack of insight • Self-destructive or aggressive behavior

✸
Expected Outcomes

Initial	*The client will:*
	• Interact appropriately with staff, visitors, and other clients • Engage in leisure activities
Discharge	*The client will:*
	• Participate in relationships without excessive clinging and avoidance • Meet dependency needs in a socially acceptable manner • Develop a social support group outside the hospital • Initiate leisure activities that he or she enjoys

✳
Therapeutic Aims

- Decrease manipulative behavior.
- Alleviate feelings of boredom.
- Facilitate development of healthy social relationships.

✳
Implementation

Nursing Interventions	Rationale
Together with the client, establish acceptable limits in relationships. Provide limits for the client if he or she is unable to do so. Do not allow the client to manipulate or take advantage of other clients or visitors. (Be aware of the client's interactions and intervene when necessary.)	Limits or controls must be supplied by you until the client is able to do so. Other clients' needs for protection must be considered and may require your intervention.
Remember: Although the client must feel that the staff members care about him or her as a person (therapeutically), it is not beneficial for the client to have your sympathy or friendship. Do not undermine the client's independence by encouraging dependence on the staff or institution.	Sympathy and friendship are only appropriate to personal or social relationships. The client's independence is a goal of a therapeutic relationship. Reliance on staff may be flattering to you but is nontherapeutic for the client.
Help the client recognize when he or she is feeling bored, and identify activities that diminish these feelings. It may be useful to help the client structure his or her time with a written schedule.	The client needs to see that boredom is his or her problem and that it is his or her responsibility to resolve it.
Help the client see that manipulation of others results in the loss of their company and subsequently boredom and loneliness for the client.	If the client dislikes boredom, he or she may diminish manipulative behavior to avoid feelings of boredom.
Help the client determine appropriate people with whom to discuss personal issues, as well as appropriate times for such discussions.	Due to the client's dependency needs and poor impulse control, he or she may disclose intimate issues to casual acquaintances or even strangers, which can lead to rejection of the client.
Encourage the client to meet others in his or her community, to begin to make acquaintances, or to contact support groups prior to discharge.	The client will need to meet relationship needs with others outside the hospital to avoid dependency on the hospital staff.

Histrionic Behavior

The terms *histrionic* and *hysterical* generally are used interchangeably. Histrionic behavior often is very dramatic and may be sensory or physical; it is frequently described as *inappropriate*. These clients may exhibit overt physical signs (typically seizure-like activity, black outs or fainting spells, and dizziness) that have no organic basis. However, it is important that the client's physical health is investigated and is determined to be sound before such episodes can be identified as histrionic and dealt with effectively by the staff. Episodes like these almost always happen when others are present (ie, with an "audience") and at a time when the client is in an unpleasant situation or wishes to avoid an anticipated situation, such as a therapy session or activity.

Histrionic behavior may be sexual or seductive. However, when the client's seductive dress or behavior results in a sexual advance or response from others, the client may be surprised and say that he or she did not expect that to happen. Clients may accuse a staff member of improper sexual comments or advances. Therefore, it is best to avoid situations in which the client could make such claims and to always work with this client within the observation of other staff members.

Clients with histrionic behavior may look and act as though they have few or no problems at times. It is easy for the staff to think the client could act appropriately "if the client wanted to." However, the client must learn appropriate behavior. Family or marital counseling may be indicated to deal with the client's problems effectively.

Nursing Diagnoses Addressed in this Care Plan

Ineffective Individual Coping
Impaired Social Interaction

Related Nursing Diagnoses

High Risk for Injury
Noncompliance
High Risk for Violence: Self-Directed or Directed at Others

Nursing Diagnosis	*Ineffective Individual Coping (5.1.1.1)*

Impairment of adaptive behaviors and problem-solving abilities of a person in meeting life's demands and roles.

Assessment Data

Defining Characteristics

- Inability to tolerate stress or deal with conflict
- Overt exaggeration or dramatization of emotions
- Emotional lability
- Low frustration tolerance
- Frequent physical complaints without organic basis
- Seductive behavior
- Attention-seeking or manipulative behavior
- Suicidal threats or gestures
- Angry outbursts or temper tantrums

Related Factors

- Lack of insight
- Unsatisfactory interpersonal relationships
- Perceived lack of coping resources

Expected Outcomes

Initial

The client will:

- Be free of injury
- Not harm others or destroy property
- Eliminate attention-seeking, seductive, and manipulative behaviors
- Express feelings verbally

Discharge

The client will:

- Demonstrate the ability to deal more effectively with frustration and stress
- Verbalize or demonstrate increased feelings of self-worth
- Express an intensity of emotion that is appropriate to the situation

Therapeutic Aims

- Decrease secondary gains from physical complaints.
- Decrease manipulative, seductive, attention-seeking behaviors.
- Promote self-esteem.

Implementation

Nursing Interventions	Rationale
Base your initial relationship with the client on establishing your consistency and reliability rather than on a discussion of the client's deep feelings.	The client will respond best to limit-setting. Clients who exhibit histrionic behavior usually are unwilling or unable to discuss deep feelings, especially initially.
Let the client know you will establish limits on acceptable and unacceptable behavior and will be consistent in enforcing these limits.	The client feels more secure and gains more self-control when the limits are clear and consistent.

(continued)
Implementation

Nursing Interventions	Rationale
Give the client honest feedback about his or her behavior. Help the client identify particular behaviors that are causing problems for him or her (seductive behavior, physical symptoms, suicidal gestures or threats). You may need to identify these for the client.	You must be concrete and specific in describing problem behavior, because the client has limited self-assessment abilities.
Accurately assess and report new physical complaints to medical personnel.	It must be determined that physical complaints or episodes are without an organic basis.
Initially it may be necessary to give the client 10 minutes per hour to discuss physical concerns. Gradually decrease the time until this behavior is totally eliminated.	The client should not be abruptly deprived of his or her physical coping strategy. The behavior can be diminished gradually while he or she learns more acceptable ways of coping.
Do not allow the client to avoid frustrating or unpleasant responsibilities or to avoid attendance at activities due to physical complaints.	If the client receives little or no reward from complaints (secondary gain), he or she is less likely to persist in complaining.
Remove the audience or the client from the situation when attention-seeking behaviors occur.	This decreases the attention given to the client's histrionic behavior.
Identify appropriate behaviors for the client in a matter-of-fact manner.	The client's insight is impaired. You must make it clear to the client which behaviors are appropriate.
Withdraw your attention from the client as long as inappropriate behavior continues.	Lack of your attention may reduce attention-seeking behaviors.
If the client begins destroying property, harming himself or herself, or threatening others, it may be necessary to place the client in a safe, secluded environment. Handle the situation swiftly, in a matter-of-fact manner. Do not argue with or chastise the client, and give as little attention to the destructive behavior as possible.	Physical safety is a priority.
When the client regains control and ceases the behavior, then attempt to talk with him or her to explore more acceptable ways of handling frustration and expressing feelings.	The client is unable to discuss feelings when he or she is out of control.
Give the client positive feedback when he or she expresses himself or herself appropriately or avoids using inappropriate behaviors when stressed or frustrated.	Positive reinforcement for appropriate behaviors will strengthen those behaviors and help extinguish unacceptable behaviors.
Point out inappropriate dress, grooming, or excessive make-up when they occur. Do so privately and without reprehension.	The client is not a child, and it is not appropriate to scold the client. The client's judgment is impaired, and he or she needs to learn appropriate grooming.
Suggest a more moderate yet attractive choice of clothes or application of make-up.	The client may not be aware of what is appropriate or socially acceptable.

❋ *(continued)*
Implementation

Nursing Interventions	Rationale
Give genuine praise when the client's appearance is suitable.	False praise or flattery is belittling to the client. Genuine, positive support will reinforce appropriate behavior.
Encourage the client's peers to give positive yet genuine feedback for improved appearance.	Peer feedback increases the attention the client receives for appropriate appearance.
Explore alternative methods of gaining attention that are not sexual or seductive. Give positive reinforcement for the client's attempts to gain appropriate attention.	The client may have limited knowledge of appropriate ways to gain attention.

❂

Nursing Diagnosis

Impaired Social Interaction (3.1.1)
The state in which an individual participates in an insufficient or excessive quantity or ineffective quality of social exchange.

❋ **Assessment Data**

Defining Characteristics	• Poor interpersonal relationships • Lack of consideration for others • Excessive quantity of verbalizations with little substance or content
Related Factors	• Low self-esteem • Shallow emotions

❋ **Expected Outcomes**

Initial	*The client will:* • Demonstrate socially acceptable behavior • Verbalize increased feelings of self-worth
Discharge	*The client will:* • Interact with others in a socially acceptable manner • Communicate effectively, both listening and speaking

❋ **Therapeutic Aims**

• Promote healthy interpersonal relationships.
• Promote increased self-esteem.

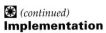 *(continued)*
Implementation

Nursing Interventions	Rationale
Teach the client social skills. Describe and demonstrate specific skills, such as eye contact, attentive listening, nodding, and so forth. Discuss the types of topics that are appropriate for casual conversation, such as the weather, news, local events, and so forth.	The client may have little knowledge of social interaction skills. Modeling provides a concrete example of the desired skills.
Teach the client a step-by-step approach to solving problems: identifying problems, exploring alternatives, evaluating consequences of alternatives, and making a decision.	The client may be unaware of a logical process for examining and resolving problems.
Give the client an opportunity to discuss his or her difficulties with interpersonal relationships; encourage the client to express feelings.	As the client gains skill with the verbal expression of feelings, inappropriate behaviors may decrease.
Encourage the client to try out alternative behaviors. Assist the client at first with short, successful, social interchanges with others. Then help the client progress to discussing feelings, problems, and more emotionally charged issues with others.	Because the client has limited abilities to deal with stress, he or she is likely to be more successful if new behaviors are practiced in order of increasing complexity or difficulty.
Teach the client about preventing transmission of human immunodeficiency virus (HIV), especially if the client remains sexually active.	Everyone needs to know how to prevent transmission of HIV. Lack of impulse control, poor judgment, excessive dependency needs, or increased sexual activity increase the need for such education.

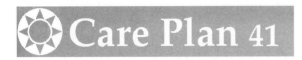

Delusional Disorders

The primary feature of a delusional disorder is the *persistence* of a *delusion* or a fixed false belief. In delusional disorders the delusion is limited to a specific area of thought and is not related to any organic or major psychiatric disorder. The different types of delusional disorders are categorized (DSM-III-R, 1987) according to the main theme of the delusional belief:

Erotomaniac. This is an erotic delusion that one is loved by another person, usually a famous person, though it may be a coworker or a complete stranger. People with this disorder may come into contact with the law as they write letters, make phone calls, or attempt to "protect" the object of their delusion.

Grandiose. This delusion usually involves a person who is convinced that he or she is uniquely talented, has created a fantastic invention, or has a religious calling. The individual may believe himself or herself to be a famous person, claiming the actual person is an imposter.

Jealous. This delusion involves the belief that the spouse or partner is unfaithful, when that is not true. The person with this delusion may follow the partner, read mail, and so forth, to find "proof" of the infidelity. The delusion can lead to demands that the partner never go anywhere alone or can even lead to physical violence.

Persecutory. This type of delusion is the most common. It involves the belief that the individual is being spied on, followed, harassed, drugged, and so forth. This individual may seek to remedy these perceived injustices through police reports, court action, and sometimes violence.

Somatic. This type of delusion involves the belief that the individual emits a foul odor from some body orifice, has infestations of bugs or parasites, or that certain body parts are ugly, deformed, or misshapen, when that is not true. These individuals most frequently seek help from medical, nonpsychiatric sources.

Delusional disorders are most prevalent in people who are 40 to 55 years old, though they can be seen in younger age groups. The client has no other symptoms of any kind and therefore can function quite well when not discussing or acting on the delusional belief. Occupational and intellectual functioning are rarely affected, but these individuals are dysfunctional in social situations and marital or partner relationships. Because the delusion persists in spite of efforts to extinguish it, the goal in therapy is not to eliminate the delusion but to contain its effect on the client's life.

Nursing Diagnosis Addressed in this Care Plan

Altered Thought Processes

Related Nursing Diagnoses

Altered Role Performance
Impaired Social Interaction
High Risk for Violence: Self-Directed or Directed at Others

Nursing Diagnosis	*Altered Thought Processes (8.3)*
	A state in which the individual experiences a disruption in cognitive operations and activities.

Assessment Data

Defining Characteristics	• Erratic, impulsive behavior
	• Poor judgment
	• Agitation
	• Feelings of distress
	• Illogical thinking
	• Irrational ideas leading to faulty conclusions
	• Extreme, intense feelings
	• Refusal to accept factual information from others
Related Factors	• Described by others as "normal" most of the time
	• Socially inappropriate or odd behavior in certain situations
	• Elicits anger from others who perceive the client's behavior to be purposeful or spiteful

Expected Outcomes

Initial	*The client will:*
	• Verbally recognize that others do not see his or her belief as real
	• Demonstrate decreased agitation and aggressive behavior
	• Express feelings about the delusion only to therapeutic staff
	• Stop acting on the delusional belief
Discharge	*The client will:*
	• Verbalize plans to maintain contact with a therapist to provide an avenue for discussing the delusional material when he or she feels a need to do so
	• Verbally validate decisions or conclusions about the delusional area before taking action
	• Refrain from any public discussion of the delusional belief

✳
Therapeutic Aims

- Identify areas of difficulty in the client's life stemming from the delusional belief.
- Provide an acceptable channel for discussion of the delusional belief and the client's feelings about the belief.
- Facilitate containment of behavior resulting from delusional belief.

✳
Implementation

Nursing Interventions	Rationale
Let the client know that all feelings, ideas, and beliefs are permissible to share with you.	The client can identify the nurse as someone who will not censure him or her for feelings and ideas, even if they are bizarre or unusual.
Do not validate the delusional ideas. Let the client know that his or her feelings are real and that the delusional ideas seem real to him or her but that the delusional ideas are not real.	The client may begin to recognize that not all people share his or her belief, but they can still respect his or her feelings.
Avoid trying to convince the client that the delusions are not real. Rather, convey that the ideas seem real to the client, but others do not share or accept that belief.	The client believes the delusions to be true and cannot intellectually be convinced otherwise. Debating this issue can damage the therapeutic relationship and is futile.
Give the client feedback that others do not share his or her perceptions and beliefs.	The feedback is reality, and it can assist the client to begin problem solving.
Assist the client to identify difficulties in daily life that are caused by or related to the delusional ideas.	If the client feels distress about life areas that are disrupted, he or she might be motivated to contain behaviors related to the delusional belief.
Have the client identify the events that led to his or her current difficulties. Discuss the relationship between these events and the delusional beliefs.	If the client can begin to see the relationship between delusions and life difficulties, he or she might be more willing to consider making some behavioral changes.
Focus interactions and problem solving on how the client can avoid further difficulties at home, work, or other situations in which problems are experienced.	The client's agreement that he or she would like to avoid further problems and distress can provide a sound basis for making changes. The "issue" of whether or not the delusion is true can be avoided.
Help the client identify people with whom it is safe to discuss the delusional beliefs, such as the therapist, nurse, psychiatrist, and so forth.	By talking with nurses, therapists, and designated others, the client has a nonthreatening outlet for expression of feelings and ideas.
Assist the client to select someone whom he or she trusts, and validate perceptions with him or her before taking any action that may precipitate difficulties.	If the client can avoid acting on the delusional beliefs by checking his or her perceptions with someone, many difficulties at home, work, and so forth can be avoided.
Contract with the client to limit the amount of time he or she will spend thinking about the delusional	It is not feasible to expect the client to forget about the delusion entirely. By limiting the time spent

(continued)
Implementation

Nursing Interventions	Rationale
area. This may be 5 minutes per hour, 15 minutes per day, or whatever the client feels able to do. Encourage the client to gradually decrease this amount of time as he or she tolerates.	focusing on the delusion, the client feels less frustrated than if he or she is "forbidden" to think about it but will not spend all of his or her time dwelling on the delusion.
Explore with the client ways he or she can redirect some of the energy or anxiety generated by the delusional ideas.	The energy from the client's anxious feelings of the client needs to be expressed in a constructive manner to prevent the client's anxiety from increasing.
Encourage the client to use his or her contact person as often as needed. It may be helpful to use telephone contact to validate perceptions, rather than always scheduling an appointment.	If the client can quickly call the person they trust and receive immediate feedback, he or she is more likely to succeed in containing behavior related to the delusional ideas.

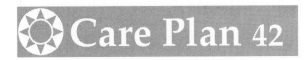

Schizoid and Schizotypal Personality Disorders

The client with a *schizoid personality disorder* manifests a "pervasive pattern of indifference to social relationships and a restricted range of emotional experience and expression" (DSM-III-R, 1987). The client with a *schizotypal personality disorder* exhibits a "pervasive pattern of peculiarities of ideation, appearance, and behavior and deficits in interpersonal relatedness" (DSM-III-R, 1987). However, many of the problems for these clients and the nursing interventions are the same. Therefore, these two disorders are addressed in the same care plan, with notations where differences exist.

Clients with a schizoid or schizotypal personality disorder frequently are isolated by their own choice. They do not have close relationships with others, nor do they desire to establish them. Their interactions usually are limited to the nuclear family or one person outside the family. Even these relationships are characterized by a cool, aloof, somewhat distant participation on the part of the client. Praise or criticism from others has little effect on the client.

In addition to the commonalities described previously, the client with a schizotypal personality disorder displays a great deal of anxiety when social situations with unfamiliar people are unavoidable. He or she generally appears odd or eccentric in a variety of ways: magical thinking; unusual perceptual experiences; silly gestures or facial expressions; beliefs in superstition, clairvoyance, or telepathy, when these beliefs are inconsistent with subcultural norms; and an unkempt, frequently unusual manner of dress (DSM-III-R, 1987).

Clients with these personality disorders do not exhibit symptoms that are severe enough to support a diagnosis of schizophrenia. However, under extreme, unavoidable stress, these clients may experience a psychotic episode. They may be able to sustain employment if working with other people is not required. Symptoms of these disorders are evident in childhood and adolescence, and persist through adulthood. Often, these individuals stay with the nuclear family or live alone if forced to leave the family unit. It is thought that many homeless people fall into these two categories.

Nursing Diagnosis Addressed in this Care Plan

Impaired Adjustment

Related Nursing Diagnoses

Self-Care Deficits
Altered Role Performance

Nursing Diagnosis

Impaired Adjustment (5.1.1.1.1)

The state in which the individual is unable to modify his/her life style/behavior in a manner consistent with a health challenge.

Assessment Data

Defining Characteristics

- Indifference to praise or criticism
- Flat, silly, or inappropriate affect
- Lack of desire for social interaction

  In addition, for clients with schizotypal personality disorder:
- Magical thinking
- Belief in telepathy, clairvoyance, superstition
- Vague, digressive, or abstract speech
- Unkempt appearance
- Bizarre mannerisms

Related Factors

- Lack of future-oriented thinking
- Preference for solitary activities
- Lack of independent behavior

Expected Outcomes

Initial

The client will:

- Identify his or her basic needs
- Verbalize any preferences, interests, or desires
- Express bizarre ideas and beliefs only to therapeutic staff
- Participate in treatment program

Discharge

The client will:

- Communicate needs appropriately to others
- Participate in vocational planning or training
- Demonstrate adequate hygiene and grooming

Therapeutic Aims

- Promote appropriate behavior.
- Maximize client's independence.
- Facilitate necessary relationships with others.
- Promote communication.
- Facilitate adjustment to the community.

Implementation

Nursing Interventions	Rationale
Direct nursing care toward changing basic or essential behaviors, that is, those that focus attention on the client in a negative manner.	The client has limited interest or desire for behavioral changes.
Give the client honest feedback about those behaviors that draw negative attention to him or her.	The client needs knowledge of behaviors that cause uncomfortable consequences for him or her.
Explain to the client that the reason to make changes is to maximize his or her freedom in the community and to avoid hospitalization. Do not attempt to give rationale for change based on what is socially acceptable or the "proper" thing to do.	The client will be indifferent to others' reactions to his or her behavior. It is possible to engage the client in behavioral changes if he or she perceives a direct, concrete benefit to be gained.
Be specific in giving feedback to the client (eg, identify the problem as making faces, talking about telepathic beliefs, and so forth).	The client lacks the ability or desire to interpret concepts or abstract ideas.
Do not expect the client to develop the ability to respond to subtleties or social cues.	The client's ability to "learn" is impaired, or he or she may lack the desire to develop these social abilities.
Encourage the client to make a checklist of people with whom communication is required. This may include a store clerk, landlord, social worker, and so forth.	A concrete written checklist is easier to manage, because the client's abstract thinking abilities are impaired.
If possible, identify one community person to coordinate services for the client. This may be a social worker, community nurse, or case manager.	The fewer people the client is required to interact with, the more successful he or she will be.
Involve the community contact person as soon as possible in the client's care.	Contact prior to discharge familiarizes the client with the community person and facilitates transferring the therapeutic relationship following discharge.
Encourage the client to write as many requests as he or she can. If that is not workable, practice the use of the telephone to make requests for what is needed.	Written requests can be prepared ahead of time and allow the client to avoid the displeasure of interaction. Telephone contact is less threatening than face-to-face interaction.
If face-to-face contact is required, the client may benefit from having a family member or the community contact person accompany him or her.	The contact person or family member can serve as a buffer for the client if needed.

✷ *(continued)*
Implementation

Nursing Interventions	Rationale
Limit expectations of client interactions to those that are necessary to obtain services that he or she truly wants or needs.	The client has a greater chance for success if he or she values the need for the service.
Assist the client's family or significant others to focus on realistic expectations for the client.	It is common for significant others to base their expectations on what they perceive to be desirable rather than the actual ability of the client, which is impaired.
Encourage the client to establish a simple daily routine for completion of hygiene.	Repetitive simple tasks and routines have a greater chance of success than changing expectations.
If the client lives with someone else, include that person in developing daily routine expectations for room care, hygiene, and so forth, that can be continued at home.	The client will be more successful in transferring skills and behaviors if they are similar to those expected or needed in the community.
Assist the client to explore any interests or activities that do not involve much contact with other people.	This type of activity is most likely to appeal to the client.
Do not attempt to promote activities "just for fun." It usually is more beneficial to explore "purposeful" activities (eg, use of a computer).	The client is unlikely to engage in activities that "serve no purpose," such as strictly recreational activities. Frequently, these clients have a high intellectual capability, which can be used if the stress of interaction with others is minimized.
Assist the client to explore alternative living arrangements if indicated. These might include a "room and board" type of facility, where meals and laundry service are provided, but little interaction is required.	If the client lives with his or her nuclear family, it is likely he or she will need to live elsewhere as family members become older or unable to care for the client at home. The most successful living situation is one that provides the maximum of services to meet basic daily needs and requires the least social participation.
Refer the client to vocational services if possible and if the client has the potential to develop a vocational or employment interest.	It is possible for the client to use intellectual abilities to increase his or her independence and decrease reliance on others to meet basic needs.

Section Twelve

Stress and Anxiety

Stress, and the anxiety it produces, is part of everyday life. Determinations about the existence of mental health or illness often are made based on a person's ability to handle stress and cope with anxiety. The overall goals of nursing care in working with stress-related illnesses are to reduce the client's anxiety to a level where he or she can again become functional in daily life and to help the client learn to deal with anxiety and stress more effectively in the future. The care plans in this section deal with the broad concept of anxious behavior as well as specific stress-related disorders.

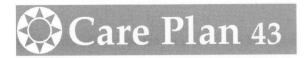

Anxious Behavior

Anxiety is a feeling of apprehension or dread that develops when the self or self-concept is threatened. Anxiety is distinct from fear, which is a response to an identifiable, external threat.

Anxiety is thought to be essential for human survival. The discomfort people feel when they are anxious provides the impetus for learning and change. Mild anxiety can cause a heightened awareness and sharpening of the senses. This type of anxiety is viewed as constructive and even necessary for growth.

Anxiety that becomes more severe can be destructive, causing the individual to become dysfunctional. This type of anxiety is believed by some theorists to be central to many psychiatric disorders. Anxious behavior and feelings of anxiety are frequently seen in conjunction with other problems.

Peplau (1963) defined four levels of anxiety:

Mild. This is normal anxiety that motivates individuals on a day-to-day basis. Stimuli are readily perceived and processed. The ability to learn and problem solve efficiently is enhanced.

Moderate. The individual's perceptual field is narrowed; he or she hears, sees, and grasps less. Learning can occur with the direction of another person. The individual may fail to attend to environmental stimuli but will notice things that are brought to his or her attention.

Severe. The individual focuses on small details or scattered details. The perceptual field is greatly reduced. The individual is unable to problem solve or use the learning process.

Panic. This is the extreme form of anxiety. The individual is disorganized and may be dangerous to himself or herself. He or she may be unable to act or speak or may be hyperactive and agitated.

Anxiety is not directly observable, it is communicated through behavior. The individual displaying anxious behavior also experiences physiologic phenomena. These include elevated blood pressure, increased pulse and respiratory rate, diaphoresis, flushed face, dry mouth, trembling, frequent urination, and dizziness. The individual also may report nausea, diarrhea, insomnia, headaches, muscle tension, blurred vision, and palpitations or chest pain. The physiologic symptoms or complaints will vary but usually become more intense as the level of anxiety increases.

Nursing Diagnoses Addressed in this Care Plan

Anxiety
Ineffective Individual Coping
Altered Health Maintenance

Related Nursing Diagnoses

High Risk for Injury
Impaired Social Interaction
Sleep Pattern Disturbance

Nursing Diagnosis	*Anxiety (9.3.1)* *A vague uneasy feeling, whose source is often nonspecific or unknown to the individual.*

Assessment Data

Defining Characteristics	• Decreased attention span • Restlessness, irritability • Poor impulse control • Feelings of discomfort, apprehension, or helplessness • Hyperactivity, pacing • Wringing hands • Perceptual field deficits • Decreased ability to communicate verbally *In addition, in panic anxiety:* • Inability to discriminate harmful stimuli or situations • Disorganized thought processes • Delusions
Related Factors	• Insomnia or excessive sleeping • History of abuse • Post-traumatic stress response

Expected Outcomes

Initial	*The client will:* • Be free of injury • Discuss feelings of dread, anxiety, and so forth • Respond to relaxation techniques with a decreased anxiety level
Discharge	*The client will:* • Reduce own anxiety level • Be free of anxiety attacks

❋
Therapeutic Aims

- Provide a safe environment.
- Decrease anxiety level.

❋
Implementation

Nursing Interventions	Rationale
Remain with the client at all times when levels of anxiety are high (severe or panic).	The client's safety is a priority. A highly anxious client should not be left alone—his or her anxiety will escalate.
Move the client to a quiet area with minimal or decreased stimuli. Using a small room or seclusion area may be indicated.	The client's ability to deal with excessive stimuli is impaired. Anxious behavior can be escalated by external stimuli. A smaller room can enhance the client's sense of security. The larger the area, the more lost and panicked the client can become.
Remain calm in your approach to the client.	The client will feel more secure if you are calm and if the client feels you are in control of the situation.
Use short, simple, and clear statements.	The client's ability to deal with abstractions or complexity is impaired.
Avoid asking or forcing the client to make choices.	The client's ability to problem solve is impaired. The client may not make sound decisions or may be unable to make decisions at all.
Use of PRN medications may be indicated if the client's level of anxiety is high or if the client is experiencing delusions, disorganized thoughts, and so forth.	Medication may be necessary to decrease the client's anxiety to a level at which he or she can listen to you and feel safe.
Be aware of your own feelings and level of discomfort or anxiety.	Anxiety is communicated interpersonally. Being with the anxious client can raise your own anxiety level.
Encourage the client's participation in relaxation exercises. These can include deep breathing, progressive muscle relaxation, meditation, guided imagery, and going (mentally) to a quiet, peaceful place.	Relaxation exercises are effective, nonchemical ways to reduce anxiety.
Teach the client to use relaxation techniques independently.	Independent use of the techniques can give the client confidence in having some conscious control over his or her anxious behavior.
Help the client see mild anxiety as a positive catalyst for change.	A frequent misconception is that anxiety itself is bad and not useful. The client does not need to avoid anxiety per se.

Nursing Diagnosis

Ineffective Individual Coping (5.1.1.1)

Impairment of adaptive behaviors and problem-solving abilities of a person in meeting life's demands and roles.

Assessment Data

Defining Characteristics	• Client-reported inability to deal with stress • Overdependence on others • Avoidance or escape patterns of behavior • Ineffective expression of feelings
Related Factors	• Lack of coping resources (actual or perceived) • Lack of confidence

Expected Outcomes

Initial	*The client will:*
	• Verbalize feelings • Identify his or her behavioral response to stress • Participate in realistic discussion of problems
Discharge	*The client will:*
	• Demonstrate alternative ways to deal with stress, including problem solving • Discuss future plans, based on realistic self-assessment

Therapeutic Aims

• Promote self-confidence.
• Promote effective problem solving.
• Facilitate verbal expression of feelings and identification of stress response.

Implementation

Nursing Interventions	Rationale
Make observations to the client about his or her anxious behavior. Help the client see the relationship between what he or she thinks or feels and the corresponding anxious behavioral response.	The client may be unaware of the relationship between emotional issues and his or her anxious behavior.
Help the client recognize early signs of his or her anxious behavior.	The sooner the client recognizes the onset of his or her anxiety, the more quickly he or she will be able to alter that response.
During the times the client is relatively calm, explore together ways in which he or she can deal with stress and anxiety.	The client will be better able to problem solve when his or her anxiety level is lower.
Encourage verbal expression of feelings. Encourage the client to identify possible threats to himself or	The more specific and concrete the client can be about anxiety-invoking stress, the better

✳ (continued)
Implementation

Nursing Interventions	Rationale
herself or possible sources of anxiety. Encourage the client to be as specific as he or she can.	he or she will be able to deal with those situations.
Teach the client a step-by-step approach to solving problems: identifying problems, exploring alternatives, evaluating consequences of each alternative, and making a decision.	The client may be unaware of a logical process for examining and solving problems.
Support the client's positive actions in viewing himself or herself and his or her abilities realistically.	Enhancing the client's confidence and abilities to self-evaluate promotes his or her sense of self-reliance.
Encourage the client to practice methods to reduce anxiety prior to approaching problems when possible.	The client will be able to better use problem solving when anxiety is at lower levels.
Encourage the client to evaluate the success of the chosen alternative. Help the client to continue to try alternatives if his or her initial choice is not successful.	The client needs to know that he or she can survive making a mistake and that making mistakes is part of the learning process.
Give the client positive feedback as he or she learns to relax, express feelings, problem solve, and so forth.	Positive feedback promotes the continuation of desired behavior.

Nursing Diagnosis

Altered Health Maintenance (6.4.2)
Inability to identify, manage, and/or seek out help to maintain health.

✳
Assessment Data

Defining Characteristics	• Frequent complaints regarding gastrointestinal (GI) distress, lack of appetite • Sleep pattern disturbances • Failure to manage stress and anxiety
Related Factors	• History of trauma or abuse • Unhealthy life-style

✳
Expected Outcomes

Initial	*The client will:* • Eat a balanced diet • Obtain restful sleep • Recognize related problems

✳ *(continued)*
Expected Outcomes

Discharge	*The client will:*
	• Maintain adequate balanced physiologic functioning
	• Verbalize intent to seek treatment for related problems, if indicated

✳
Therapeutic Aims

• Promote homeostasis.
• Minimize physical complaints.
• Seek treatment for related conditions, if necessary.

✳
Implementation

Nursing Interventions	Rationale
Help the client channel energy constructively. Participation in activities using gross motor skills is best (running, cleaning, exercising).	Physical activities can provide an outlet for the client's excess energy. Use of large muscles, followed by relaxation, also can facilitate sleep.
Promote development of a bedtime routine. Try to include activities that have been successful for the client in the past (tepid bath, warm milk, reading).	Relaxing, routine activities facilitate sleep and rest.
Encourage the client to eat nutritious foods. Provide a quiet atmosphere at meal times. Avoid discussing emotional issues before, during, and immediately after meals.	Relaxation around meal times promotes digestion and avoids GI distress. The client may have used eating (or not eating) as a way to deal with anxiety.
Encourage continued treatment for any related problems the client has identified (eg, eating disorders, post-traumatic stress, abuse) or refer the client to support groups.	History of a traumatic experience can be associated with high levels of anxiety; treatment for these problems often is long term.

Phobias

The primary response of the client with a phobic disorder is anxiety. The distinguishing difference between anxiety related to a phobia and other anxiety responses is the client's awareness of a specific trigger for the anxiety in the phobic response. A *phobia* is an irrational, persistent fear of an event, situation, activity, or object. The client recognizes this fear as irrational but is unable to prevent it. Many times the client can avoid the source of the phobic response and does not seek treatment. When the phobic behavior is in response to something that is very general or unavoidable or the avoidance behavior becomes so extreme that it interferes with the client's daily life, the client usually seeks treatment.

The DSM-III-R (1987) categorizes phobic attacks into three types:

Agorophobia is a fear of being in public places. The individual feels he or she may become "trapped," that is, unable to escape or obtain help if needed. This phobia usually manifests in the person's 20s and may persist throughout his or her life. In severe cases people have been reported to stay in their houses or apartments for months or even years, sending out for and having food and other necessities delivered to them.

Social phobia is a person's fear that he or she will be publicly embarrassed or humiliated by his or her own behavior. This may result in the individual's inability to eat in the company of others, use a public restroom, answer simple questions, or engage in social conversation.

Simple phobia is described as a "specific" phobia; the stimulus is easily identifiable, such as a fear of heights, animals, water, and so forth. With simple phobias it often is easier to avoid the stimulus, and treatment is not seen as necessary. Treatment is sought only if the irrational fear interferes with daily life or the person experiences a great deal of distress about having the fear.

Phobic people experience intense anxiety when confronted with the object of the phobia and may have a *panic anxiety attack*. There also is marked *anticipatory anxiety* when the individual contemplates the necessity of confronting the phobic situation. It is this intense anticipatory anxiety that leads to avoidance of the situation.

Typically, phobic behavior is treated with a behavioral technique called *systematic desensitization*. This technique is easier to use and most effective when working with clients with simple phobias. Medications rarely are useful in treating people with phobic behavior.

Nursing Diagnosis Addressed in this Care Plan

Fear

Related Nursing Diagnoses

Ineffective Individual Coping
Altered Role Performance
Impaired Social Interaction

Nursing Diagnosis	*Fear (9.3.2)*
	Feeling of dread related to an identifiable source which the person validates.

Assessment Data

Defining Characteristics	• Anticipatory anxiety (when thinking about the phobic object) • Panic anxiety (when confronted with the phobic object) • Avoidance behaviors that interfere with relationships or social or occupational functioning
Related Factors	• Recognition of the phobia as irrational • Embarrassment over the phobic fear • Sufficient discomfort to seek treatment

Expected Outcomes

Initial	*The client will:* • Verbalize feelings of fear and discomfort • Effectively demonstrate relaxation techniques
Discharge	*The client will:* • Effectively decrease own anxiety level • Eliminate avoidance behaviors • Demonstrate effective functioning in social and occupational roles

Therapeutic Aims

• Decrease anxiety response through systematic desensitization.
• Facilitate expression of feelings.

Implementation

Nursing Interventions	Rationale
Allow the client to express feelings openly. Initially, it may be beneficial to focus on the client's feeling embarrassed, need to seek treatment, and so forth without discussing the phobic situation specifically.	The client often experiences additional anxiety because he or she has been unable to handle the situation alone, especially because the client knows that the phobia is irrational.

✽ *(continued)*
Implementation

Nursing Interventions	Rationale
Teach the client and his or her family or significant others about phobic reactions. Dispel any myths that may be troubling the client. For example, it is common for others to tell the phobic individual that all they have to do is face up to [the phobic situation] and they will get over it.	The client and his or her family or significant others may have little or no knowledge related to phobias or anxiety. Myths often are a barrier to the success of treatment. Support from the client's significant others can enhance the chances of successful and lasting treatment.
Reassure the client that he or she can learn to decrease the anxiety and gain control over the anxiety attacks.	The client can feel greater self-confidence, which will enhance chances for success.
Reassure the client that he or she will not be forced to confront the phobic situation until he or she is prepared to do so.	The client can feel more comfortable knowing he or she will not be asked to confront a situation that produces extreme anxiety until equipped to handle it.
Assist the client to distinguish between the phobic trigger and those problems related to avoidance behaviors that are interfering with his or her daily life.	The phobic situation has usually existed for some time before the client seeks treatment. The client may have been experiencing such pervasive anxiety that he or she is unclear about the problem.
Instruct the client in progressive relaxation techniques. These include deep breathing, focusing on specific muscles to decrease tenseness, and imagining himself or herself in a quiet, peaceful place.	The client must have the ability to decrease his or her anxiety to participate in treatment.
Encourage the client to practice relaxation until he or she is comfortable and successful.	The client must feel well prepared with the techniques to be able to use them when anxiety does occur.
Explain the steps of the procedure thoroughly to the client (see below).	Unknown situations can produce added anxiety.
Reassure the client that you will allow him or her as much time as needed at each step.	This will increase the client's sense of control and help lessen his or her anxiety.
Have the client develop a hierarchy of situations that relate to the phobia. Have the client rank the list in order from the least anxiety producing to the most anxiety producing situation for the client. (For example, a client with a phobia of dogs might rank situations beginning with looking at a picture of a dog, up to actually petting a dog.)	Creating a hierarchy is the beginning step of systematic desensitization.
Begin with the least anxiety-producing situation. Have the client use progressive relaxation in that situation until he or she is able to decrease the anxiety. When the client is comfortable with that situation, go to the next item on the list, and repeat the procedure.	The client will be most successful initially in the least anxiety-producing situation. The client will be unable to progress to more difficult situations until he or she can master the current one.

✳ *(continued)*
Implementation

Nursing Interventions	Rationale
If the client becomes excessively anxious or begins to feel out of control, return to the former step with which the client was comfortable and successful, and proceed slowly to subsequent steps.	Staying too long with a step with which the client feels out of control will undermine his or her confidence. It is important for the client to feel confident in his or her ability to manage the anxiety.
Give positive feedback for the client's efforts at each step. Convey the idea that he or she is succeeding at each step. Avoid equating success only with mastery of the entire process.	This increases the number of times the client can experience success and gain self-confidence, which enhances the overall chance for mastery of the anxiety.
Discuss the previously identified avoidance behaviors with the client to determine if there is a corresponding decrease as the client progresses in systematic desensitization.	Avoidance behaviors should decrease as the client successfully copes with the phobia and resulting anxiety.
It may be necessary to address specific avoidance behavior(s) if any persist after the client has completed the desensitizing process.	Avoidance behaviors that interfere with daily life will require further work if they have not been eliminated with mastery over the phobic situation. It also is possible that the client is experiencing difficulties that were not related to the phobic situation as he or she believed.

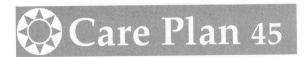

Obsessive Thoughts or Compulsive Behavior

Obsessive thoughts are persistent thoughts that usually are troublesome to the client. *Compulsions* are ritualistic behaviors, usually repetitive in nature, and may be attempts to contain or diminish obsessive thoughts. Obsessive thoughts and compulsive behaviors are a means of dealing with excessive anxiety; the client engages in repetitive acts to control anxiety and deal with the obsessive thoughts. Compulsive behavior is a defense that is perceived by the client as necessary to protect himself or herself from anxiety or impulses that are unacceptable (Simoni, 1991).

In early treatment do not prevent the client from performing compulsive acts. Intervention should be limited at first to harmful or dangerous situations or practices. Drawing undue attention to or attempting to forbid compulsive behaviors increases the client's anxiety. Initial nursing care should allow the client to be undisturbed in performing his or her rituals (unless they are harmful). Nursing care should reduce anxiety and build self-esteem.

The particular obsessive thoughts and compulsive behaviors may be symbolic of the client's anxieties or conflicts. Many obsessive thoughts are religious or sexual in nature. The obsessive thoughts also may be destructive or delusional. (The client may be obsessed with the thought of killing his or her significant other, may be convinced that he has cancer, or may be convinced that she is pregnant.) The client also may be placing unrealistic rigid standards on himself or herself and others. Many people have some obsessive thoughts or compulsive behaviors without seeking treatment. However, clients come to treatment when the thoughts or behaviors impede or inhibit their overall ability to function.

Nursing Diagnoses Addressed in this Care Plan

Anxiety
Ineffective Individual Coping

Related Nursing Diagnoses

Altered Health Maintenance
Altered Thought Processes
High Risk for Injury
High Risk for Trauma
Ineffective Denial
Impaired Social Interaction

Nursing Diagnosis

Anxiety (9.3.1)

A vague uneasy feeling whose source is often nonspecific or unknown to the individual.

Assessment Data

Defining Characteristics	• Obsessive thoughts (may be destructive or delusional)
	• Compulsive, ritualistic behavior (eg, repeated hand washing)
	• Self-mutilation or other physical problems (such as damage to skin from excessive washing)
	• Overemphasis on cleanliness and neatness
	• Fears
	• Guilt feelings
	• Denial of feelings

Related Factors	• Aggression toward others
	• Rigidity or extremely high standards
	• Unmet needs
	• Lack of control over events
	• Self-destructive behavior

Expected Outcomes

Initial	*The client will:*
	• Be free of self-inflicted harm
	• Demonstrate decreased anxiety, fears, guilt, rumination, or aggressive behavior

Discharge	*The client will:*
	• Verbalize feelings of fear, guilt, anxiety, and so forth
	• Express feelings nonverbally in a safe manner

Therapeutic Aims

- Provide a safe environment.
- Promote expression of feelings.
- Alleviate anxiety, fear, and guilt.

Implementation

Nursing Interventions	Rationale
The client may need to be secluded or restrained or otherwise protected from self-mutilation or harm.	The client's physical safety, health, and well-being are priorities.
Try to substitute a physically safe behavior for harmful practices, even if the new behavior is compulsive or ritualistic. If the client is cutting himself or herself, direct him or her toward tearing paper.	Substitute behaviors may satisfy the client's need for compulsive behaviors but protect the client's safety and provide a transition toward decreasing these behaviors.
If the client's behaviors are not harmful, try not to call attention to the compulsive acts initially.	Preventing or attending to compulsive acts may increase the client's anxiety.
Encourage the client to verbally identify his or her concerns, life stresses, anxieties, fears, and so forth.	Addressing feelings directly may help diminish the client's anxiety and thus diminish obsessive thoughts, rumination, and compulsive acts.
Encourage the client to express his or her feelings in ways that are acceptable to the client (through talking, crying, physical activities, and so forth).	The client may be uncomfortable with some ways of expressing emotions or find them unacceptable initially.
If the client is ruminating (eg, on his or her worthlessness), acknowledge the client's feelings, but then try to redirect the interaction in a positive direction. Disucss the client's specific perceptions of his or her feelings and possible ways to deal with these feelings. If the client continues to ruminate, withdraw your attention at that time. (Tell the client that you will discuss other things, and state when you will return or when you will be available for interaction again.)	Withdrawing attention may help decrease rumination by not reinforcing that behavior. Redirecting the client to focus directly on emotions may help diminish anxiety and rumination.
If the client has delusional fears, do not argue with him or her about the logic of these fears. Acknowledge the client's feelings, interject reality briefly (like "Your tests show that you are not pregnant"), and move on to a concrete subject for conversation.	Delusions are intense (though false) beliefs; often the client can give seemingly logical support for them. Arguing about delusions can reinforce delusional beliefs and may be futile. Providing a concrete subject for interactions can reinforce reality for the client.
At first, allot specific time periods, such as 10 minutes every hour, when the client can focus on his or her obsessive thoughts or ritualistic behaviors. Require the client to attend to other feelings, problems, or activities for the rest of the hour. Gradually decrease the time allowed (for example, from 10 minutes per hour to 10 minutes every 2 hours).	Setting time limits recognizes the significance of these thoughts and acts in the client's life but still encourages him or her to focus on other feelings or problems.

Nursing Diagnosis

Ineffective Individual Coping (5.1.1.1)

Impairment of adaptive behaviors and problem-solving abilities of a person in meeting life's demands and roles.

Assessment Data

Defining Characteristics	

- Ambivalence regarding decisions or choices
- Disturbances in normal functioning due to obsessive thoughts or compulsive behaviors (loss of job, loss of or alienation of family members, and so forth)
- Inability to tolerate deviations from standards
- Rumination
- Low self-esteem
- Feelings of worthlessness
- Lack of insight
- Difficulty or slowness completing daily living activities because of ritualistic behavior

Related Factors

- Inadequate support system
- Financial, relationship, or employment problems
- Unanticipated or undesired life or role changes
- Self-destructive behavior

Expected Outcomes

Initial

The client will:

- Identify stresses, anxieties, and conflicts
- Verbalize realistic self-evaluation
- Establish adequate nutrition, hydration, and elimination
- Establish a balance of rest, sleep, and activity
- Identify alternative methods of dealing with stress and anxiety
- Complete daily routine activities

Discharge

The client will:

- Demonstrate a decrease in obsessive thoughts or ritualistic behaviors to a level at which the client can function independently
- Demonstrate alternative ways of dealing with stress, anxiety, and life situations
- Maintain adequate physiologic functioning
- Verbalize knowledge of illness, treatment plan, and safe use of medications, if any
- Verbalize plans to continue with therapy, if indicated

Therapeutic Aims

- Decrease or eliminate obsessive thoughts or compulsive behaviors.
- Promote self-esteem.
- Promote independent functioning.
- Facilitate physiologic functioning.

※
Implementation

Nursing Interventions	Rationale
Observe the client's eating, drinking, and elimination patterns, and assist the client as necessary.	The client may be unaware of physical needs or may ignore feelings of hunger, thirst, the urge to defecate, and so forth.
Assess and monitor the client's sleep patterns, and prepare him or her for bedtime by decreasing stimuli, giving a backrub, and other comfort measures or medications.	Limiting noise and other stimuli will encourage rest and sleep. Comfort measures and sleeping medications will enhance the client's ability to relax and sleep.
You may need to allow extra time, or the client may need to be verbally directed to accomplish activities of daily living (personal hygiene, preparation for sleep, and so forth).	The client's thoughts or ritualistic behaviors may interfere with or lengthen the time necessary to perform tasks.
As the client's anxiety decreases (by identifying and expressing feelings) and as a trust relationship builds, talk with the client about his or her thoughts and behavior and about the client's feelings regarding them. Help the client identify alternative behaviors and methods for dealing with anxiety.	The client may need to learn ways to manage anxiety so he or she can deal with it directly. This will increase his or her confidence in managing anxiety and other feelings.
Encourage the client to attempt to gradually decrease the frequency of compulsive behaviors. The client (or staff members) may identify a baseline frequency and then keep a record of the decrease.	Gradually reducing the frequency of compulsive behaviors and replacing them with new behaviors will minimize the client's anxiety in the transition and encourage success and independence.
Convey honest interest and concern for the client. (Do not flatter the client or be otherwise dishonest.)	Your presence and interest in the client conveys your acceptance of the client as a worthwhile person. Clients with low self-esteem do not benefit from flattery or undue praise. Sincere and genuine praise that the client has earned can foster self-esteem.
Support the client for participation in activities, treatment, and interactions. Provide opportunities for the client to participate in activities that are easily accomplished or enjoyed by the client.	The client may be limited in his or her ability to deal with complex tasks, activities, or stimuli and in his or her ability to relate to others. Activities that the client can accomplish and enjoy can enhance self-esteem.
Teach the client and his or her family or significant others about the client's illness, treatment, or medications, if any.	The client and his or her family or significant others may have little or no knowledge regarding the client's illness, treatment, or medications.
Encourage the client to participate in follow-up therapy, if indicated.	Clients often experience long-term difficulties in dealing with obsessive thoughts.

Post-Traumatic Behavior

Post-traumatic behavior occurs as a response to the experience of an unusually traumatic event or situation, one that would be expected to produce significant distress in most people. The traumatic event may be due to natural causes or to human activity; distress following human activity seems to be more severe than that following a natural event. Experiences that evoke post-traumatic behavior include violent crimes, such as rape or assault, combat experiences, incest or other abuse, earthquakes, floods, hurricanes, or other natural disasters, and major accidents, injuries, and so forth (Petit, 1991). Post-traumatic behavior has been described in terms of specific experiences such as *rape trauma syndrome* following a rape; *post-traumatic stress disorder* (PTSD), usually following a combat experience in the Vietnam War (Gerlock, 1991); or as part of the *survivor theory* (Mejo, 1990), which is based on the behaviors of the survivors of the Hiroshima and Nagasaki bombings and of concentration camps in World War II.

Behavior following a trauma resembles a grief reaction, and much of the post-traumatic behavior observed in hospital settings can be described in terms of delayed grief or a failure to grieve. As in grief, there is a period of shock or denial immediately following the trauma. People who exhibit delayed post-traumatic behaviors (beginning 6 months or more after the event) or who experience chronic post-traumatic behaviors (continuing for more than 6 months) seem to have prolonged this initial phase of denial and have repressed or supressed feelings evoked by the original event. This delay in grieving can last many years or even be lifelong. These people exhibit symptoms that include reexperiencing the event through recurrent dreams, memories, or behaviors (flashbacks) and decreased emotional involvement with others or the world. Other distressing symptoms include guilt, sleep disturbances, and difficulty concentrating (Petit, 1991). Anger often is a dominant symptom in post-traumatic behavior; it may occur overtly as violent or abusive behavior or covertly, internalized and manifested as depression. This, too, can be seen as a delay in the grieving process. A major focus of nursing interventions in working with clients who exhibit post-traumatic behavior is facilitation of the grief process.

PTSD, manifested by Vietnam veterans, may occur in as many as half of the men who had direct combat experience and may include many of the symptoms described previously. A number of factors have been identified as contributing to the development of PTSD in Vietnam veterans, including the guerilla nature of the war, the social ostracism of the veterans, the lack of a hero's welcome, and the sociopolitical climate of the United States on their return home. Other factors discussed in the development of PTSD include substance use, minority status, level and duration of combat experience, age (in combat), educational level, and support (or lack of) from significant others on return from combat and in present life (Mejo, 1990).

Some women who have been raped experience rape trauma syndrome, which also may be prolonged or delayed. It has been described as consisting of three stages: *acute, outward adjustment,* and *reorganization* (during which denial, fear, anger, guilt, and depression may occur). Rape victims also may experience flashbacks or dreams of the event, sleep disturbances, emotional withdrawal, and other symptoms of post-traumatic behavior. As in PTSD, factors involved in the responses of rape victims include presence or absence or emotional support, age (at the time of the rape), and educational level (Lenox and Gannon, 1983).

Rape victims, Vietnam veterans, incest survivors, and other trauma survivors have experienced events that would be expected to cause a significant distress response in a normal, healthy person. Their progression through the grief and related feelings following such an event are influenced by the amount of understanding and support they receive from others, both in personal relationships and in encounters with professionals. Unfortunately, too often those others are frightened by their own feelings (for example, survivors of trauma remind others that such experiences can happen to them, too, thus threatening their feelings of safety, well-being, and control). Others may lack understanding of the event itself, and do not offer the support that is needed. Therefore, an important primary nursing intervention is to provide education to the client, to his or her family or significant others, and to the community to dispel myths about the nature of such experiences as rape, incest, and combat and about the responses and grief that follow them.

Nursing Diagnoses Addressed in this Care Plan

Post-Trauma Response
High Risk for Violence: Self-Directed or Directed at Others

Related Nursing Diagnoses

Dysfunctional Grieving
Rape Trauma Syndrome
Anxiety
Ineffective Individual Coping
Sleep Pattern Disturbance
Altered Health Maintenance
Sexual Dysfunction
Social Isolation
Self-Esteem Disturbance
Altered Role Performance

Nursing Diagnosis	*Post-Trauma Response (9.2.3)*

The state of an individual experiencing a sustained painful response to an overwhelming traumatic event(s).

Assessment Data

Defining Characteristics

- Flashbacks or reexperiencing the traumatic event(s)
- Nightmares or recurrent dreams of the event or other trauma
- Sleep disturbances (eg, insomnia, early awakening, crying out in sleep)
- Depression
- Denial of feelings or emotional numbness
- Projection of feelings
- Difficulty in expressing feelings
- Anger (may not be overt)
- Guilt or remorse
- Low self-esteem
- Frustration and irritability
- Anxiety, panic, or separation anxiety
- Fears—may be displaced or generalized (as in fear of men in rape victims)
- Decreased concentration
- Difficulty expressing love or empathy
- Difficulty experiencing pleasure
- Difficulty with interpersonal relationships, marital problems, divorce
- Abuse in relationships
- Sexual problems
- Substance use
- Employment problems
- Physical symptoms

Related Factors

- History of experiencing traumatic event(s)
- Preexisting emotional problems
- Limited community resources

Expected Outcomes

Initial

The client will:

- Identify the traumatic event
- Demonstrate decreased physical symptoms
- Verbalize need to grieve loss(es)
- Establish an adequate balance of rest, sleep, and activity
- Identify strengths and weaknesses realistically
- Demonstrate decreased anxiety, fear, guilt, and so forth
- Participate in treatment program

Discharge

The client will:

- Begin the grieving process
- Express feelings directly and openly in nondestructive ways
- Demonstrate an increased ability to cope with stress

- Eliminate substance use
- Demonstrate initial integration of the traumatic experience into his or her life outside the hospital

Discharge	

- Identify support system in the community
- Verbalize realistic future plans, including plans for follow-up or ongoing therapy, if indicated
- Verbalize knowledge of illness, treatment plan, or safe use of medications, if any

✸ Therapeutic Aims

- Build a trust relationship.
- Facilitate progress through the grief process.
- Promote self-esteem.
- Decrease fears, guilt, and anxiety.
- Facilitate communication.

✸ Implementation

Nursing Interventions	Rationale
When you approach the client, be nonthreatening and professional.	The client may have difficulty with authority figures (PTSD client), may fear men (rape survivor), or may feel threatened easily.
Initially, assign the same staff members to the client if possible; try to respect the client's feelings regarding gender issues at this time. Gradually increase the number and variety (including gender) of staff members interacting with the client.	Limiting the number of staff members who interact with the client at first will facilitate familiarity and trust. The client may have strong feelings of fear or mistrust about working with male staff members (if a rape survivor) or female staff members (if a PTSD client). These feelings may have been reinforced in previous encounters with professionals and in any case interfere with the therapeutic relationship if not respected.
Educate yourself and other staff members about the client's experience and about post-traumatic behavior.	Learning about the client's experience will help dispel myths and prepare you for both the client's feelings and the details of his or her experience.
Examine and remain aware of your own feelings regarding both the client's traumatic experience and his or her feelings and behavior at the present time. Talk with other staff members to ventilate and work through your feelings.	Events such as combat experiences and sexual assault engender strong feelings in others and may be quite threatening. These feelings may be related to issues of sexuality or morality, safety, or well-being. You may be reminded of a related experience or of your own vulnerability. It is essential that you remain aware of your feelings so that you do not unconsciously project feelings, avoid issues, or be otherwise nontherapeutic with the client.
Remain nonjudgmental in your interactions with the client.	It is important not to reinforce blame that the client may have internalized related to his or her experience.
Be consistent with the client; convey acceptance of him or her as a person while setting and maintaining limits regarding behaviors.	The client may test limits or the therapeutic relationship. Problems with acceptance, trust, or authority often occur with post-traumatic behavior.

✳ (continued)
Implementation

Nursing Interventions	Rationale
Assess the client's history of chemical use (information from significant others might be helpful).	Clients often have a history of chemical dependence or presently use chemicals to help repress (or release) emotions.
Be aware of the client's use or abuse of chemicals while hospitalized. Determine and enforce consequences for this behavior; it may be helpful to allow the client or client group to have input into these decisions.	Chemical use in the hospital undermines therapy and limits and may endanger the client's health. Allowing input from the client or group may help minimize power struggles and the use of chemicals as a factor in such struggles.
If chemical use is a major problem for the client, referral to a chemical dependence treatment program may be appropriate.	The problem of chemical use must be dealt with directly, because it may affect all other areas of the client's life and behaviors.
Encourage the client to talk about his or her experience(s); be accepting and nonjudgmental of the client's accounts and perceptions.	Retelling the experience can help the client to identify the reality of what has happened and help to identify and work through related feelings.
Encourage the client to express his or her feelings through talking, writing, crying, or other ways in which the client is comfortable.	Identification and expression of feelings is central to the grieving process.
Especially encourage the expression of anger, guilt, and rage.	In general these feelings often are dominant in clients who have experienced trauma. Specifically, they may feel survivor's guilt that they have survived when others did not or guilt about the behavior they undertook to survive (killing others in combat, enduring a rape).
Teach the client and his or her family or significant others about post-traumatic behavior and treatment.	The client and his or her family or significant others may have little or no knowledge of post-traumatic behavior. This knowledge may help alleviate anxiety or guilt and may increase hope for recovery.
As tolerated, encourage the client to share his or her feelings and experiences in group therapy, in a support group related to post-trauma, or with other clients informally.	The client needs to know that his or her feelings are acceptable to others and can be shared. Peer or support groups can offer understanding, support, and the opportunity for sharing experiences.
Give the client positive feedback for expressing feelings and sharing experiences. Remain nonjudgmental toward the client.	The client may feel that he or she is burdening others with his or her problems. It is important not to reinforce the client's internalized blame.
If the client has a religious or spiritual orientation, referral to a member of the clergy or a chaplain may be appropriate.	Guilt and forgiveness often are religious or spiritual issues for the client.
Encourage the client to make realistic plans for life outside the hospital and to make appropriate changes integrating his or her traumatic experience.	Integrating traumatic experiences and making future plans are important resolution steps in the grief process.

(continued)
Implementation

Nursing Interventions	Rationale
Provide education about and practice with stress reduction or stress management techniques, relaxation techniques, assertiveness training, self-defense training (for rape survivors), and development of other skills as appropriate.	The client's traumatic experience may have resulted in a loss of self-confidence or sense of safety or a decreased ability to deal with stress.
Provide social skills and leisure time counseling, or refer the client to a recreational therapist as appropriate.	Social isolation and lack of interest in recreational activities are common problems for clients with post-traumatic behavior.
Talk with the client about employment, including his or her history of employment, job-related stress, problems with authority figures, and so forth. Refer the client to vocational services as needed.	Problems with employment frequently occur in clients with post-traumatic behavior.
Help the client arrange for follow-up therapy as needed. Referral to a therapist or groups that specialize in PTSD, rape or incest survival, sexual issues, and so forth may be indicated.	Recovering from trauma may be a long-term process, even though the client no longer needs to be hospitalized. Follow-up therapy can offer continuing support in the client's recovery.

Nursing Diagnosis	*High Risk for Violence: Self-Directed or Directed at Others (9.2.2)* *A state in which an individual experiences behaviors that can be physically harmful either to the self or others.*

Risk Factors

- Anger or rage (may be persistent, generalized, or sporadic; may not be overt)
- Hyperalertness, feelings of being endangered (may keep weapons)
- Paranoid behavior, suspiciousness, mistrust of others
- Abuse in relationships, especially with significant others (spouse or partner or children)
- Hostility
- Verbal abuse
- Violence, aggressive behavior
- Suicidal ideation or behavior
- Homicidal ideation
- Legal problems, history of criminal activity
- Difficulty with authority figures
- Substance use
- Lack of impulse control
- Thrill-seeking behavior

Expected Outcomes

Initial	*The client will:*
	• Not harm self or others
	• Refrain from hostile, abusive, or violent behavior
Discharge	*The client will:*
	• Express feelings in a safe manner

Therapeutic Aims

- Protect the client and others from injury.
- Provide a safe environment.
- Assist client to use internal control.

Implementation

Nursing Interventions	Rationale
Provide a safe environment for the client. Remove items that can be used to harm himself or herself or others. Ask the client if he or she has a weapon; it may be necessary to search the client or his or her belongings with the client present.	The client's safety and the safety of others is a priority. The client may be mistrustful of others or feel so threatened that he or she keeps concealed weapons.
Encourage the client to engage in physical exercise or to substitute safe physical activities for aggressive behaviors (eg, punching bag, lifting weights).	Physical activity can help release tension in a nondestructive manner. The client may be able to ventilate aggression by using substitute behaviors as a step in learning to express feelings verbally.
Assure the client that staff members will provide control if he or she is not able to use internal controls effectively. Encourage the client to talk about feelings when he or she is not agitated.	The client may feel overwhelmed by the intensity of his or her feelings and may fear loss of control if he or she releases those feelings.
Be firm and consistent in setting and maintaining limits, enforcing hospital and unit policies, and so forth. Do not take the client's hostility personally. Protect other clients from abusive behaviors.	Clients who exhibit post-traumatic behavior may displace or act out anger in destructive ways.
See Care Plan 52: Aggressive Behavior.	
Talk with the client and his or her family or significant others about abusive behavior. It may be necessary to obtain this information from significant others if the client is not able or willing to discuss abuse issues.	Abusive behavior occurs frequently in the post-traumatic client's relationships. The client may be too angry, overwhelmed, or ashamed to deal with these issues initially, but the client's significant others need attention immediately.
Refer the client's family or significant others to a therapist, treatment center, or appropriate support groups. It may be necessary for the client's significant others to participate without the client initially.	Abuse in interpersonal relationships often requires treatment for longer periods, beyond the length of the client's hospitalization. The client's significant others can begin therapy even if he or she is not ready or able to participate immediately.
See Care Plan 53: Sexual, Emotional, or Physical Abuse.	

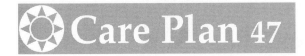

Adjustment Disorders in Adults

An *adjustment disorder* involves a maladaptive reaction to an identified psychosocial stressor. The problem occurs within 3 months after the onset of the stressor but does not persist for longer than 6 months. The reaction is expected to remit when the stressor is no longer present or when the client reaches a new level of adaptation (DSM-III-R, 1987).

Adjustment disorders can occur at any age and can be related to developmental milestones, such as graduation from high school or college, beginning a career, getting married, retiring, and so forth. Not all stressors are "negative" life events. In fact, some are generally perceived as happy occasions and many have been awaited with great anticipation, such as a promotion or the birth of a child.

Clients who are experiencing adjustment disorders typically cope with day-to-day life effectively, provided there are no major changes in their roles or in the expectations placed on them. However, major life changes or the culmination of several smaller stressors result in the client's inability to deal with the stress or changes.

The severity of the client's adjustment disorder may not be proportional to the observed severity of the stressor and may be described as excessive. Also, the client experiences an impairment in his or her social or occupational functioning.

Adjustment disorders are further specified according to the primary feature or predominant manifestation. Examples are adjustment disorders with anxious mood, depressed mood, physical complaints, withdrawal, and so forth. Although some of the primary behaviors or complaints are similar to other diagnoses, they are not severe enough to be diagnosed as anxiety, depression, or other such disorders.

Nursing Diagnosis Addressed in this Care Plan

Ineffective Individual Coping

Related Nursing Diagnoses

Self-Esteem Disturbance
Altered Role Performance
Anxiety

Nursing Diagnosis

Ineffective Individual Coping (5.1.1.1)

Impairment of adaptive behaviors and problem-solving abilities of a person in meeting life's demands and roles.

Assessment Data

Defining Characteristics	• Feelings of inadequacy or being overwhelmed • Difficulty with problem solving • Loss of control over life situation • Mild mood alterations • Low self-esttem • Emotional reactions that are disproportional to life stressors • Difficulty fulfilling occupational or social role expectations
Related Factors	• History of successful coping skills • Imminent or recent change in life status • Occurrence of a significant life event within the past 3 months

Expected Outcomes

Initial	*The client will:* • Express relief of feelings of anxiety, fear, or helplessness • Identify difficulties of current life change or stress • Identify personal strengths
Discharge	*The client will:* • Demonstrate the ability to solve problems effectively • Demonstrate successful resolution of the current crisis • Demonstrate integration of the change or new situation into day-to-day functioning • Verbalize feelings of self-worth

Therapeutic Aims

• Identification of feelings and thoughts about life change or crisis.
• Promote return of self-confidence.
• Reestablish and mobilize successful coping skills.

Implementation

Nursing Interventions	Rationale
Assist the client to identify aspects of the change that he or she likes and the aspects that he or she dislikes.	The client may need help viewing the change objectively as having positive and negative aspects. Identifying dislikes may be particularly important if the change is supposed to be a happy one, such as retirement.

✪ (continued)
Implementation

Nursing Interventions	Rationale
Have the client make a written list of the aspects identified.	A written list may provide a more concrete way of specifying positive and negative aspects, when the client can see them. Also, once a negative aspect is written, the client can move on to identify others, rather than getting stuck and dwelling on one particular aspect.
Explore with the client things he or she might do to view the change more constructively, such as "It sounds like you have more time with your son at college. What are some of the things you have always wanted to do if only you had the time?"	Many times the client is focused on the change or loss that is occurring. Exploration of positive alternatives can help broaden the client's perspective.
Avoid giving the client specific suggestions, such as "Wouldn't you like to . . . " or "How about trying . . . . "	If the client is having negative feelings about the change, he or she will probably respond to your suggestions with reasons why they won't work. Allowing the client to develop the suggestions puts the responsibility for ideas on the client, not you.
Encourage the client to express feelings openly. Help the client clarify vague feelings. For example, if the client feels overwhelmed, ask if he or she is scared, angry, and so forth.	Outward expression of feelings is a way of acknowledging the feelings and beginning to deal with them. The more specific and descriptive the feelings, the easier it is for the client to accept them and deal with them.
Give positive feedback for expressing feelings, particularly negative ones.	Your acceptance helps the client feel better about his or her feelings. It helps the client see that negative feelings are normal, not necessarily "good" or "bad."
Help the client identify his or her areas of strengths and areas of difficulty in dealing with problems or changes. Have the client make written lists.	The client may have difficulty recognizing strengths. Written lists provide a concrete method for seeing assets.
Teach the client a step-by-step problem-solving process. For example, identify the problem, examine alternatives, weigh the pros and cons of each alternative, and select an approach.	The client may not know the steps of a logical, orderly process to solve problems.
Help the client evaluate the success or failure of a new approach. Encourage the client to select another approach if the previous one was unsuccessful.	The client needs to know that he or she can make a mistake without it being a tragedy. The client needs support to take a risk and try again.
Help the client identify past ways of coping or methods of problem solving that were successful for him or her. Encourage the client to apply past successful methods of coping to the present situation.	The client can build on his or her successful coping skills to deal with the current situation.
Encourage the client to work with his or her family or significant others to gain their help in dealing with aspects of the life change.	The client's family or significant others working with the client to deal with the change have a greater chance for success than the client working alone.

(continued)
Implementation

Nursing Interventions	Rationale
Help the client and his or her significant others to identify or anticipate future changes. Encourage them to talk about ways to deal with the change before it occurs when possible.	Once the client identifies that change is difficult for him or her, it is helpful to preplan for dealing with future changes.

Section Thirteen

Other Behaviors or Problems

The behaviors and disorders addressed in this section may occur in concert with each other and with various other problems in other sections of this *Manual*. Some of these problems may be manifested by a client who exhibits psychotic behavior or other psychiatric disorders; others may be found to be a client's primary problem or a significant contributing factor to that problem (such as abusive or paranoid behavior). These care plans are especially suited to choosing specific nursing diagnoses or elements of care for an individual care plan according to the client's specific behaviors and problems.

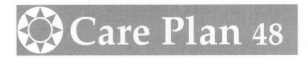

Sleep Disturbances

Sleep disturbances are a common complaint that can be associated with a variety of emotional or physical disorders or can occur as a primary symptom. Transient sleep disturbances can be a normal part of life sometimes associated with an identifiable psychosocial stressor. According to the DSM-III-R (1987), the diagnosis of a sleep disorder is made only if the problem exceeds 1 month in duration. Sleep disturbances are commonly seen in depressive disorders, in conditions that cause chronic pain, or as an effect of medication.

Sleep disorders can involve a decreased amount of sleep, sleeping at times other than the individual's desired time for sleep, or feeling unrefreshed when awakening, regardless of the amount of sleep obtained. It is common for people to attempt self-medication with prescription or over-the-counter drugs or alcohol. Though this may have a beneficial effect temporarily, prolonged use of these remedies may result in further sleep problems.

When sleep disturbances are related to an identifiable cause, such as depression or chronic arthritis pain, it is common for primary treatment to focus on relief of the depression or the pain. However, it can enhance the therapeutic effects of treatment to assist the client with other measures to facilitate restful sleep. These measures become even more important when an underlying cause cannot be identified or when that cause fails to respond fully to treatment.

Nursing Diagnosis Addressed in this Care Plan

Sleep Pattern Disturbance

Related Nursing Diagnoses

Fatigue
Anxiety
Knowledge Deficit (Specify)

Nursing Diagnosis	*Sleep Pattern Disturbance (6.2.1)*
	Disruption of sleep time causes discomfort or interferes with desired life-style.

Assessment Data

Defining Characteristics	• Amount of sleep
	• Unrefreshing sleep
	• Difficulty falling asleep
	• Periods of wakefulness during desired hours of sleep
	• Fragmented sleep pattern
	• Nightmares, night terrors
	• Preoccupation with not obtaining restful sleep

Related Factors	• Use of prescription or over-the-counter drugs or alcohol to obtain restful sleep
	• Excessive caffeine intake
	• Neurologic or physical problems or effects of medications that disrupt sleep pattern
	• Psychiatric problems or increased stress
	• Lack of an identifiable psychosocial stressor or physiologic reason for sleep disturbance

Expected Outcomes

Initial	*The client will:*
	• Eliminate or minimize factors that inhibit restful sleep
	• Identify factors that facilitate sleep
	• Establish regular hours for sleeping
	• Verbalize decreased anxiety about sleep difficulties

Discharge	*The client will:*
	• Fall asleep within 30 minutes after going to bed
	• Sleep an adequate number of hours (considering age, activity level, previous sleeping patterns) each night
	• Report feeling refreshed when awakening
	• Verbalize diminished fatigue, anxiety
	• Participate in or verbalize plans for treatment of related problems
	• Verbalize knowledge about sleep disturbance and effects of activity, medications, or chemicals on sleep

Therapeutic Aims

• Provide education about the effects of food, fluids, or chemicals on sleep.
• Promote development of a bedtime routine.
• Facilitate relaxation.
• Promote maintenance of successful sleep.

❂
Implementation

Nursing Interventions	Rationale
Provide accurate information about the effects of alcohol on sleep. The client should refrain from any alcohol intake until restful sleep patterns are well established.	Alcohol intake can produce initial drowsiness that the client may believe to be beneficial; however, when the effects wear off, fragmented sleep will result. The greater the alcohol intake, the more fragmented the sleep will be.
Substitute decaffeinated products for the client's coffee, tea, or soda intake. Discourage use of chocolate and cocoa products.	Chemical stimulants, such as caffeine, will interfere with sleep.
Provide a light bedtime snack for the client.	Hunger can awaken people if they sleep lightly or have difficulty sleeping.
Offer milk as a substitute for other bedtime beverages.	Milk products contain L-tryptophan, which is a natural sedative.
Avoid full meals at least 3 hours prior to bedtime. Foods also should be avoided if they cause gastric distress for the client.	After 3 hours the stomach has emptied, and the client will not feel full or uncomfortable. Any foods known to cause distress will interfere with the ability to maximize relaxation.
Limit fluid intake for 4 to 5 hours before bedtime.	Limiting fluid intake can eliminate awakening due to a full bladder.
If the client smokes, advise him or her to have the last cigarette at least 30 minutes before bedtime.	Nicotine is a stimulant.
Educate the client about the effects of sleeping medications. If the client has been using sleep medications regularly, it may be best to decrease the frequency and dosage of such medications gradually.	Sleep-inducing medications can become ineffective when used regularly. The client also may feel unrefreshed after sleep due to a decrease in rapid eye movement (REM) sleep that results from some medications. Abrupt cessation of sleep medications may increase the client's sleep difficulties.
Assist the client to determine the desired number of sleeping hours each night, then designate a time to retire and a regular time to rise to obtain that amount of sleep.	Regular hours help establish a routine. If the client waits until he or she "feels sleepy," sleep patterns may be erratic.
Encourage the client to avoid naps, unless indicated by age or physical condition.	Daytime napping interferes with the ability to sleep an adequate number of hours at night, unless there is a physiologic need for additional sleep.
Limit the client's attempts to sleep to his or her bed; that is, he or she should never try to fall asleep on the couch or in a recliner. Also, the client should only use the bed for sleep-related activities; that is, not have snacks, talk on the telephone, or work while in bed.	The client will establish the expectation that going to bed facilitates sleep.

✸ *(continued)*
Implementation

Nursing Interventions	Rationale
Provide an atmosphere conducive for sleeping (that is, dim or no lighting, quiet, a nondisruptive roommate or single room, and so forth).	External stimuli or disturbances interfere with sleep.
Encourage the client to maintain the bedtime routine for at least 2 weeks or longer if the sleep disturbance has been of extended duration.	It will take regular practice to establish a routine that will be effective in facilitating sleep.
Assist the client to identify factors that produce relaxation for him or her. These may be former habits that were effective, or the client may have to initiate new behaviors.	The client may have neglected to do things that have been purposefully relaxing or may never have had a need to purposefully relax before retiring.
Offer education and practice of progressive relaxation techniques. The use of a cassette tape relaxation program may be helpful.	Relaxation techniques frequently are helpful in facilitating sleep. These techniques need to be practiced to achieve full effectiveness.
Encourage the client to increase physical activity during waking hours, even though he or she may feel fatigued.	Physical activity is frequently avoided because the client may experience a lack of energy. Activity during the day will promote a healthy feeling of physical "tiredness," which can facilitate sleep.
Limit vigorous activity for 2 hours prior to bedtime.	The stimulating effects of physical activity last for several hours and interfere with efforts to relax prior to bedtime.
Suggest that the client experiment with a warm bath, soft music, reading, or other nonstimulating activities for relaxation.	The client may have to try several activities to determine which ones are effective for him or her.
If the client is unable to feel drowsy in 20 minutes after retiring, suggest that he or she get up and engage in 15 to 20 minutes of a quiet activity that is boring for the client (eg, reading, sorting papers, or knitting), then return to bed. This should be repeated until the client begins to feel ready for sleep.	Lying in bed for extended periods can increase the client's focus on and frustration with sleeping difficulties. Monotonous activities can facilitate drowsiness.
Encourage the client to practice these techniques consistently for a minimum of 2 weeks, even if there seems to be no benefit.	A minimum of 2 weeks may be needed to determine the effectiveness of newly initiated sleep-promoting activities.
Educate the client's family or significant others about sleep, relaxation, and the need for the previous routines. Enlist their support for the client's efforts.	The client's family or significant others may have little or no knowledge about these areas and may unwittingly interfere with the client's sleep.
Encourage the client to seek treatment for problems that may adversely affect sleep.	Sleep disturbances are associated with many physical and psychiatric problems and may not entirely be resolved without treatment of the associated problem.

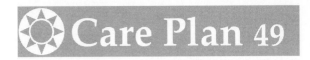

Withdrawn Behavior

Withdrawn behavior is a type of "disruption in relatedness" (Stuart and Sundeen, 1991) in which the client retreats from the external world. The degree of the client's withdrawal can range from mild to severe and represents a disruption in his or her relatedness to the self, others, or the environment.

Withdrawn behavior that is mild or transitory, such as a stunned or dazed period following trauma, is thought to be a self-protecting defense mechanism. This brief period of "emotional shock" allows the individual to rest and gather internal resources with which to cope with the trauma. Withdrawal of this nature is considered to be normal, healthy behavior because it can be expected and does not extend beyond a brief period.

Withdrawn behavior can be protracted or severe, however, and can interfere with the client's ability to function in activities of daily living, relationships, work, or other aspects of life. Seemingly total withdrawal, such as *catatonic stupor*, involves mutism, physical immobility, and no food or fluid intake. Without treatment, it can lead to coma and death. Severely withdrawn behavior often occurs in conjunction with other behaviors and problems addressed elsewhere in this manual, such as depression or suicidal behavior (see other care plans as appropriate).

Nursing Diagnoses Addressed in this Care Plan

Altered Thought Processes
Altered Health Maintenance
Ineffective Individual Coping

Related Nursing Diagnoses

Self-Care Deficits (Bathing/Hygiene, Feeding, Toileting, and/or Dressing/Grooming)
Impaired Physical Mobility
Impaired Verbal Communication
Social Isolation
Altered Nutrition: Less than Body Requirements
Sleep Pattern Disturbance
Constipation
High Risk for Injury
Self-Esteem Disturbance

Nursing Diagnosis

Altered Thought Processes (8.3)

A state in which an individual experiences a disruption in cognitive operations and activities.

Assessment Data

Defining Characteristics

- Psychologic immobility
- Hallucinations, delusions, other psychotic symptoms
- Inability to attend
- Lack of spontaneity
- Apathy
- Decreased or absent verbal communication
- Lack of awareness of surroundings
- Decreased motor activity or physical immobility
- Fetal position, eyes closed, teeth clenched, muscles rigid
- Anergy (lack of energy)
- Changes in body posture
- Fear
- Anxiety, panic
- Depression
- Muteness

Related Factors

- Post-traumatic behavior
- History of abuse
- Sleep disturbances
- Psychosis

Expected Outcomes

Initial

The client will:

- Demonstrate increased psychomotor activity
- Demonstrate decreased hallucinations, delusions, or other psychotic symptoms
- Begin to interact with others
- Participate in the treatment program

Discharge

The client will:

- Maintain contact with reality
- Interact with others nonverbally and verbally
- Demonstrate improvement in associated problems (eg, depression)
- Be free of hallucinations, delusions, or other psychotic symptoms
- Function at his or her optimal level

Therapeutic Aims

- Establish contact and rapport with the client.
- Promote a supportive and secure environment.
- Help the client maintain contact with the environment.

❀ *(continued)*
Therapeutic Aims

- Provide sensory stimulation.
- Promote increased physical activity.
- Promote interaction with others.

❀
Implementation

Nursing Interventions	Rationale
Assess the client's current level of functioning and communication, and begin to work with the client at that level.	To make contact with the client, you must begin where he or she is now.
Sit with the client for regularly scheduled periods of time.	Your physical presence conveys caring and acceptance to the client.
Tell the client your name and that you are there to be with him or her.	By telling the client you are there to be with him or her, you convey interest without making demands on the client.
Remain comfortable with periods of silence; do not overload the client with verbalization.	The client's ability to deal with verbal stimulation is impaired.
Use physical touch with the client (holding the client's hand, laying your hand on his or her shoulder) as the client tolerates. If the client responds to touch negatively, remove your hand at that time, but continue attempts to establish physical touch.	Your physical touch presents reality and conveys acceptance.
Talk with the client in a soft voice to express your caring and interest in him or her. If the client remains unresponsive, continue to do this with the positive expectation of a response from the client.	A soft voice can be comforting and nonthreatening. Expecting the client to respond increases the likelihood that he or she will do so.
Be alert for nonverbal cues from the client; the client's response usually will not be dramatic but rather very gradual and subtle (hand movement, eyes opening).	The client will probably be able to respond nonverbally before verbal communication is possible.
Give the client positive feedback for any response to your attempted interaction or to the external environment, and encourage him or her to continue to respond and reach out to others.	Your encouragement can foster the client's attempts to reestablish contact with reality.
Initially encourage or help the client to spend short periods of time with one other person. (For example, have the client sit with one person for 15 minutes of each hour during the day.)	At first, the client will deal more readily with minimal stimulation (eg, interactions for short time periods) and minimal changes (eg, interacting with the same staff member).
Ask the client to open his or her eyes and look at you when you are speaking to him or her.	You will facilitate reality contact and the client's ability to attend by encouraging eye contact.

✳ *(continued)*
Implementation

Nursing Interventions	Rationale
Use a radio, tape player, or television in the client's room to provide stimulation.	Media can provide stimulation during times that staff are not available to be with the client.
Avoid allowing the client to isolate himself or herself in a room alone for long periods of time.	Isolation will foster continued withdrawal.
Gradually increase the amount of time the client spends with others and the number of people with whom the client interacts.	A gradual increase in stimulation can foster the client's tolerance in a nonthreatening manner.
Assess the client's level of tolerance of stimuli; do not force too much stimulation too fast.	Increasing stimuli too rapidly could result in the client's further withdrawal.
Talk with the client as though he or she will respond: avoid rapidly chattering at the client, and continue to expect a response from him or her. Allow adequate time for the client to respond to you, either verbally or physically.	A positive expectation on your part increases the likelihood of the client's response. A withdrawn client may need more time to respond due to slowed thought processes.
Refer to other people, objects in the immediate environment, the weather, and so forth as you interact with the client.	You are furthering the client's contact with current reality and the external environment by calling the client's attention to things and people in his or her immediate environment.
At first, walk slowly with the client. Progress gradually from gross motor activity (walking, gestures with hands) to activities requiring fine motor skills (jigsaw puzzles, writing).	The client will be able to use gross motor skills first. Fine motor skills require more of the client's skill and attention.
Initially, encourage the client to express himself or herself nonverbally (eg, by writing or drawing).	Nonverbal communication usually is less threatening to the client than verbalization.
Encourage the client to verbalize about these nonverbal communications, and progress to more direct verbal communication as the client tolerates. Encourage the client then to express feelings as much as possible.	By talking about his or her writing or drawing rather than asking the client to speak directly about himself or herself or emotional issues, you minimize the perception of threat by the client. Gradually, direct verbal communication becomes tolerable to the client.
Interact with the client on a one-to-one basis initially, then help the client progress to small groups and to larger groups as tolerated.	Gradual introduction of other people minimizes the threat perceived by the client.
See Basic Concepts: Nurse–Client Interactions and other care plans as indicated.	Withdrawn behavior frequently is encountered with psychotic symptoms, depression, organic pathology, abuse, and post-traumatic behavior.
Teach the client and his or her significant others about withdrawn behavior, safe use of medications, and other disease process(es) if indicated.	The client and his or her significant others may have little or no knowledge of the client's illness, caregiving responsibilities, or safe use of medications.

Nursing Diagnosis

Altered Health Maintenance (6.4.2)

Inability to identify, manage, and/or seek out help to maintain health.

Assessment Data

Defining Characteristics	• Inattention to grooming and personal hygiene • Inadequate food or fluid intake; refusal to eat • Retention of urine or feces • Incontinence of urine or feces
Related Factors	• Decreased motor activity or physical immobility • Delusions, hallucinations, or other psychotic symptoms

Expected Outcomes

Initial	*The client will:* • Be physically safe • Establish adequate nutrition, hydration, and elimination • Establish an adequate balance of rest, sleep, and activity • Begin to perform activities of daily living and personal hygiene
Discharge	*The client will:* • Maintain adequate nutrition, hydration, and elimination • Maintain an adequate balance of rest, sleep, and activity • Demonstrate independence in performing activities of daily living, personal hygiene, and meeting other self-care needs

Therapeutic Aims

• Promote adequate food and fluid intake.
• Promote adequate elimination.
• Promote an adequate balance of rest, sleep, and activity.
• Promote independence in self-care activities.

Implementation

Nursing Interventions	Rationale
Remain with the client during meals.	Your physical presence can stimulate the client and promote reality contact.
Feed the client if necessary.	The client needs to reestablish nutritional intake, without intravenous or tube feeding therapy if possible.
Monitor the client's bowel elimination pattern.	Constipation may occur due to decreased food and fluid intake, decreased motor activity, or the client's inattention to elimination.

(continued)

Implementation

Nursing Interventions	Rationale
If the client is immobile or in the fetal position, provide passive range of motion exercises. Turn the client at least every 2 hours (more frequently would be better); provide skin care and observe for pressure areas and skin breakdown.	Range of motion exercises will maintain joint mobility and muscle tone. You must be alert to the prevention of physical complications due to immobility.
At first, walk slowly with the client. Progress gradually from gross motor activity (walking, gestures with hands) to activities requiring fine motor skills (jigsaw puzzles, writing).	The client will be able to use gross motor skills first. Fine motor skills are added later because they require more of the client's skill and attention.
Encourage the client to take gradually increasing levels of responsibility for hydration, nutrition, elimination, sleep, activity, and other self-care needs. See Care Plan 28: The Client Who Will Not Eat and Care Plan 48: Sleep Disturbances.	Initially, the client may be totally passive regarding basic physical and self-care needs, and you may need to provide total care. Asking the client to perform self-care as his or her general behavior improves will help the client assume more responsibility for himself or herself. Your positive expectations of the client will promote independence in these activities.

Nursing Diagnosis

Ineffective Individual Coping (5.1.1.1)

Impairment of adaptive behaviors and problem-solving abilities of a person in meeting life's demands and roles.

Assessment Data

Defining Characteristics	• Decreased or absent verbal communication • Lack of energy or spontaneity • Difficulty in interpersonal relationships • Apathy • Denial • Psychologic immobility • Fear • Anxiety, panic
Related Factors	• Depression • Low self-esteem • Social isolation • Post-traumatic behavior • History of having been abused • Psychosis

Expected Outcomes

Initial	*The client will:*
	• Demonstrate decreased psychotic symptoms
	• Participate in the treatment program
Discharge	*The client will:*
	• Maintain contact with reality
	• Demonstrate improvement in associated problems (eg, depression)
	• Demonstrate alternative methods of dealing with stress
	• Demonstrate or verbalize increased feelings of self-worth
	• Verbalize plans for continued therapy after discharge, if indicated

Therapeutic Aims

• Establish contact and rapport with the client.
• Promote interaction with others.
• Encourage expression of emotions.
• Prepare the client for discharge.

Implementation

Nursing Interventions	Rationale
Initially encourage or help the client spend short periods of time with one other person. (For example, have the client sit with one person for 15 minutes of each hour during the day.)	At first the client will deal more readily with minimal stimulation (eg, interactions for short time periods) and minimal changes (eg, interacting with the same staff member).
Initially encourage the client to express himself or herself nonverbally (eg, by writing or drawing).	Nonverbal communication usually is less threatening than verbalization.
Encourage the client to verbalize about these nonverbal communications and progress to more direct verbal communication as the client tolerates. Encourage the client then to express feelings as much as possible.	By talking about his or her writing or drawing rather than asking the client to speak directly about himself or herself or emotional issues, you minimize the perception of threat by the client. Gradually, direct verbal communication becomes tolerable to the client.
Interact on a one-to-one basis initially, then help the client progress to small groups, and to larger groups as tolerated.	Gradual introduction of other people minimizes the threat perceived by the client.
Teach the client about using the problem-solving process: identifying the problem, identifying and evaluating alternative solutions, choosing and implementing a solution, and evaluating its success.	The client may be unaware of a logical, step-by-step approach to problem resolution.
Give the client positive feedback for attempts to learn and use the problem-solving process.	Positive feedback encourages desired behavior.
Teach the client social skills, and encourage the client to practice these skills with staff members and other	Increasing the client's social skills and confidence can help decrease social isolation.

✳ *(continued)*
Implementation

Nursing Interventions	Rationale
clients. Give the client feedback regarding social interactions.	
Encourage the client to identify supportive people outside of the hospital environment and to develop those relationships. See Care Plan 2: Discharge Planning, Care Plan 5: Supporting the Caregiver, and Section 2: Chronic Mental Illness.	Increasing the client's support system may help prevent withdrawn behavior in the future.

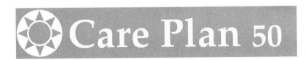

Paranoid Behavior

Paranoid behavior is characterized by lack of trust, suspicion, grandiose or persecutory delusions, hallucinations, and hostility. Paranoid ideation or behaviors may be rooted in an earlier experience of loss, pain, or disappointment that was denied by the client (unconsciously). The client uses the defense mechanism of projection to ascribe to others the feelings he or she has (as a result of those earlier experiences and denial) and attempts to protect himself or herself with suspiciousness or paranoia.

The client may have extremely low self-esteem or feel very powerless in his or her life and therefore compensates with delusions to bolster self-esteem or to decrease feelings of powerlessness. The delusions may be *grandiose* (the client believes he or she is a prominent religious or political figure), *destructive,* or *conspiratorial* (groups of people are watching, following, torturing, or controlling the client). This may involve *ideas of reference*—the client thinks that statements by others or certain events are caused by, controlled by, or specifically meant for him or her (eg, that a television program was produced to send the client a message).

Many paranoid clients have average or greater intelligence, and their delusional systems may be very complex and appear to be logical on some level. Different psychiatric disorders may include paranoid behavior, for example, paranoid schizophrenia, delusional disorder, psychotic depression, organic mental syndrome, sensory deprivation, sleep deprivation, and substance use. Caffeine, especially in large quantities, is suspected of contributing to anxiety or paranoid feelings (or both) in some clients.

Nursing Diagnoses Addressed in this Care Plan

Altered Thought Processes
Defensive Coping
Impaired Social Interaction
Ineffective Management of Therapeutic Regimen

Related Nursing Diagnoses

Altered Health Maintenance
Sleep Pattern Disturbance
High Risk for Violence: Self-Directed or Directed at Others
Anxiety

Nursing Diagnosis

Altered Thought Processes (8.3)

A state in which the individual experiences a disruption in cognitive operations and activities.

Assessment Data

Defining Characteristics	• Non–reality-based thinking • Disorganized, illogical thoughts • Impaired judgment • Impaired problem solving • Alterations in perceptions (hallucinations, ideas of reference) • Delusions, especially grandiose and persecutory
Related Factors	• Suicidal ideation • Rumination • Hostility, aggression, or homicidal ideation • Sensory deprivation or overload

Expected Outcomes

Initial	*The client will:* • Be free of self-inflicted harm • Not harm others • Demonstrate decreased psychotic symptoms: hallucinations, delusions, and so forth
Discharge	*The client will:* • Demonstrate reality-based thinking

Therapeutic Aims

• Decrease rumination, delusions, and other psychotic symptoms.
• Decrease hostile, aggressive, or suicidal ideation.
• Provide a safe environment for the client and others.

Implementation

Nursing Interventions	Rationale
Search the client's belongings carefully for weapons. If the client has a vehicle at the facility, consider that there may be weapons in it.	Paranoid clients may carry or conceal weapons.
Be calm and nonthreatening in all your approaches to the client. Approach the client with a quiet voice. Do not surprise the client.	If the client is feeling threatened, he or she may perceive any person or stimulus as a threat.
Observe the client closely for agitation, and decrease stimuli or move the client to a less stimulating area or seclusion area if indicated.	Whenever possible, it is best to intervene before the client loses control. The client's ability to deal with stimuli may be impaired.

⚙ *(continued)*
Implementation

Nursing Interventions	Rationale
Observe the client's interactions with his or her visitors. The lengths, number, or frequency of visits may need to be limited.	The client's ability to deal with other people may be impaired.
Do not argue with the client about delusions or ideas of reference, but interject reality when appropriate. Do not give any indication that you believe as the client does. (You might say "I don't see it that way.")	Introducing and reinforcing reality may help diminish psychotic symptoms.
Do not joke with the client regarding his or her beliefs.	The client's ability to understand and use abstractions, such as humor, is impaired.
Do not enter into political, religious, or other controversial discussions with the client.	Controversial discussions may precipitate arguments and increase hostility or aggression.
Encourage the client to discuss topics other than delusions such as home life, family, work, or school.	Concrete or familiar topics may be helpful in directing the client's attention to reality.
Do not allow the client to ruminate or to ramble about delusions; if the client refuses to discuss other topics, talk with the client about his or her feelings regarding the delusions, fears, and so forth. If the client refuses to do this, withdraw your attention, stating your intent to return.	It is important to minimize reinforcement of psychotic symptoms. Talking about feelings may help the client begin to deal with emotional issues. It must be clear to the client that you are rejecting his or her behavior, while accepting the client as a person.
If the client's delusions or ruminations are religious, a referral to the facility chaplain may be indicated (if the chaplain has special education or experience in this area).	Areas beyond nursing's scope require referral to appropriate people or agencies.
You may need to reassure the client that the origin of his or her fears is internal and that the fears are not based on external reality.	Reassurance of the safety of the environment may help diminish the client's fears.
Observe the client for expression of symptoms, and try to note environmental factors that precipitate or exacerbate symptoms. Then try to manipulate the environment to decrease or control these factors (noise level, the number of other people). See Care Plan 52: Aggressive Behavior.	Assessment provides information on which to base interventions. The client's ability to deal with stimuli or other people is impaired.

Nursing Diagnosis

Defensive Coping (5.1.1.1.2)

The state in which an individual repeatedly projects falsely positive self-evaluation based on a self-protective pattern that defends against underlying perceived threats to positive self-regard.

Assessment Data

Defining Characteristics	
	• Lack of trust
	• Low self-esteem
	• Suspicion
	• Fears
	• Feelings of powerlessness
	• Projection of blame on others
	• Rationalization
	• Superior attitude toward others

Related Factors	
	• Psychomotor disturbances, such as pacing
	• Ineffective interpersonal relationships

Expected Outcomes

Initial	
	The client will:
	• Demonstrate decreased suspicious behavior
	• Verbalize realistic feelings of self-worth

Discharge	
	The client will:
	• Verbalize realistic self-assessment
	• Demonstrate more direct, constructive ways to deal with stress, pain, loss, feelings of powerlessness, and so forth

Therapeutic Aims

- Decrease suspicion and fears.
- Promote self-esteem.
- Promote expression of feelings.

Implementation

Nursing Interventions	Rationale
Introduce yourself, and identify yourself as a staff member on your first approach to the client and thereafter if it is necessary to remind the client. Be nonthreatening in all your approaches to the client.	The client may be fearful, suspicious, or not in contact with reality.
Give the client clear information regarding his or her personal safety on the unit, confidentiality, identify and function of staff members, equipment, and so forth.	Giving matter-of-fact information will help to reassure and reorient the client.

�֎ *(continued)*
Implementation

Nursing Interventions	Rationale
If the client is pacing, walk with the client to converse, if necessary.	You must meet the client at his or her level of functioning. Your presence and willingness to walk with the client indicates interest and caring.
If the client is experiencing hallucinations or illusions, try to talk with him or her in an area of decreased stimuli.	The client is unable to deal with excess stimuli. External stimuli may be misperceived by the client.
Include the client in the formulation of a treatment plan when possible and appropriate.	Including the client may help build trust and decrease suspicion and feelings of powerlessness.
Do not be secretive with the client. Do not whisper to others in the presence of the client.	Secretive behavior will reinforce the client's suspicion.
Let the client see the notes that you take during interviews. Answer questions honestly with little or no hesitation.	Open and direct behavior on your part may help decrease suspicion.
Be aware of the client's presence around the nursing station when discussing the client (or other clients).	Because the client fears that others are discussing him or her, the client may listen to others' conversations, particularly staff members.
Assure the client that the hospital is a safe and protective environment and that the staff will help the client maintain control—that the client will not be "in trouble" for having feelings.	The client may fear that personal feelings may be overwhelming, that they are unacceptable, or that experiencing feelings may cause him or her to lose control.
Encourage the client to express feelings. Approach the client for interaction at least once per shift. (Determine the length of interactions by the client's tolerance.)	Expression of feelings can help the client identify, accept, and work through his or her feelings, even if these feelings are painful or otherwise uncomfortable for him or her.
When the client appears to be experiencing intense emotions, point this out to the client, and explain what leads you to think this (the situation, the client's facial expression, or fidgeting). Ask for the client's feelings and feedback regarding your observations.	The client may be unaware of emotions he or she is experiencing. Giving the client feedback in a nonthreatening way may help the client recognize emotional cues.
Encourage the client to verbalize or express feelings in other outward ways (such as physical activity) at the time the client is experiencing them.	Physical exercise and expression of feelings can help the client decrease tension and deal with feelings directly.
Use limited role playing with the client to elicit the expression of feelings. ("Pretend that I'm your [husband, wife, etc.]. What would you like to say to me right now?")	Role playing allows the client to explore feelings and try out new behaviors in a nonthreatening situations.
Demonstrate honest interest in and concern for the client; do not flatter the client or be otherwise dishonest.	Clients with low self-esteem do not benefit from flattery or undue praise. Unwarranted flattery can be recognized as dishonest and interpreted as belittling by the client.

❄ (continued)

Implementation

Nursing Interventions	Rationale
Support the client for his or her participation in activities, treatment, and interactions.	Positive feedback can reinforce desired behaviors.
Provide opportunities for the client to perform activities that are easily accomplished or that the client likes to do, and give support for their completion or success.	The client's abilities to deal with complex tasks may be impaired. Any task that the client can complete provides an opportunity for positive feedback to the client.

Nursing Diagnosis

Impaired Social Interaction (3.1.1)

The state in which an individual participates in an insufficient or excessive quantity or ineffective quality of social exchange.

❄ **Assessment Data**

Defining Characteristics

- Avoidance of others
- Limited or monosyllabic responses
- Discomfort around others
- Refusal to communicate with others

Related Factors

- Altered thought processes
- Mistrust of others
- Social isolation
- Hostile or aggressive behavior

❄ **Expected Outcomes**

Initial

The client will:

- Interact with staff
- Attend small group activities

Discharge

The client will:

- Communicate effectively with family or significant others

❄ **Therapeutic Aims**

- Promote participation in the milieu.
- Promote social interaction.

❄ **Implementation**

Nursing Interventions	Rationale
Initially, the staff may need to protect the client from the anger he or she may elicit from other clients by his or her paranoid or grandiose behavior.	The client may be hostile, abusive, or ridiculing to other clients who may not recognize this behavior as part of the client's illness.

❋ *(continued)*
Implementation

Nursing Interventions	Rationale
After the client's initial days on the unit, begin assigning different staff members to the client, and encourage other staff members to approach this client for brief interactions.	Limiting the number of new contacts initially will provide consistency and promote familiarity and trust. However, the number of people interacting with the client should increase as soon as possible to facilitate the client's abilities to communicate and the building of trust relationships with a variety of people.
Initially, help the client make individual contacts (with staff members and other clients); progress to small informal groups and then larger or more formal groups as the client can tolerate.	The client's ability to respond to others may be impaired. It is easier initially to interact with a single person, then progress to more difficult situations as the client's comfort and skills increase.
Observe the client's interactions with other clients, and encourage the development of appropriate relationships with others.	The client may be unaware of interpersonal dynamics. Feedback can help increase insight and give support to the client's efforts to develop relationships.
Give the client support for any interactions and attempts to interact with others.	Positive feedback may reinforce desired behaviors.
Try to involve the client in activities and tasks that are noncompetitive at first, and then help the client progress to larger and more competitive groups as tolerated.	Competition may reinforce the client's low self-esteem or hostile feelings.
Build the client's socialization skills through the previous interventions, leisure-time counseling, and through the use of and referral to other facility and community resources (occupational or recreational therapy, outpatient social clubs or groups).	The client's relationships with others in the community may be impaired and need to be reestablished.

Nursing Diagnosis

Ineffective Management of Therapeutic Regimen (Individuals) (5.2.1)

A pattern of regulating and integrating into daily living a program for treatment of illness and the sequelae of illness that is unsatisfactory for meeting specific health goals.

❋
Assessment Data

Defining Characteristics	• Reluctance or refusal to take medications
	• Inability to carry out responsibilities at work, home, and so forth
	• Inadequate attention to need for nutrition, rest, or sleep
	• Inability to carry out activities of daily living
Related Factors	• Mistrust and suspicion
	• Altered thought processes
	• Low neuroleptic levels

❋
Expected Outcomes

Initial	*The client will:*

- Ingest medications as given
- Establish an adequate balance of nutrition, hydration, and elimination
- Establish an adequate balance of rest, sleep, and activity

Discharge	*The client will:*

- Maintain adequately balanced physiologic functioning
- Comply with continuing therapy, including medications

❋
Therapeutic Aims

- Ensure ingestion of medications.
- Promote adequate nutrition, hydration, rest, and sleep.
- Promote completion of activities of daily living.

❋
Implementation

Nursing Interventions	Rationale
Give the liquid form of a medication when possible if the client is reluctant to take medication or if there is a question whether the client is ingesting medication.	Giving medication in liquid form helps to ensure that the client will ingest the medication. Note: Some liquid medications are irritable to oral membranes. Observe precautions in administration as indicated.
Tell the client you expect him or her to take medications as prescribed. Check the client's mouth if necessary after giving oral medications (have the client open mouth, raise tongue, and so forth). Point out to the client that the medications are a part of the treatment plan and that he or she is expected to take them.	It is important to know if the client is ingesting medications. Being direct with the client will help him or her know what is expected.
Be straightforward and specific with the client when giving information about his or her medications; tell the client the name of the medication and its desired effects (eg, "to help clear your thinking," or "to decrease your fears," or "to make the voices go away").	Clear information will help build trust and decrease suspicion.
Observe the client's eating, drinking, and elimination patterns, and assist the client as necessary. See Care Plan 28: The Client Who Will Not Eat.	The client may be unaware of physical needs or may ignore feelings of thirst, hunger, the urge to defecate, and so forth.
If the client is overactive or pacing, frequently offer small amounts of juice, milk, or finger foods that can be ingested while walking.	If the client is unable or unwilling to sit and eat, providing highly nutritious foods that require little effort to eat may be effective.
Assess and record the client's caffeine intake and limit it if necessary.	Caffeine consumption, especially in large amounts, may increase anxiety or paranoid feelings.
Assess and monitor the client's sleep patterns, and prepare him or her for bedtime by decreasing stimuli, giving a backrub (if tolerated), and administering comfort measures or medications. See Care Plan 48:	Limiting noise and other stimuli will encourage rest and sleep. Comfort measures and sleeping medications will enhance the client's ability to relax and sleep.

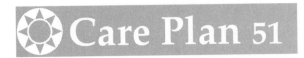
Care Plan 51

Hostile Behavior

Hostile behavior, or *hostility*, is characterized by verbal abuse, threatened aggressive or violent behavior, uncooperativeness, and in the therapeutic milieu, behaviors that have been defined as undesirable, unacceptable, or in violation of established limits. Much hostility is the result of feelings that are unacceptable to the client, which the client then projects on others, particularly staff members, other authority figures, or significant others. Often the client is afraid to express anger appropriately, fearing a loss of control. Also, hostile behavior may be the result of the client's inability to express other feelings directly, such as shame, fear, or anxiety.

Although anger and hostility often may be seen as similar, hostility may be considered different from anger in that hostility is characterized as destructive, while anger can be seen as constructive (Wilson and Kneisl, 1988). Remember that all anger in a client is not necessarily hostility and therefore may not be in need of control or modification. A client's anger may be justified and often is a healthy response to circumstances, feelings, or hospitalization itself (that is, with an accompanying loss of civil rights or dignity). It is important to examine the client's feelings with him or her and to support the expression of anger when the client expresses it in ways that are not injurious to himself or herself or others (physically or verbally) and are acceptable to the client. The goal of therapy is not to control the client or to eliminate anger, but to protect the client and others from injury and to help the client develop and use healthy ways of expressing and dealing with feelings.

Hostile behavior can lead to aggressive behavior. In assessing clients with hostile behavior, it is important to be aware of the client's past behavior: How has the client exhibited hostile behavior in the past? What has the client threatened to do? What are the client's own limits for himself or herself? Also, be aware of the medications the client is taking. Some medications (like the benzodiazepines) may agitate the client or precipitate outbursts of rage by suppressing inhibitions.

It is extremely important in working with these clients to be aware of your own feelings. If you are angry with the client, you may want to tell the client that you are angry and explain the reason(s) for your anger, thereby showing the client an appropriate expression of anger. However, do *not* act out your anger by reacting to the client in a hostile or punitive way.

Nursing Diagnoses Addressed in this Care Plan

High Risk for Violence: Self-Directed or Directed at Others
Noncompliance with treatment plan or prescribed medications
Ineffective Individual Coping

Related Nursing Diagnoses

Self-Esteem Disturbance
Impaired Social Interaction

| **Nursing Diagnosis** | ***High Risk for Violence: Self-Directed or Directed at Others* (9.2.2)** *A state in which the individual experiences behaviors that can be physically harmful either to the self or others.* |

Risk Factors

- Feelings of anger or hostility
- Verbal aggression or abuse
- Agitation
- Restlessness (figeting, pacing)
- Inability to control voice volume (shouting)
- Outbursts of anger or hostility
- Uncooperative or belligerent behavior
- Physical combativeness, homicidal ideation, or destruction of property
- Lack of impulse control
- Suicidal thoughts or behavior
- Delusions or hallucinations
- Personality disorder, such as borderline or antisocial personality
- Behavioral or conduct disorder
- Manic behavior
- Substance use
- Post-traumatic behavior

Expected Outcomes

Initial

The client will:

- Not harm self or others
- Demonstrate decreased agitation, restlessness, other risk factors

Discharge

The client will:

- Not harm self or others
- Express angry feelings in a safe way
- Be free of hostile behavior
- Verbalize knowledge of hostile behavior and alternatives to hostile behavior
- Verbalize plans to continue with long-term therapy if appropriate

⊛
Therapeutic Aims

- Prevent harm to the client and others.
- Decrease hostile or aggressive behavior.
- Build a trust relationship.
- Promote the client's ability to control his or her behavior.
- Decrease verbal abuse.

⊛
Implementation

Nursing Interventions	Rationale
Be consistent and firm yet gentle and calm in your approach to the client.	Your behavior as you provide limits is a role model for the client.
Set and maintain firm limits.	Limits must be established by others when the client is unable to use internal controls effectively.
Make it clear that you accept the client as a person, but certain behaviors are unacceptable (specify unacceptable behaviors).	The client is acceptable as a person regardless of his or her behaviors, which may or may not be acceptable.
Give the client support and positive feedback for controlling aggression, assuming and fulfilling responsibilities, expressing angry and hostile feelings appropriately, and verbalizing feelings in general.	Positive feedback provides reinforcement for the client's growth and can enhance self-esteem. It is essential that the client be supported in positive ways and not given attention only for unacceptable behaviors.
If the client is agitated, do not attempt to discuss feelings at this time, especially anger.	Talking about anger or hostilities when the client is agitated may increase the client's agitation.
See Care Plan 1: Building a Trust Relationship and Care Plan 52: Aggressive Behavior.	
Encourage the client to seek a staff member when he or she is becoming upset or having strong feelings.	Seeking staff assistance allows intervention before the client can no longer control his or her behavior and encourages the client to recognize feelings and seek help.
As early as possible in the treatment program, give the client the responsibility for recognizing and appropriately dealing with his or her feelings. Expect the client to take responsibility for himself or herself and his or her actions; make this expectation clear to the client.	Assuming responsibility for his or her feelings and actions may help the client to develop or increase insight or internal controls. It may diminish the client's blaming others or feeling victimized.
If necessary, withdraw your attention (ignore the client) as much as possible when the client is verbally abusive. Tell the client that you are doing this and that you will give attention for appropriate behavior. If the client becomes physically abusive, provide for the safety of the client and others, and then withdraw your attention from the client.	Withdrawing attention can be more effective than negative reinforcement in decreasing unacceptable behaviors. The client may be seeking attention with this behavior. It is important to reinforce positive behaviors rather than unacceptable ones.

✳ *(continued)*
Implementation

Nursing Interventions	Rationale
Do not become insulted or defensive in response to the client's behavior.	Remember it is not necessarily desirable for the client to like you. It may help to view verbal abuse as a loss of control or as projection on the client's part.
Do not argue with the client.	Arguing with the client can reinforce adversarial attitudes and undermine limits.
Give support to others who are targets of the client's abuse (other clients, visitors, significant others, staff members), rather than giving attention to the client for abusive behavior.	Other clients may not understand the client's behavior and may need support. If the client is seeking attention with hostile behavior, withdrawing your attention and giving it to others may be effective in decreasing hostile behavior in the client.
Remain calm. Be in control of your own behavior, and communicate that control. If you are becoming upset, leave the situation in the hands of other staff members if possible.	Your behavior provides a role model for the client.
Remain aware of your own feelings. It may be helpful if staff members express their feelings in a client care conference or informally to each other in private (away from the client and other clients).	A client who is hostile may be difficult to work with and may engender feelings of anger, frustration, and resentment in staff members. These feelings need to be identified and expressed so that they are not denied and subsequently acted out with the client. They should be discussed with other staff members to avoid reinforcing the client's hostility. It may not be therapeutic for the client to have to respond to or deal with the staff's feelings.
Be alert for a build-up of anxiety or hostility in the client, such as increased verbal abuse or restless behavior.	Outbursts of hostility or aggression often are preceded by a period of increasing tension.
Be aware of and note the situation and progression of events carefully, including the general situation, precipitating factors, ward tension, level of stimuli, degree of structure in the environment, time, staff members present, and others present (clients, visitors).	Identifying patterns of behavior can be helpful in the anticipation of and early intervention in destructive behaviors.
Discuss with the client alternative ways of expressing emotions and releasing physical energy or tension.	The client may need to learn other ways to express feelings and release tension.

Nursing Diagnosis

Noncompliance with Treatment Plan or Prescribed Medications (5.2.1.1)

A person's informed decision not to adhere to a therapeutic recommendation.

Assessment Data

Defining Characteristics	• Refusal to take medications • Refusal to participate in treatment program • Refusal to observe limits on behavior
Related Factors	• Lack of trust • Lack of insight • Denial of problems • Denial and projection of feelings • Personality disorder

Expected Outcomes

Initial	*The client will:* • Begin to participate in treatment plan
Discharge	*The client will:* • Demonstrate compliance with treatment plan and medications • Verbalize plans to continue with long-term therapy if appropriate

Therapeutic Aims

• Build a trust relationship.
• Decrease or eliminate psychotic symptoms or suicidal behavior.
• Decrease resentment of staff members or of the treatment program.
• Facilitate the client's cooperation in the treatment program.

Implementation

Nursing Interventions	Rationale
Involve the client in treatment planning and in decision making regarding his or her treatment as much as possible.	Participation in planning treatment can help reinforce the client's participation in his or her treatment program, give the client some control over his or her treatment, and help prevent the client from assuming a victim role or feeling that he or she has no choice (and no responsibility) in the treatment program.
One staff member may review with the client the limits, rationale, and other aspects of the treatment program, but this explanation should be given only once and should not be negotiated after limits have been set. You may want to write down the plan (or elements of it), and give a copy to the client.	The client is entitled to an explanation of the treatment program, but justification or repeated discussions may undermine the credibility and limits of the program.

(continued)
Implementation

Nursing Interventions	Rationale
Set and maintain firm limits. Do not argue with the client regarding treatment, rules, expectations, or responsibilities. Be specific and consistent regarding expectations of the client; do not make exceptions.	Setting clear, specific limits lets the client know what is expected of him or her. Arguing with the client interjects doubt and undermines limits.
It may be helpful to have one staff person per shift designated for decision making regarding the client and special circumstances. (See Care Plan 36: Passive–Aggressive or Manipulative Behavior and Basic Concepts: Therapeutic Milieu.)	Having one person designated as responsible for decisions minimizes the chance of manipulation by the client.
As the client's hostile behavior diminishes, talk with the client about his or her underlying problems and feelings, and continue to include the client in treatment planning as his or her behavior changes.	When the client is less agitated, he or she will be better able to focus on feelings and other problems and more receptive to participation in treatment.
Withdraw your attention if possible (and safe) when the client refuses to participate or exceeds limits. Give attention and positive support for the client's efforts to participate in treatment planning and his or her treatment program.	Withdrawing attention from unacceptable behavior can help diminish such behavior. However, you also must give attention for desired behaviors so that the client does not receive attention only for unacceptable behavior.

Nursing Diagnosis

Ineffective Individual Coping (5.1.1.1)
Impairment of adaptive behaviors and problem-solving abilities of a person in meeting life's demands and roles.

Assessment Data

Defining Characteristics

- Inability to deal with feelings of anger or hostility
- Lack of insight
- Denial and projection of feelings that are unacceptable to the client

Related Factors

- Underlying feelings of anxiety, guilt, or shame
- Disordered thoughts
- Delusions
- Low self-esteem
- Personality disorder, such as borderline or antisocial personality
- Behavioral disorder, such as manipulative behavior
- Suicidal thoughts or behavior
- Substance use
- Post-traumatic behavior

Expected Outcomes

Initial	*The client will:*
	• Identify and verbalize feelings in a nonhostile manner
Discharge	*The client will:*
	• Identify and demonstrate nonhostile ways to deal with feelings, stress, and problems
	• Express feelings to staff, other clients, or significant others, in a nonhostile manner

Therapeutic Aims

- Build a trust relationship
- Facilitate appropriate expression of angry, hostile feelings.
- Promote verbalization of feelings, insight into behaviors, and feelings of self-worth.
- Promote treatment of psychiatric problems.
- Prepare the client for discharge.

Implementation

Nursing Interventions	Rationale
When the client is not agitated, discuss the client's feelings with him or her and different ways to express and deal with them.	The client may need to learn how to identify feelings and ways to express them.
Use role playing and groups (formal and informal) to facilitate the client's expression of feelings.	The client can practice new behaviors in a nonthreatening, supportive environment.
Discuss the client's feelings about his or her hostile behavior, including past experiences with hostile behaviors, consequences of those behaviors, and so forth, in a matter-of-fact and nonjudgmental manner.	The client may be ashamed of his or her behavior, feel guilty, or lack insight into his or her behavior.
Encourage the client to seek a staff member when he or she is becoming upset or having strong feelings.	Seeking staff assistance allows intervention before the client can no longer control his or her behavior and encourages the client to recognize feelings and seek help.
Discuss with the client alternative ways of expressing angry feelings and releasing physical energy or tension.	The client may need to learn other ways to express feelings and release tension.
Try to make physical activities available on a regular basis and when the client is becoming upset (eg, running laps in a gymnasium, using a punching bag). Encourage the client to develop a regular exercise program and to exercise when he or she feels the need to release tension.	Physical activity provides the client with a way to relieve tension in a healthy, nondestructive manner.

⊛ *(continued)*
Implementation

Nursing Interventions	Rationale
Provide opportunities for the client to succeed at activities, tasks, and interactions. Give positive feedback, and point out the client's demonstrated abilities and strengths.	Activities within the client's abilities will provide opportunities for success. Positive feedback provides reinforcement for the client's growth and can enhance self-esteem.
Help the client set goals for his or her behavior; give positive feedback when the client achieves these goals.	Achieving goals can foster self-confidence and self-esteem. Allowing the client to set goals promotes the client's sense of control and teaches goal-setting skills.
Be realistic in your feedback to the client; do not flatter the client or be otherwise dishonest.	Honesty promotes trust. Clients with low self-esteem do not benefit from flattery or undue praise.
Teach the client and his or her family or significant others about hostile behavior, other psychiatric problems, and medication use, if any.	Information about psychiatric problems and medications can promote understanding, compliance with treatment regimen, and safe use of medications.
Encourage the client to follow through with continuing treatment for chemical dependence or other psychiatric problems, if appropriate.	Problems associated with hostile behavior may require long-term treatment.

See Care Plan 2: Discharge Planning.

Aggressive Behavior

Aggressive behavior is the acting out of aggressive or hostile impulses in a violent or destructive manner. Aggressive behavior may be directed toward objects, other people, or the self. The behavior may be related to feelings of anger or hostility, homicidal ideation, fears, delusions, hallucinations, or other psychotic processes; to substance use; to a personality disorder; or to other factors (see other care plans as appropriate). Aggressive behavior may develop gradually or occur suddenly, and it may involve significant danger to staff and others.

There are important ethical and legal issues involved in the care of clients who exhibit aggressive behavior. Because the client is not in control of his or her own behavior, it is the staff's responsibility to provide control to protect the client and others. Control of the client's behavior is not done to punish the client, nor is it done for the convenience of the staff. The client who displays aggressive behavior may be difficult to work with, because this behavior may invoke feelings of anger, fear, frustration, and so forth in staff members. It is essential to be aware of such feelings in yourself so that you do not act them out in your treatment of the client in nontherapeutic or dangerous ways. *Remember:* Clients who are aggressive continue to have feelings, dignity, and human and legal rights. The principle of treating the client safely with the least degree of restriction is important when working with aggressive clients. Do not overreact to a situation (eg, if the client does not need to be restrained, do not restrain him or her). Because of legal considerations, accurate observation and documentation are essential.

Clients who exhibit aggressive behavior may pose real danger to others, sometimes life threatening. Because of the possibility of sustaining an injury that may involve being exposed to blood or other body fluids, nursing staff must be cautious when attempting to physically control or restrain a client. Appropriate precautions should be taken to avoid exposure to blood or other body substances, such as taking extreme care to avoid a needlestick injury (when medicating an agitated client) and to avoid scratches and bites (see Basic Concepts: HIV Disease and AIDS). If a situation progresses beyond the ability of nursing staff to control the client's behavior safely, the nurse in charge may decide to seek outside assistance, such as the hospital security people or the police. If this occurs, the nursing staff will completely relinquish the situation to them. The other clients then become the sole nursing responsibility until the crisis is over.

Nursing Diagnoses Addressed in this Care Plan

High Risk for Violence: Self-Directed or Directed at Others
Ineffective Individual Coping
High Risk for Injury

Related Nursing Diagnoses

Noncompliance with treatment plan or prescribed medications
Impaired Social Interaction
Self-Esteem Disturbance

**Nursing
Diagnosis**

High Risk for Violence: Self-Directed or Directed at Others (9.2.2)
A state in which an individual experiences behaviors that can be physically harmful either to the self or to others.

Risk Factors

- Actual or potential physical acting out of violence
- Destruction of property
- Homicidal or suicidal ideation
- Physical danger to self or others
- History of assaultive behavior or arrests
- Neurologic illness
- Disordered thoughts
- Agitation or restlessness
- Lack of impulse control
- Delusions, hallucinations, or other psychotic symptoms
- Personality disorder or other psychiatric disorder
- Manic behavior
- Conduct disorders
- Post-traumatic stress syndrome
- Substance use

Expected Outcomes

Initial

The client will:

- Not harm others or destroy property
- Be free of self-inflicted harm
- Decrease acting out behavior
- Experience decreased restlessness or agitation
- Experience decreased fear, anxiety, or hostility
- Participate in therapy for underlying or associated psychiatric problems

(continued)
Expected Outcomes

Discharge	*The client will:*

- Demonstrate the ability to exercise internal control over his or her behavior
- Be free of psychotic behavior
- Identify ways to deal with tension and aggressive feelings in a nondestructive manner
- Express feelings of anxiety, fear, anger, or hostility verbally or in a nondestructive manner
- Verbalize an understanding of aggressive behavior, associated disorder(s), and medications, if any

Therapeutic Aims

- Prevent physical aggression or acting out that can cause danger to the client or others.
- Provide a nonthreatening, therapeutic environment.
- Deal safely and effectively with the client's physical aggression or acting out.
- Provide safe transportation of the client from one area to another (eg, into seclusion).
- Provide for the client's safety and needs while the client is in restraints or seclusion.
- Provide for the safety and needs of other clients.
- Deal safely with the client who has a weapon.
- Provide an outlet for the client's feelings, physical tension, and agitation.
- Decrease psychotic symptoms.

Implementation

Nursing Interventions	Rationale
Build a trust relationship with this client as soon as possible, ideally well in advance of aggressive episodes.	Familiarity with and trust in the staff members can decrease the client's fears and facilitate communication.
Be aware of factors that increase the likelihood of violent behavior or that signify a build-up of agitation. Use verbal communication or PRN medication to intervene before the client's behavior reaches a destructive or violent point, and physical restraint becomes necessary.	A period of building tension often precedes acting out or violent behavior. A client who is intoxicated or psychotic may become violent without warning. Signs of increasing agitation include increased restlessness; verbal cues ("I'm afraid of losing control."); threats; increased motor activity (pacing, tremors); increased voice volume; decreased frustration tolerance; frowning; clenching fists.
Decrease environmental stimulation by turning stereo or television off or lowering the volume; lowering the lights; asking other clients, visitors, or others to leave the area (or you can go with the client to another room).	If the client is feeling threatened, he or she can perceive any stimulus as a threat. The client is unable to deal with excess stimuli when agitated.

(continued)

Implementation

Nursing Interventions	Rationale
If the client tells you (verbally or nonverbally) that he or she is beginning to feel hostile, aggressive, or destructive, try to help the client express these feelings, verbally or physically, in nondestructive ways (remain with the client and listen; use communication techniques; or take the client to the gym or outside with adequate supervision for physical exercise).	The client may need to learn nondestructive ways to express feelings. The client can try out new behaviors with you in a nonthreatening environment and learn to focus on emotions rather than acting out.
Assure the client that you (the staff) will provide control if he or she cannot control himself or herself.	The client may fear loss of control and will be reassured that control will be provided. The client may be afraid of what he or she may do if he or she begins to express anger. Show that you are in control without competing with the client and without lowering his or her self-esteem.
Be aware of PRN medication, seclusion, or restraint orders. If you feel there is a need for such orders, discuss this with the physician in advance of agressive episodes.	In an aggressive situation you will need to make decisions and act quickly. If the client is severely agitated, medication may be necessary to decrease the agitation.
Be familiar with restraint, seclusion, and staff assistance procedures and legal requirements.	You must be prepared to act and direct other staff in the safe management of the client. You are legally accountable for your decisions and actions.
Always maintain control of yourself and the situation; remain calm. If you do not feel competent in dealing with a situation, obtain assistance as soon as possible.	Your behavior provides a role model for the client and communicates that you can and will provide control.
Notify the charge nurse and supervisor as soon as possible in a (potentially) aggressive situation; give them pertinent information: your assessment of the situation and need for help, the client's name, the client's care plan, and orders for medication, seclusion, or restraint.	You may need assistance from staff members who are unfamiliar with this client. They will be able to help more effectively and safely if they are aware of this information.
Follow the hospital staff assistance plan (eg, use intercom system to page "Code _____," area), and then if possible have one staff member meet the additional help at the unit door with necessary information (the client's name, situation, goal, plan, and so forth).	The need for help may be immediate in an emergency situation. Any information that can be given to arriving staff will be helpful in ensuring safety and effectiveness in dealing with this client.
Do not use physical restraints or techniques without sufficient reason.	The client has a right to the fewest restrictions possible within the limits of safety and prevention of destructive behavior.
Remain aware of the client's body space or territory; do not trap the client.	Potentially violent people have a body space zone much larger than that of other people (up to four times as large). That is, you need to allow them more space and stay farther away from them for them to not feel trapped or threatened.

✸ *(continued)*
Implementation

Nursing Interventions	Rationale
Allow the client freedom to move around (within safety limits) unless you are trying to restrain him or her.	Interfering with the client's mobility without the intent of restraint may increase the client's frustration, fears, or perception of threat.
Talk with the client in a low, calm voice. You may need to reorient the client: Call the client by name, tell the client your name and where you are, and so forth.	Using a low voice may help calm the client or prevent increasing agitation. The client may be disoriented or unaware of what is happening.
Tell the client what you are going to do and what you are doing. Use simple, clear, direct speech; repeat if necessary. Do not threaten the client, but state limits and expectations.	The client's ability to understand the situation and to process information is impaired. Clear limits let the client know what is expected of him or her.
When a decision has been made to subdue or restrain the client, act quickly and cooperatively with other staff members. Tell the client in a matter-of-fact manner that he or she will be restrained, subdued, or secluded; allow no bargaining after the decision has been made. Reassure the client that he or she will not be hurt and that restraint or seclusion is to ensure safety.	Firm limits must be set and maintained. Bargaining interjects doubt and will undermine the limit.
While subduing or restraining the client, talk with other staff members to ensure coordination of effort (eg, don't attempt to carry the client until you are sure that everyone is ready).	Direct communication will promote cooperation and safety.
Do not strike the client.	Physical safety of the client is a priority.
Do not help to restrain or subdue the client if you are angry (if enough other staff members are present). Do not restrain or subdue the client as a punishment.	Staff members must maintain self-control at all times and act in the client's best interest. There is no justification for being punitive to a client.
Develop and practice consistent techniques of restraint as part of nursing orientation and continuing education.	Consistent techniques let each staff person know what is expected and what to do in advance of this highly stressful situation and will increase safety and effectiveness.
Obtain or develop instructions in safe techniques for carrying clients, to provide consistency among all staff members. Obtain additional staff assistance when needed. Have someone clear furniture and so forth from the area through which you will be carrying the client.	Consistent techniques increase safety and effectiveness. Transporting a client who is agitated can be dangerous if attempted without sufficient help and sufficient space.
When placing the client in restraints or seclusion, tell the client what you are doing, the reason for this (to regain control or to protect the client from injuring himself, herself, or others). Use simple, concise language in a nonjudgmental, matter-of-fact manner. (See Nursing Diagnosis: High Risk for	The client's ability to understand what is happening to him or her may be impaired.

⊛ *(continued)*
Implementation

Nursing Interventions	Rationale
Injury" in this care plan for restraint safety interventions and rationale.)	
Tell the client where he or she is and that he or she will be safe. Assure the client that staff members will check on him or her, and if possible, tell the client how to summon the staff.	Being placed in seclusion or restraints can be terrifying to a client. Your assurances may help alleviate the client's fears.
Reassess the client's need for continued seclusion or restraint as you observe him or her. Reorient the client or remind him or her of the reason for restraint if necessary. Release the client or decrease restraint as soon as it is safe and therapeutic to do so. Base your decisions and actions on the client's, not the staff's, needs.	The client has a right to the least restrictions possible within the limits of safety and prevention of destructive behavior.
Remain aware of the client's feelings (including fear), dignity, and rights.	The client is a worthwhile person regardless of his or her unacceptable behavior.
Carefully observe the client, and promptly complete charting and reports in keeping with hospital or unit policy. Bear in mind possible legal implications or problems.	Accurate recording of information is essential in situations that may later be reviewed in court. Restraint, seclusion, assault, and so forth are situations that may involve legal action.
If you are not properly trained or skilled in dealing safely with a client who has a weapon, do not attempt to intervene. Keep something (like a pillow, mattress, or a blanket wrapped around your arm) between you and the weapon.	Avoiding personal injury, summoning help, leaving the area, or protecting other clients may be the only things you can realistically do. You may risk further danger by attempting to remove a weapon or subdue an armed client.
If it is necessary to remove the weapon, try to kick it out of the client's hand. (Never reach for a knife with your hand.)	Reaching for a weapon increases your physical vulnerability.
Distract the client momentarily to remove the weapon (throw water in the client's face, or yell suddenly).	Distracting the client's attention may give you an opportunity to remove the weapon or subdue the client.
You may need to summon outside assistance (especially if the client has a gun). When this is done, total responsibility for decisions and actions is delegated to the outside authorities.	Exceeding your abilities may place you in grave danger. It is not necessary to try to deal with a situation beyond your control or to assume personal risk.
Do not recruit or allow other clients to help in restraining or subduing a client.	Physical safety of all clients is a priority. Clients should not assume a staff role; other clients are not responsible for controlling the behavior of a client.
Administer medications safely; take care to prepare correct dosage, identify correct sites for intramuscular administration, withdraw plunger to aspirate for blood, and so forth.	When the client is agitated, you are in a stressful situation and under pressure to move quickly, which increases the possibility of making an error in dosage or administration of medication.

(continued)
Implementation

Nursing Interventions	Rationale
Take care to avoid needlestick injury and other injuries that may involve exposure to the client's blood or body fluids.	Human immunodeficiency virus (HIV) and other diseases are transmitted by exposure to blood or body fluids.
Monitor the client for effects of medications, and intervene as appropriate.	Psychoactive drugs can have adverse effects, such as allergic reactions, hypotension, and pseudoparkinsonian symptoms.
If at all possible, do not allow other clients to watch the situation of staff subduing or restraining the client. Take them to a different area, and involve them in activities or discussion.	Other clients may be frightened, agitated, or endangered by an aggressive client. They need safety and reassurance at this time.
Talk with the other clients, especially after the situation is resolved; allow them to ventilate their feelings related to the situation.	The other clients have their own needs and problems. Be careful not to give attention only to the client who is acting out.

Nursing Diagnosis

Ineffective Individual Coping (5.1.1.1)
Impairment of adaptive behaviors and problem-solving abilities of a person in meeting life's demands and roles.

Assessment Data

Defining Characteristics	• Lack of problem-solving skills • Destructive behavior • Feelings of anger or hostility • Feelings of anxiety, fear, or panic • Feelings of worthlessness or guilt • Inability to deal with feelings
Related Factors	• Low self-esteem • Post-traumatic stress syndrome • Substance use

Expected Outcomes

Initial	*The client will:* • Express feelings of anxiety, fear, anger, or hostility verbally or in a nondestructive manner • Verbalize feelings of self-worth • Experience decreased fear, anxiety, or hostility • Participate in therapy for underlying or associated psychiatric problems

✷
Expected Outcomes

Discharge	*The client will:*

- Demonstrate or verbalize increased feelings of self-worth
- Verbalize feelings of anxiety, fear, anger, hostility, worthlessness, and so forth
- Identify ways to deal with tension and aggressive feelings in a nondestructive manner
- Verbalize plans to continue with long-term therapy if appropriate

✷
Therapeutic Aims

- Provide a nonthreatening, therapeutic environment.
- Provide an outlet for the client's feelings, physical tension, and agitation.
- Promote the client's ability to deal with feelings in a nonaggressive manner.
- Help the client develop or increase feelings of self-worth.

✷
Implementation

Nursing Interventions	Rationale
Approach the client in a calm, matter-of-fact manner. Speak in a quiet, steady voice.	Your calm demeanor will communicate your confidence and sense of control to the client.
If the client tells you (verbally or nonverbally) that he or she is beginning to feel hostile, aggressive, or destructive, try to help the client express these feelings, verbally or physically in nondestructive ways. Remain with the client and listen; use communication techniques; or take the client to the gym or outside for physical exercise.	A period of building tension often precedes acting out or violent behavior. A client who is intoxicated or psychotic may become violent without warning. Signs of increasing agitation include increased restlessness, verbal cues ("I'm afraid of losing control."), threats, increased motor activity (pacing, tremors), increased voice volume, decreased frustration tolerance, frowning, clenching fists.
When the client is not agitated, encourage him or her to express feelings verbally, in writing, or in other nonaggressive ways.	The client will be most able to discuss emotional issues when he or she is not agitated. If the client is agitated, attempts to discuss emotional problems may increase his or her agitation.
Teach the client about aggressive behavior, including feelings or behaviors that may precede this behavior, such as increasing tension, restlessness, and anxiety. Encourage the client to recognize these feelings before aggressive behavior begins. Help the client identify strategies that may help him or her avoid aggressive behavior in future situations.	The client may be unaware of the dynamics of aggressive behavior and feelings associated with it. Gaining this knowledge may help prevent aggressive behavior in the future.
Encourage the client to identify and use nondestructive ways to express feelings or deal with physical tension in the future.	The client may be able to avoid aggressive behavior using these techniques.
Teach the client (and family or significant others) about other disease process(es) and medication use, if any.	The client's family or significant others can benefit from understanding the client's behavior and how to deal with it; they also can be supportive to the client in his or her attempts to change behavior.

❋ *(continued)*
Implementation

Nursing Interventions	Rationale
Include the client's family or significant others in teaching, goal-setting, and planning strategies for change, as appropriate.	Information about disease process(es) and medications can promote understanding, compliance with treatment regimen, and safe use of medications.
Teach the client about use of the problem-solving process: identifying the problem, identifying and evaluating possible solutions, choosing and implementing a possible solution, and evaluating the process.	The client may never have learned a systematic, effective approach to solving problems.
Provide opportunities for the client to succeed at activities, tasks, and interactions. Give positive feedback, and point out the client's demonstrated abilities and strengths.	Activities within the client's abilities will provide opportunities for success. Positive feedback provides reinforcement for the client's growth and can enhance self-esteem.
Help the client set goals for his or her behavior; give positive feedback when the client achieves these goals.	Achieving goals can foster self-confidence and self-esteem. Allowing the client to set goals promotes the client's sense of control and teaches goal-setting skills.
Be realistic in your feedback to the client; do not flatter the client or be otherwise dishonest.	Honesty promotes trust. Clients with low self-esteem do not benefit from flattery or undue praise.

Nursing Diagnosis

High Risk for Injury (1.6.1)
A state in which the individual is at risk of injury as a result of environmental conditions interacting with the individual's adaptive and defensive resources.

❋
Risk Factors

- Actual or potential physical acting out of violence
- Destructive behavior toward objects or other people
- Agitation or restlessness
- Neurologic illness
- Delusions, hallucinations, or other psychotic symptoms
- Disordered thoughts
- Transportation of the client by staff under duress
- Confinement of the client in restraints

❋
Expected Outcomes

Initial	*The client will:*
	- Be free of self-inflicted harm
	- Be free of accidental injury

❇
Expected Outcomes

Discharge	*The client will:*
	• Remain free of injury
	• Be free of psychotic behavior

❇
Therapeutic Aims

• Prevent physical aggression or acting out that can cause danger to the client or others.
• Deal safely and effectively with the client's physical aggression or acting out.
• Provide safe transportation of the client from one area to another (eg, into seclusion).
• Provide for the client's safety and needs while the client is in restraints or seclusion.

❇
Implementation

Nursing Interventions	Rationale
Follow the hospital staff assistance plan (eg, use intercom system to page "Code _____," area), and then if possible have one staff member meet the additional help at the unit door with necessary information (the client's name, situation, goal, plan, and so forth).	The need for help may be immediate in an emergency situation. Any information that can be given to arriving staff will be helpful in ensuring safety and effectiveness in dealing with this client.
While subduing or restraining the client, talk with other staff members to ensure coordination of effort. (For example, don't attempt to carry the client until you are sure that everyone is ready.)	Direct communication will promote cooperation and safety.
Obtain or develop instructions in safe techniques for carrying clients to provide consistency among all staff members. Obtain additional staff assistance when needed. Have someone clear furniture and so forth from the area through which you will be carrying the client.	Consistent techniques increase safety and effectiveness. Transporting a client who is agitated can be dangerous if attempted without sufficient help and sufficient space.
Apply mechanical restraints safely: Do not restrain the client lying on his or her back, but position the client on his or her stomach or side. Check extremities for color, temperature, and pulse distal to the restraints.	Placing the client on his or her stomach or side decreases the chances of aspiration or muscle strain and is not as psychologically vulnerable a position as lying on one's back. Mechanical restraints applied too tightly can impair circulation of blood.
Perform passive range of motion on restrained limbs, and reposition the client at least every 2 hours.	These actions minimize the deleterious effects of immobility.
If necessary, loosen the restraints one at a time to exercise limbs or change the client's position.	The client may continue to be agitated while in restraints. Loosening one restraint and reapplying it before loosening another can minimize chances of injury to you and the client.

✳ *(continued)*
Implementation

Nursing Interventions	Rationale
Check extremities at least every 30 minutes for color, temperature, and pulse distal to the restraints.	The client may change position and increase the pressure of restraints against limbs.
Monitor the client by checking or observing him or her at least as often as specified in hospital or unit policy (eg, every 15 minutes). Assess the client with regard to safety, effects of medications, nutrition, hydration, and elimination. Offer fluids, food, and opportunities for hygiene and elimination; assist the client as necessary.	The client's safety is a priority. The client is in a helpless position and needs assistance with activities of daily living. The client's nutrition and hydration needs may be increased due to the physical exertion of his or her agitation.
Administer medications safely; take care to prepare correct dosage, identify correct sites for intramuscular administration, withdraw plunger to aspirate for blood, and so forth.	When the client is agitated, you are in a stressful situation and under pressure to move quickly, which increases the possibility of making an error in dosage or administration of medication.
Monitor the client for effects of medications, and intervene as appropriate.	Psychoactive drugs can have adverse effects, such as allergic reactions, hypotension, and pseudoparkinsonian symptoms.

Care Plan 53

Sexual, Emotional, or Physical Abuse

Abusive behavior, also known as *family violence, battering,* or *abuse,* is the physical, sexual, or psychologic maltreatment of one person by another (or others). This behavior can range from the infliction of minor to life-threatening injuries to homicide to sexual abuse (including *incest, date rape,* and *marital rape*) to refusal to provide needed care or emotional nurturing to a dependent person. Emotional abuse may be perceived by the victim as more devastating than even severe physical abuse, and the emotional consequences of any kind of abuse may be lifelong. Abusive behavior can occur in many different relationships, but it often takes place in intimate, family, or caregiving relationships, such as between parent and minor child, spouses or partners (heterosexual and homosexual), or adult child and elderly parent. Abuse is a major problem in the United States: The annual cost of family violence in the United States is conservatively estimated to be $44 million in medical costs alone, which includes 100,000 hospital days and 30,000 emergency room visits (these numbers may underestimate the actual costs by as much as 10 to 40 times) (Hammers, 1993). Other estimates of family violence include the following: 15% to 38% of adults reported having experienced sexual abuse in childhood; 23% to 39% of adult women reported having experienced rape or attempted rape; and 28% to 31% of wives reported having been beaten by their husbands (Sampselle, 1992). Other information regarding domestic abuse in the United States includes estimates that 1.8 to 4 million wives are beaten by their husbands annually; people who are related to their victims commit 25% of all violent acts, and 95% of victims of domestic violence are female (Hammers, 1993).

Abusive behavior is characterized by a pattern of abusive episodes over time; without intervention, abuse is likely to continue, with episodes increasing in severity. An abusive episode has been identified as a cycle with three stages: (1) a build-up of tension; (2) an outburst of physical or emotional assault; and (3) a period of contrition, when the abuser demonstrates remorse and loving behavior toward the victim. People involved in abusive behavior often deny that abuse is occurring and may be quite resistant to change. The abuser, in addition to denying abusive behavior to others, also may deny it to himself or herself and is likely to justify the behavior and to blame it on others, especially the victim. Adult victims of abuse often seek help in crisis situations and return to the abusive relationship when the crisis is past. Reasons for this return include economic dependence, fear of increasing abuse or retribution, and love for the abusive person. Child abuse must be reported by health care workers (and others) to appropriate authorities, but adult victims of abuse often must agree to reporting and intervention (except under certain circumstances that may vary from state to state, especially with regard to abuse of the elderly). People who experienced incest as children may not recall incestuous behavior until well into their adult lives, if at all. Behavior related to abuse or incest often resembles post-traumatic behavior. (See Care Plan 46: Post-Traumatic Behavior.) Both abusers and adult victims of abuse may have witnessed or been the victims of abuse as children. The behavior of abuse victims has been described as "learned helplessness," in that they come to see themselves as totally powerless (because their actions have no effect on the abuser's behavior), and they become extremely passive and feel they have no control over the situation. The abuser and the adult victim of abuse often share certain characteristics, such as low self-esteem, dependency needs, social isolation, lack of trust, and dysfunctional personal relationships. Domestic abuse may be seen as a dysfunctional family behavior, and family therapy may be indicated as a part of intervention.

Cultural values may underlie or support abusive behaviors, such as ideas of personal ownership (that is, that a child is the property of his or her parents, a wife is the property of her husband), masculinity, discipline, traditional marriage roles, and so forth. For example, a battered woman may be reluctant to face her abusive relationship because she feels that *she* has failed at making a successful marriage, which she sees as her responsibility and which is central to her self-concept. Certain myths, too, persist in our society that increase the difficulty of recognizing the problem of abuse. Two of these myths are that abuse happens only in low-income, alcoholic families, and that the victim enjoys or provokes the abuse. *Remember:* There is *never* any justification for beating or other abuse.

Abusive behavior may be a factor in a number of other psychiatric problems, such as depression, suicidal behavior, hostility, aggressive behavior, withdrawn behavior, conduct disorders, eating disorders, substance abuse, and personality disorders. Abusive behavior, or the possibility that a client has been abused, should be considered when you assess any client, especially those who present with any of the previous problems.

Nursing Diagnoses Addressed in this Care Plan

Post-Trauma Response
Ineffective Individual Coping
Self-Esteem Disturbance

Related Nursing Diagnoses

Rape Trauma Syndrome
Powerlessness
High Risk for Violence: Self-Directed or Directed at Others
Ineffective Denial
Altered Role Performance
Anxiety
Fear
Hopelessness
Impaired Social Interaction
Social Isolation
Sleep Pattern Disturbance
Sexual Dysfunction
Knowledge Deficit regarding illness

Nursing Diagnosis	*Post-Trauma Syndrome (9.2.3)*

The state of an individual experiencing a sustained painful response to an overwhelming traumatic event(s).

Assessment Data

Note: These parameters may be appropriate in the assessment of the abuser, the victim of the abuse, or both.

Defining Characteristics

- Reexperience of trauma (abuse) through flashbacks, dreams or nightmares, intrusive thoughts, and so on
- Feelings of helplessness or powerlessness
- Denial of abuse
- Fatigue
- Apathy
- Poor grooming
- Excessive or inadequate body weight
- Sleep disturbances (nightmares, insomnia)
- Stress-related physiologic problems, such as headaches, ulcers, and gastrointestinal disturbances
- History of repeated hospitalizations or emergency room visits
- Substance abuse
- Fear, anxiety
- Feelings of shame or humiliation
- Feelings of guilt or remorse
- Depressive behavior
- Anger or rage (may not be overt)
- Difficulty in interpersonal relationships, such as lack of trust, dependency needs, economic or physical dependence, manipulative behavior, social isolation
- Poor impulse control
- History of assaultive behavior
- Anhedonia (inability to experience pleasure)
- Sexual problems
- Suicidal ideas or feelings or history of suicidal attempts or gestures
- Low self-esteem

Related Factors

- History of recent abuse
- History of having witnessed abuse or of having been abused as a child
- Economic stress
- Personality disorder or other psychiatric problems

Expected Outcomes

Initial

The client will:

- Identify the abusive behavior
- Be free of self-inflicted harm
- Demonstrate decreased abusive behavior

(continued)
Expected Outcomes

Initial	

- Express feelings of helplessness, fear, anger, guilt, anxiety, and so forth
- Demonstrate decreased withdrawn, depressive, or anxious behaviors
- Demonstrate a decrease in stress-related or psychosomatic symptoms
- Participate in self-care for basic needs (eg, personal hygiene, nutrition, and so forth)
- Participate in treatment for associated problems

Discharge

The client will:

- Verbalize acceptance of losses related to the abusive relationship(s)
- Be free of abusive behavior
- Identify support systems outside the hospital
- Identify choices available for future plans
- Make future plans integrating an awareness of the abusive relationship patterns
- Complete self-care for basic needs and activities of daily living independently
- Verbalize knowledge of abusive behavior and recovery process

Therapeutic Aims

- Promote recognition of the abusive situation.
- Assess the potential for injury to the client or others.
- Protect the client from harm.
- Decrease withdrawn, depressive, aggressive, or suicidal behavior.
- Promote self-care and participation in the treatment program.
- Promote expression of feelings.
- Promote the client's ability to deal with stress.
- Help the client identify choices and make future plans.

Implementation

Nursing Interventions	Rationale
Assure the client of confidentiality and that any decisions made will be his or hers to make (if the client is an independent adult).	The client may feel pressured to make a change he or she does not feel ready to make and may fear that the abuser will find out that he or she has identified abuse.
Report abuse to the authorities if child abuse is involved. Remain aware that adult victims of abuse usually must decide whether or not to report abuse. (If abuse of an elderly or dependent person is involved, check state laws for reporting information.)	The law requires that child abuse be reported. In some states health care workers are encouraged or required to report abuse of the elderly. The adult victim of abuse may place himself or herself in greater danger by reporting abuse if he or she has continued contact with the abuser.
Allow the client to give his or her perceptions of the situation. Initially, you may ask if the client feels he or she is the victim of abuse or point out your observations that may indicate an abusive situation, but do not pressure the client at this time.	Victims of abuse may be seen as experiencing multiple losses and grieving for those losses. Denial is a part of this grief process.

Implementation

Nursing Interventions	Rationale
With the client's consent, you may want to limit the client's visitors, or the client may wish to have a staff member present during visits.	The client may not feel safe if the abuser is present; your presence minimizes the likelihood of an abusive outburst.
Be nonjudgmental with the client, whether he or she is an abuser or a victim of abuse. Be aware of your own feelings of anger, frustration, blaming, and your attitudes about abuse.	The abuser may be in denial or defensive about his or her behavior and needs to receive help, not blame. The victim may feel very powerless in the situation, even if you disagree. You may have attitudes and feelings about abuse from your own experiences and from cultural values.
Encourage the client to tell you the extent of the abuse and his or her perception of the need for protection.	The client may need to be referred to a shelter or other safe sanctuary after hospitalization.
Document information accurately, carefully, and objectively. Do not put your opinions in the client's record.	Legal proceedings may develop, perhaps at a much later time, for which documentation will be required.
Encourage the client to take care of himself or herself by meeting basic needs and performing activities of daily living. Give the client positive support for caring for himself or herself. (See Care Plan 23: Depressive Behavior, Care Plan 28: The Client Who Will Not Eat, and Care Plan 48: Sleep Disturbances.)	The client may have neglected his or her own needs and self-care due to distress or low self-esteem or may have suffered abuse for meeting his or her own needs in the past.
Remain aware of the client's potential for self-destructive or aggressive behavior, and intervene as necessary. (See Care Plan 24: Suicidal Behavior and Care Plan 52: Aggressive Behavior.)	Clients who are in abusive situations are at increased risk for aggressive or self-destructive behavior, including homicide and suicide.
Spend time with the client, and encourage the client to express his or her feelings through talking, writing, crying, and so forth. Be accepting of the client's feelings, including guilt, anger, fear, and caring for the abuser.	Abusive situations engender a variety of feelings that the client needs to express, including grief for the loss of an ideal or healthy relationship, trust, health, hope, plans, financial security, and home. In addition, victims of abuse often feel that they deserved abuse, or it would not have happened. Finally, abuse in a relationship does not preclude feelings of caring.
If the client has been abused, encourage him or her to talk about experiences involving abusive behavior; however, do not probe or push the client to recall experiences. Maintain a nonjudgmental attitude when talking with the client about his or her experiences.	Recalling and retelling traumatic experiences are part of the grieving process and recovery from such experiences. However, the feelings engendered by such recall may create extreme anxiety, and the client may not be ready to face these feelings. Long-term supportive therapy may be indicated.
Involve the client in group therapy if possible, such as groups of other victims of abuse, groups of abusers, or mixed groups of abusers and victims.	Support groups can help abusers and victims decrease their sense of isolation and shame, increase their self-respect, examine their behaviors, and

✳ *(continued)*
Implementation

Nursing Interventions	Rationale
Refer the client to resources outside the hospital if necessary.	receive support for change. The client may feel alone in the abusive situation.
Teach the client about abusive behavior.	Learning about abuse can give the client a framework within which to begin to identify and express feelings and face the reality of the abusive situation.
Teach the client about the stress of being in an abusive situation and about the relationship between stress and physical symptoms. Teach the client relaxation and other stress management techniques.	The client may need to learn to recognize stress and develop skills that deal effectively with stress.
Help the client identify and contact support systems, crisis centers, shelters, and other community resources. Provide written information to the client (such as telephone numbers of these resources), especially if he or she chooses to return to an abusive situation.	Clients in abusive relationships often are isolated and unaware of support or resources available. Contacting people or groups before discharge can be effective in ensuring continued contact.
Encourage the client to identify and list options for the future. Help the client identify positive and negative aspects and consequences of these options. Encourage the client to discover what he or she would like and to explore choices.	Clients in abusive relationships often see themselves as powerless, with no options, desires, or choices.
Help the client arrange follow-up care or therapy. Make referrals to therapists, support groups, or other community resources as appropriate.	Family or individual therapy may be indicated; marital therapy may be appropriate provided the therapist is knowledgeable about abuse, dynamics within an abusive relationship, and so forth. Support or therapy groups are available in many communities, including groups for battered women (through shelters or abuse and assault centers), survivors of child abuse or incest, child abusers (eg, Parents Anonymous groups), men who are abusive (men's groups to prevent violence against women), and groups for lesbians or gay men in abusive situations.
Provide the client with information regarding legal issues and options. Make referrals as appropriate.	The client may wish to obtain legal protection, pursue prosecution, or retain information for future consideration.
Remember that an adult client needs to make his or her own decisions about changes in relationships and so forth. Be aware of your own feelings, such as frustration, disappointment, and fear for the client's safety. Remain nonjudgmental about the client's decisions.	Realizing and grieving for the losses involved in abusive relationships can be a long process. The client may not feel ready to make major changes at the present time. The support and information you give, along with your nonjudgmental attitude, may help motivate the client to seek help again or make other changes in the future.

Nursing Diagnosis	*Ineffective Individual Coping (5.1.1.1)* *Impairment of adaptive behaviors and problem-solving abilities of a person in meeting life's demands and roles.*

Assessment Data

Defining Characteristics	• Verbalization of inability to cope • Inability to problem solve • Difficulty in interpersonal relationships • Lack of trust • Self-destructive behavior • Denial of abuse • Guilt • Fear • Anxious, withdrawn, or depressive behavior • Manipulative behavior
Related Factors	• Low self-esteem • Excessive or inadequate body weight • Social isolation • Substance use

Expected Outcomes

Initial	*The client will:* • Express feelings of helplessness, fear, anger, guilt, anxiety, and so forth • Demonstrate decreased withdrawn, depressive, or anxious behaviors • Demonstrate a decrease in stress-related or psychosomatic symptoms • Participate in treatment for associated problems
Discharge	*The client will:* • Identify support systems outside the hospital • Continue to express feelings directly • Verbalize plans for continued therapy if indicated

Therapeutic Aims

• Decrease withdrawn, depressive, aggressive, or suicidal behavior.
• Promote expression of feelings.
• Promote the client's ability to deal with stress.

Implementation

Nursing Interventions	Rationale
Spend time with the client, and encourage the client to express his or her feelings through talking, writing, crying, and so forth. Be accepting of the client's feelings, including guilt, anger, fear, and caring for the abuser.	Abusive situations engender a variety of feelings that the client needs to express, including grief for the loss of an ideal or healthy relationship, trust, health, hope, plans, financial security, and home. In addition, victims of abuse often feel that they deserved abuse, or it would not have happened. Finally, abuse in a relationship does not preclude feelings of caring.
When interacting with the client point out and give support for decision making, seeking assistance, expressions of strengths, problem solving, and successes. Recognize the client's efforts in interactions, activities, and his or her treatment plan.	The client may not see his or her strengths or work as valuable and may have suffered abuse when displaying strengths in the past. Positive support may help reinforce the client's efforts and promote the client's growth and self-esteem.
Give the client choices as much as possible. Structure some activities at the client's present level of accomplishment to provide successful experiences.	Offering choices to the client conveys that the client has the right to make choices and is capable of making them. Achievement at any level is an opportunity for the client to receive positive feedback.
Use role playing and group therapy to explore and reinforce effective behaviors.	The client can try out new or unfamiliar behaviors in a nonthreatening, supportive environment.
Teach the client problem-solving and coping skills. Support his or her efforts at decision making; do not make decisions for the client or give advice.	The client needs to learn effective skills and to make his or her own decisions. When the client makes a decision, he or she can enjoy the achievement of a successful decision or learn that he or she can survive a mistake and identify alternatives.
Encourage the client to pursue educational, vocational, or professional avenues as desired. Refer the client to a vocational rehabilitation or educational counselor, to a social worker, or to other mental health professionals as appropriate.	Development of the client's strengths and abilities can increase self-confidence and enable the client to see and work toward independence from the abusive relationship and self-sufficiency.
Encourage the client to interact with other clients and staff members and to develop relationships with others outside the hospital. Assist the client, or facilitate interactions as necessary.	Clients in abusive relationships often are socially isolated and lack social skills or confidence.
Refer the client to appropriate resources and professionals to obtain child care, economic assistance, and other social services.	Abusive behavior often occurs when economic or other stressors are present or increased.
Help the client identify and contact support systems, crisis centers, shelters, and other community resources. Provide written information to the client (eg, telephone numbers of these resources), especially if he or she chooses to return to an abusive situation.	Clients in abusive relationships often are isolated and unaware of support or resources available. Contacting people or groups before discharge can be effective in ensuring continued contact.

Nursing Diagnosis	*Self-Esteem Disturbance (7.1.2)*

Negative self-evaluation/feelings about self or self capabilities, which may be directly or indirectly expressed.

Assessment Data

Defining Characteristics

- Verbalization of low self-esteem, negative self-characteristics, or low opinion of self
- Verbalization of guilt or shame
- Feelings of worthlessness, hopelessness, or rejection
- Feelings of helplessness, powerlessness, or despair

Related Factors

- History of having witnessed abuse or of having been abused as a child
- History of recent abuse
- Denial of abuse
- Social isolation

Expected Outcomes

Initial

The client will:

- Express feelings related to self-esteem and self-worth issues
- Verbalize increased feelings of self-worth

Discharge

The client will:

- Demonstrate increased self-esteem and self-confidence or verbalize plans to continue therapy regarding self-esteem issues if needed

Therapeutic Aims

- Promote increased self-esteem and self-confidence.
- Help the client prepare for discharge.

Implementation

Nursing Interventions	Rationale
Convey that you care about the client and that you believe the client is a worthwhile human being.	Often, feedback received by clients in abusive situations is negative and demeaning; the client may not have experienced direct acceptance from significant others of himself or herself as a person.
Encourage the client to ventilate his or her feelings; convey your acceptance of the client's feelings.	Ventilation of feelings can help the client to identify, accept, and work through his or her emotions, even if these are painful or otherwise uncomfortable for the client. Feelings are not inherently bad or good. You must remain nonjudgmental about the client's feelings and express this attitude to the client.

✿ *(continued)*
Implementation

Nursing Interventions	Rationale
In interacting with the client, point out and give support for decision making, seeking assistance, expressing strengths, solving problems, and achieving successes. Recognize the client's efforts in interactions, activities, and his or her treatment plan.	The client may not see his or her strengths or work as valuable and may have suffered abuse when displaying strengths in the past. Positive support may help reinforce the client's efforts and promote the client's growth and self-esteem.
Initially, provide activities at the client's present level of accomplishment to provide successful experiences. Give the client positive feedback for even very small accomplishments.	Positive feedback provides reinforcement for the client's growth and can enhance self-esteem. The client's abilities to concentrate, to complete tasks, and to interact with others may be impaired.
Encourage the client to take on progressively more challenging and rewarding activities. Give the client positive support for any efforts made to participate in activities or interact with others.	As the client's abilities to accomplish activities increase, he or she may be able to feel increasing self-regard related to these accomplishments. Your direct verbal feedback can help the client recognize his or her active role in accomplishments and take credit for them.
Help the client identify positive aspects about himself or herself and his or her behavior or activities. You may point out positive aspects of the client as observations without arguing with the client about his or her feelings.	The client may see only his or her negative self-evaluation; his or her ability to recognize the positive may be impaired. The client's feelings of low self-esteem are very real and valid to him or her. Your positive observations, however, present a different point of view that the client can examine and begin to integrate.
Give the client acknowledgment and support for his or her efforts to interact with others, participate in the treatment program, and express emotions.	Regardless of the level of accomplishment or "success" of a given activity, the client is making an effort and can benefit from acknowledgment of his or her efforts.
Do not flatter the client or be otherwise dishonest. Give honest, genuine, positive feedback to the client whenever possible.	The client will not benefit from insincerity; dishonesty undermines trust and the therapeutic relationship.
Encourage the client to pursue personal interests, hobbies, and recreational activities. Consultation with a recreational therapist may be indicated.	Recreational activities can help increase the client's social interaction and provide enjoyment.
Referral to a clergy member or spiritual advisor of the client's faith may be indicated.	The client's feelings of shame or guilt may be related to his or her religious beliefs.
Teach the client problem-solving and coping skills. Support his or her efforts at decision making; do not make decisions for the client or give advice.	The client needs to learn effective skills and to make his or her own decisions. When the client makes a decision, he or she can enjoy the achievement of a successful decision or learn that he or she can survive a mistake and identify alternatives.
Encourage the client to pursue long-term therapy for self-esteem issues if indicated.	Self-esteem problems can be deeply rooted and require long-term therapy.

References

Ackerman, R. J. (1987). A new perspective on adult children of alcoholics. *EAP Digest, 2*, 25–29.

Agras. W. S. (1991). Nonpharmacologic treatments of bulimia nervosa. *Journal of Clinical Psychiatry, 52*(10, Suppl.), 29–33.

American Psychiatric Association. (1987). *DSM-III-R: Diagnostic and statistical manual of mental disorders-revised* (4th ed.). Washington, D.C.: American Psychiatric Association.

Antai-Otong, D. (1991). The patient with schizophrenia: Helping you stay in touch with reality. *Advancing Clinical Care, 1,* 16–18.

Armitage, P., & Morrison, P. (1991). Changing behaviour. *Nursing Times, 87*(9), 33–35.

Arnold, L. J. (1990). Codependency, part I: Origins, characteristics. *AORN Journal, 51*(5), 1341–1348.

Arnold, L. J. (1990). Codependency, part II: The hospital as a dysfunctional family. *AORN Journal, 51*(6), 1581–1584.

Aro, H., Hanninen, V., & Paronen, O. (1989). Social support, life events and psychosomatic symptoms among 14–16-year-old adolescents. *Social Science Medicine, 29*(9), 1051–1056.

Beck, C. M., Rawlins, R. P., & Williams, S. R. (1988). *Mental health—Psychiatric nursing.* St. Louis: Mosby.

Bentley, K. J., Rosenson, M. K., & Zito, J. M. (1990). Promoting medication compliance: Strategies for working with families of mentally ill people. *Social Work,* 274–277.

Boyd, M. A. (1990). Polydipsia in the chronically mentally ill: A review. *Archives of Psychiatric Nursing, 4*(3), 166–175.

Britnell, J. (1990). The family as client: Nursing families who have relatives with dementia. *Perspectives,* 18–20.

Bronheim, H., Strain, J.J., & Biller, H.F. (1991). Psychiatric aspects of head and neck surgery: Part II: Body image and psychiatric intervention. *General Hospital Psychiatry, 13,* 225–232.

Brusecker, R. (1991). Attitudes and behaviour of chronic schizophrenia. *The Lamp, 33*–36.

Bunting, L. K., & Fitzsimmons, B. (1991). Depression in Parkinson's disease. *Journal of Neuroscience Nursing, 23*(3), 158–164.

Byers, P. H. (1991). Family members' perceptions of care of institutionalized patients with Alzheimer's disease. *Applied Nursing Research, 4*(3), 135–140.

Cadieux, R. J. (1989). Early differentiation of senile dementias. *Hospital Practice, 24*(12), 77–94.

Calabretta-Caprini, T. (1989). Contracting with patients diagnosed with borderline personality disorder. *Canadian Journal of Occupational Therapy, 56*(4), 179–184.

Carino, C. M., & Chmelko, P. (1983). Disorders of eating in adolescence: Anorexia nervosa and bulimia. *Nursing Clinics of North America, 18*(343).

Carter, S. L. (1989). Themes of grief. *Nursing Research, 38*(6), 354–358.

Clare, J. (1991). Understanding schizophrenia. *Nursing Times, 87*(5), 43–45.

Coggins, C. (1990). Myths and facts about suicide. *Nursing 90, 20*(9), 27.

Dennison, P. D., & Kelling, A. W. (1989). Clinical support for eliminating the nursing diagnosis of Knowledge Deficit. *Image, 21*(3), 142–144.

Drew, N. (1991). Combating the social isolation of chronic mental illness. *Journal of Psychosocial Nursing, 29*(6), 14–17.

DuBrul, T. (1989). Separation-individuation roller coaster in the therapy of a borderline patient. *Perspectives in Psychiatric Care, 25*(3,4), 10–14.

Farberow, N.L. (Ed.) (1980). *The many faces of suicide: Indirect self-destructive behavior.* New York: McGraw-Hill.

Fariello, D., & Scheidt, S. (1989). Clinical case management of the dually diagnosed patient. *Hospital and Community Psychiatry, 40*(10), 1065–1067.

Fleming, K. (1990). Knowledge deficit (letter). *Image, 22*(1), 61–62.

French, C. (1991). Individual fears. *Nursing Times, 87*(9), 37–38.

Freud, A. (1961). Adolescence. *Psychoanalytic Study of the Child, 16,* 225–278.

Gerlock, A. A. (1991). Vietnam: Returning to the scene of the crime. *Journal of Psychosocial Nursing, 29*(2), 5–8.

Gibson, D. (1990). Borderline personality disorder issues of etiology and gender. *Occupational Therapy in Mental Health, 10*(4), 63–77.

Giles, G. M., & Shore, M. (1989). A rapid method for teaching severely brain injured adults how to wash and dress. *Archive of Physical Medicine Rehabilitation, 70,* 156–158.

Goldblum, K. (1992). Knowledge deficit in the ophthalmic surgical patient. *Nursing Clinics of North America, 27*(3), 715–725.

Gomez, G. E., & Gomez, E. A. (1991). Chronic schizophrenia: The major mental health problem of the century. *Perspectives in Psychiatric Care, 27*(1), 7–9.

Haack, M. (1989). Anxiety disorders and alcoholism: Seeking connections in ACOAs. *Addictions Nursing Network, 1*(1), 19–20.

Hall, J. M., Koehler, S. L., & Lewis, A. (1989). HIV-related mental health nursing issues. *Seminars in Oncology Nursing, 5*(4), 276–283.

Hamera, E. K., Peterson, K. A., Handley, S. M., Plumlee, A. A., & Frank-Ragan, E. F. (1991). Patient self-regulation and functioning in schizophrenia. *Hospital and Community Psychiatry, 42*(6), 630–631.

Hammers, M. (1993). Domestic violence: Facing the epidemic. *NurseWeek, 6*(1), 6–8.

Harbert, K. H., & Hunsinger, M. (1991). The impact of traumatic stress reactions on caregivers. *Journal of the American Academy of Physician Assistants, 4*(5), 384–394.

Hartman, D., & Boerger, M. J. (1989). Families of borderline clients: Opening the door to therapeutic interaction. *Perspectives in Psychiatric Care, 25*(3,4), 15–17.

Hilton, B. (1991). Demystifying schizophrenia. *Nursing Times, 87*(28), 30–31.

Hofland, S. L., & Dardis, P. O'B. (1992). Bulimia nervosa: Associated physical problems. *Psychosocial Nursing, 30*(2), 23–27.

Houseman, C., & Pheifer, W. G. (1988). Potential for unresolved grief in survivors of persons with AIDS. *Archives of Psychiatric Nursing, 2*(5), 296–301.

Janosik, E. H., & Davies, J. L. (1989). *Psychiatric mental health nursing* (2nd ed.). Boston: Jones and Bartlett Publishers.

Jed, J. (1989). Social support for caretakers and psychiatric rehospitalization. *Hospital and Community Psychiatry, 40*(12), 1297–1299.

Jenny, J. L. (1987). Knowledge deficit: Not a nursing diagnosis. *Image, 19*(4), 184–185.

Johnson, L. B., Cline, D. W., Marcum, J. M., & Intress, J. L. (1992). Effectiveness of a stress recovery unit during the Persian Gulf War. *Hospital and Community Psychiatry, 43*(8), 829–833.

Keltner, B., Keltner, N. L., & Farren, E. (1990). Family routines and conduct disorders in adolescent girls. *Western Journal of Nursing Research, 12*(2), 161–174.

Kennedy, S. H., & Goldbloom, D. S. (1991). Current perspectives on drug therapies for anorexia nervosa and bulimia nervosa. *Drugs, 41*(3), 367–377.

Killeen, M. R. (1990). Challenges and choices in child and adolescent mental health-psychiatric nursing. *Journal of Child and Adolescent Psychiatric Mental Health Nursing, 3*(4), 113–119.

Kim, M. J., McFarland, G. K., & McLane, A. M. (1991). *Pocket guide to nursing diagnoses* (4th ed.). St. Louis: Mosby.

Kübler-Ross, E. (1969). *On death and dying.* New York: McGraw-Hill.

Lachance, R., & Coles, E. M. (1989). Management of disturbed and aggressive behaviour in psychopaths. *Psychiatric Nursing, 9,* 13–16.

Lenox, M. C., & Gannon, L. R. (1983). Psychological consequences of rape and variables influencing recovery: A review. *Women and Therapy, 2,* 37.

Leonardelli, C. A. (1989). Specification of daily living skills for persons with chronic mental illness. *The Occupational Therapy Journal of Research, 9*(6), 323–333.

Leverett, M. (1991). Approaches to problem behaviors in dementia. *The Mentally Impaired Elderly,* 93–106.

Lindgren, C. L. (1990). Burnout and social support in family caregivers. *Western Journal of Nursing Research, 12*(4), 469–487.

Marks, S. F., & Millard, R. W. (1990). Nursing assessment of positive adjustment for individuals with multiple sclerosis. *Rehabilitation Nursing, 15*(3), 147–151.

Marshall, C., & Demmler, J. (1990). Psychosocial rehabilitation as treatment in partial care settings: Service delivery for adults with chronic mental illness. *Journal of Rehabilitation,* 27–31.

Marshall, L. (1992). Eating disorders: Caring for patients with anorexia and bulimia. *NurseWeek, 5*(8/10), 16–17.

Martin, T. L. (1989). The study of grief: An in-depth look at a response to loss. *The American Journal of Hospice Care, 6*(4), 27–33.

Mason, S. E., Gingerich, S., & Siris, S. G. (1990). Patients' and caregivers' adaptation to improvement in schizophrenia. *Hospital and Community Psychiatry, 41*(5), 541–544.

McFarland, G. K., & McFarlane, E. A. (1989). *Nursing diagnosis & intervention: Planning for patient care.* St Louis: C. V. Mosby.

McFarland, G. K., & Thomas, M. D. (1991). *Psychiatric mental health nursing: Application of the nursing process.* Philadelphia: JB Lippincott.

Mejo, S. L. (1990). Post-traumatic stress disorder: An overview of three etiological variables, and psychopharmacologic treatment. *Nurse Practitioner, 15*(8), 41–45.

Mitchell, J. E., Specker, S. M., & de Zwaan, M. (1991). Comorbidity and medical complications of bulimia nervosa. *Journal of Clinical Psychiatry, 52*(10, Suppl.), 13–20.

Morency, C. R. (1990). Mental status change in the elderly: Recognizing and treating delirium. *Journal of Professional Nursing, 6*(6), 356–365.

Newell, R. (1991). Body image disturbance: Cognitive behavioral formulation and intervention. *Journal of Advanced Nursing, 16,* 1400–1405.

Norris, J., Kunes-Connell, M., Stockard, S., Ehrhart, P. M., & Newton, G. R. (1987). *Mental health-psychiatric nursing: A continuum of care.* New York: John Wiley & Sons.

Palmer, T. A. (1990). Anorexia nervosa, bulimia nervosa: Causal theories and treatment. *Nurse Practitioner, 15*(4), 13–21.

Peplau, H. E. (1963). A working definition of anxiety. In S. F. Burd & M. A. Marshall (Eds.), *Some clinical approaches to psychiatric nursing.* New York: MacMillan.

Perkins, K. A., Simpson, J. C., & Tsuang, M. T. (1986). Ten-year follow-up of drug abusers with acute or chronic psychosis. *Hospital and Community Psychiatry, 37*(5), 481–484.

Petit, M. (1991). Recognizing post-traumatic stress. *RN, 3,* 56–58.

Piotrowski, M. M. (1982). Body image after a stroke. *Rehabilitation Nursing, 7*(1), 11.

Plylar, P. A. (1989). Management of the agitated and aggressive head injury patient in an acute hospital setting. *Journal of Neuroscience Nursing, 21*(6), 353–356.

Powers, P. S. (1990). Anorexia nervosa: Evaluation and treatment. *Comprehensive Therapy, 16*(12), 2434.

Puskar, K. R., Lamb, J., & Martsolf, D. S. (1990). The role of the psychiatric/mental health nurse clinical specialist in an adolescent coping skills group. *Journal of Child and Adolescent Psychiatric Mental Health Nursing, 3*(2), 47–51.

Robinson, K. M. (1989). Predictors of depression among wife caregivers. *Nursing Research, 38*(6), 359–363.

Robinson, L. (1989). Stress and anxiety. *Nursing Clinics of North America, 25*(4), 935–943.

Sampselle, C. M. (Ed.) (1992). *Violence against women: Nursing research, education, and practice issues.* New York: Hemisphere.

Scahill, L. (1991). Nursing diagnosis vs. goal-oriented treatment planning in inpatient child psychiatry. *IMAGE: Journal of Nursing Scholarship, 23*(2), 95–98.

Simoni, P. S. (1991). Obsessive-compulsive disorder: The effect of research on nursing care. *Journal of Psychosocial Nursing, 29*(4), 19–23.

Sladyk, K. (1990). Teaching safe sex practices to psychiatric patients. *The American Journal of Occupational Therapy, 44*(3), 284–286.

Smith, G. R., & Knice-Ambinder, M. K. (1989). Promoting medication compliance in clients with chronic mental illness. *Holistic Nursing Practice, 4*(1), 70–77.

Smitherman, C. H. (1990). A drug to ease attention deficit-hyperactivity disorder. *MCN, 15,* 362–365.

Snider, K., & Boyd, M. A. (1991). When they drink too much: Nursing interventions for patients with disordered water balance. *Journal of Psychosocial Nursing, 29*(7), 10–16.

Sparadeo, F. R., Strauss, D., & Barth, J. T. (1990). The incidence, impact, and treatment of substance abuse in head trauma rehabilitation. *Journal of Head Trauma Rehabilitation, 5*(3), 1–8.

Steiner, J. F. (1991). Anxiety: An update on pharmacologic therapy. *Journal of the American Academy of Physician Assistants, 4*(5), 421–426.

Stillion, J. M., McDowell, E. E., & May, J. H. (1989). *Suicide across the lifespan—Premature exits.* New York: Hemisphere.

Stuart, G. W., & Sundeen, S. J. (1991). *Principles and practice of psychiatric nursing* (4th ed.). St. Louis: Mosby.

Tanka, K. (1988). Development of a tool for assessing posttrauma response. *Archives of Psychiatric Nursing, 2*(6), 350–356.

Tennant, K. F. (1990). Knowledge deficit (letter). *Image, 22*(1), 62.

Tomaselli, N., Jenks, J., & Morin, K. H. (1991). Body image in patients with stomas: A critical review of the literature. *Journal of ET Nursing, 18,* 95–99.

Vasquez, C., & Javier, R. A. (1991). The problem with interpreters: Communicating with Spanish-speaking clients. *Hospital and Community Psychiatry, 42*(2), 163–165.

Walding, M. F. (1991). Pain, anxiety, and powerlessness. *Journal of Advanced Nursing, 16,* 388–397.

Waller, D. A., Newton, P. A., Hardy, B. W., & Svetlik, D. (1990). Correlates of laxative abuse in bulimia. *Hospital and Community Psychiatry, 41*(7), 797–799.

Walsh, B. T. (1991). Psychopharmacologic treatment of bulimia nervosa. *Journal of Clinical Psychiatry, 52*(10, Suppl.), 34–38.

Weber, G. (1991). Nursing diagnosis: A comparison of nursing textbook approaches. *Nurse Educator, 16*(2), 22–27.

Weber, G. (1991). Making nursing diagnosis work for you and your client: A step-by-step approach. *Nursing and Health Care, 12*(8), 424–430.

Wester, J. M. (1991). Rethinking inpatient treatment of borderline clients. *Perspectives in Psychiatric Care, 27*(2), 17–20.

Westermeyer, J. (1990). Working with an interpreter in psychiatric assessment and treatment. *The Journal of Nervous and Mental Disease, 178*(12), 745–749.

Whitley, G. G. (1991). Ritualistic behavior: Breaking the cycle. *Journal of Psychosocial Nursing, 29*(10), 31–35.

Wilson, H. S., & Kneisl, C. R. (1992). *Psychiatric nursing* (4th ed.). Redwood City, CA: Addison-Wesley.

Wolfelt, A. D. (1991). Toward an understanding of complicated grief: A comprehensive overview. *The American Journal of Hospice and Palliative Care, 8*(2), 28–30.

Young, S. M. (1986). Strategies for improving compliance. *Topics in Clinical Nursing, 7,* 31–39.

Glossary

Acquired Immunodeficiency Syndrome: see *AIDS.*

Acting out: Behavior that occurs as a means of expressing feelings. It may be acceptable (crying when sad) or unacceptable, even destructive (throwing chairs or hitting another person when angry).

Adaptation: The adjustment that occurs in response to a change in the environment, in a static sense. Dynamically, the process by which the adjustment is made. An adjustment that occurs but does not meet the individual's needs constructively is called maladaptation.

Adult child of an alcoholic: An adult who was raised in an environment in which at least one parent was an alcoholic.

Affect: The behavioral expression of an individual's mood.

Aggressive behavior: Behavior that is violent or destructive, ranging from threatening verbalizations to striking other persons or throwing objects. This behavior often is associated with anger, hostility, or intense fear.

Agitation: A state of restlessness characterized by hyperactivity, increased response to stimuli, and an inability to relax or become calm.

AIDS, acquired immunodeficiency syndrome: A condition caused by infection with human immunodeficiency virus (HIV) that results in severe, life-threatening impairment of the immune system.

Alzheimer's disease: An organic mental disorder characterized by cerebral atrophy, plaque deposits in the brain, and enlargement of the third and fourth ventricles. It results in loss of speech and motor function, profound changes in behavior and personality, and death, usually over a 5-year period.

Amyotrophic lateral sclerosis: A motor neuron disease that causes progressive muscular atrophy, weakness, and death.

Anergy: The lack of normal levels of energy, ambition, or drive.

Anhedonia: The inability to experience pleasure.

Anorexia nervosa: An eating disorder characterized by refusal to eat or eating only minimal amounts of food.

Anticipatory guidance: A process used to assist people to cope with an impending event or situation prior to its occurrence. The process includes identification of the future event and identification and evaluation of possible responses to the event.

Antisocial behavior: Behavior frequently in conflict with society's social, moral, and/or legal mores.

Anxiety: Feelings of apprehension cued by a threat to a person's self-esteem, values, or beliefs.

Apathy: A seeming lack of feelings or emotional response; apparent indifference to surroundings, circumstances, or situation.

Appropriate: Fitting the circumstances, situation, or environment at a given time.

ARC, AIDS-Related Complex: A term given to conditions that involve a variety of illnesses that are associated with human immunodeficiency virus (HIV) but are not diagnostic for AIDS.

Attention-seeking behavior: Actions that occur for the primary purpose of gaining another's attention. Attention-seeking behavior is frequently a type of behavior (such as throwing dishes when upset) that attempts to force another person to become engaged or to intervene. See also *Manipulative behavior.*

Bipolar affective disorder: An affective disorder characterized by periods of manic behavior and periods of depressive behavior, formerly called "manic depressive illness."

Body image: The individual's perception of his or her physical self, although it also may include non-physical attributes.

Bulimia nervosa, bulimia, buliminarexia: An eating disorder characterized by food consumption binges usually followed by purging or vomiting.

Catatonic: A state of disrupted relatedness and withdrawal that is characterized by physical and psychological immobility.

Chemical dependence: The taking of any element into the body to produce a specific effect to the extent that, in time, achieving this effect gains priority over any or all major life concerns. Chemicals (eg, alcohol, glue, medication) are frequently the elements used. The substance is desired and used even when overall effects to physical or emotional health are deleterious.

Commitment: The legal detainment of a person without his or her consent, in a facility for mental health treatment. Usually, the person must meet one of the following criteria to be committed: (1) dangerous to self, (2) dangerous to others, (3) incapable of caring for self in a reasonable manner. (Specific laws vary from state to state.)

Compulsive behaviors: Ritualistic acts, usually repetitive and purposeless in nature, used in an effort to deal with anxiety or unacceptable thoughts.

Confrontation: The technique of presenting a person with one's perception of that person's behavior, or with conflicts one sees between what the person says and what he or she does. The goal of confrontation is for the client to gain insight or to progress in the problem-solving process.

Conversion reaction: The expression of an emotional conflict through a physical symptom, which is usually sensorimotor in nature.

Coping strategy: The means used by an individual in an effort to achieve adaptation to events or situations in one's life.

Date rape: Sexual assault by an individual with whom the victim agreed to have a social engagement or date. The victim declines sexual activity but is assaulted regardless of his or her wishes.

Defense mechanism: An unconscious process that functions to protect the self or ego from anxiety; a coping mechanism.

Delirium tremens: The most severe result of alcohol withdrawal, characterized by disorientation, hallucinations, combative behavior and/or suicidal behavior, or life-threatening physical sequelae.

Delusion: A false belief that has no base in reality.

Delusion, fixed: A false belief that persists over time and does not respond to psychotropic medications or treatment.

Delusion, transient: A false belief that diminishes in response to psychotropic medications, treatment, or time.

Dementia: A progressive, deteriorating condition caused by organic brain pathology, characterized by losses in the areas of memory, judgment, affect, orientation, and comprehension.

Denial: The unconscious process of putting aside ideas, conflicts, problems, or any source of emotional discomfort. This is sometimes a healthy response (eg, as a stage in the grief process) to give the person a chance to organize thoughts and align resources to deal with the current crisis. However, if this is a person's only response, or if it is prolonged, it becomes an unhealthy response and a means of avoiding problems and conflicts. These may then be acted out in other nonproductive ways.

Depression: An affective state characterized by feelings of sadness, guilt, and low self-esteem, often related to a loss.

Disorientation: A state in which the individual has lost the ability to recognize or determine his or her position with respect to time, place, and/or identity.

Dual diagnosis: Coexisting diagnoses of a major mental illness and chemical dependence. (Note: Some authors define dual diagnosis as mental illness and mental retardation, or any two coexisting primary diagnoses.)

Ego boundary: In the differentiation of the self from the not-self or environment, the point or boundary of the self.

Feedback: Information provided to a person to increase insight, facilitate the problem-solving process, or give an external interpretation of behavior.

Gratification: The meeting of one's needs in a satisfactory or pleasing manner.

Grief, grieving, grief work: Behavior associated with mourning a loss, whether observable or perceived. It can be viewed as tasks necessary for adaptation to the loss (identification of loss, expression of related feelings, making lifestyle changes that incorporate the loss).

Hallucination: A sensory experience that is not the result of external stimuli. It may be visual, auditory, tactile, olfactory, or gustatory in nature.

Histrionic, hysterical: The appearance of physical (sensory or motor) symptoms in the absence of organic pathology, or behavior that is dramatic, not appropriate to place or situation.

HIV, human immunodeficiency virus: The virus that causes ARC and AIDS.

HIV positive or seropositive: Having had a positive HIV or HIV antibody test.

Homeostasis: A tendency toward stability and balance among the individual's bodily processes.

Homicidal ideation: Thoughts about killing other people.

Hostility: Feelings of animosity and resentment that are similar to anger but are destructive in nature.

Huntington's chorea: An inherited disorder involving cerebral atrophy, demyelination, and ventricle enlargement. It is characterized by choreiform movements, loss of motor control, and progressive mental deterioration.

Hypochondriacal: Exhibiting physical symptoms that have no organic pathology; caused by or influenced by psychological stress.

Hysterical: See *Histrionic.*

Illusion: The misinterpretation of sensory stimulation.

Incest: Sexual contact or activity between family members.

Insight: Understanding or self-awareness that occurs when connections between conscious behavior and feelings, desires, or conflicts are recognized.

Intellectualization: A defense mechanism that separates and denies or ignores the emotions associated with an event from ideas and opinions about the event. The rational discussion of facts devoid of the feelings aroused by the person, event, or situation.

Interpersonal: Involving a dynamic interchange between two or more people.

Intrapersonal: Occurring as an internal process; occurring within one's self.

Knowledge deficit: Lack of information or understanding; may be related to a lack of prior education, impaired ability to understand or retain information, resistance to learning, or other problems.

Labile: Unstable; quickly and easily changed, frequently from one extreme to another.

Loose associations: A symptom of disordered thought processes in which successive ideas are expressed in an unrelated or only slightly related manner.

Manic behavior: Hyperactive behavior characterized by excessive response to stimuli, push of speech, short attention span, lack of impulse control, low frustration tolerance, inability to impose internal controls, and possibly aggressive and/or self-destructive actions.

Manipulative behavior: Actions designed to indirectly influence another person's response. It frequently helps the person avoid the logical consequences of his or her negative actions. See also *Attention-seeking behavior.*

Marital rape: Sexual assault by a legal spouse.

Milieu: Any specific environment, including a group of persons.

Milieu therapy: A group of persons interacting in a given environment, usually with a mental health orientation, with specific goals of problem-solving, improved mental health, and resolution of difficulties achieved by the interaction within the milieu.

Multiple sclerosis: Demyelination of the central nervous system causing muscle weakness, loss of motor control, irritability, and mood changes.

Myasthenia gravis: A neurological disease characterized by remissions and exacerbations of muscle weakness, fatigue, and respiratory difficulties.

Negativism: A pervasive mood resulting in perceptions and responses that are pessimistic in nature.

Noncompliance: Failure to accurately adhere to therapeutic recommendations.

Nursing diagnosis: A statement of an actual or potential problem or situation amenable to nursing intervention.

Obsessive thoughts: Ideas that occupy the individual's time and energy to the point of interfering with daily life. The thoughts are often ruminative, deprecatory, or persecutory in nature.

One-to-one: Involving one client and one nurse (staff member). This may be for the purpose of interaction or for observation, as with *Suicide precautions.*

Optimal level of functioning: The highest level of mental and physical wellness attained by a given individual. This is influenced by the person's inherent capabilities, the environment, coping mechanisms, and internal and external stressors.

Panic: An extreme, disabling state of acute anxiety.

Paranoia: Behavior characterized by mistrust and suspicion. It may involve delusions of grandiosity or persecution.

Parkinson's disease: A progressive neurological disease characterized by tremor, muscle rigidity, and loss of postural reflexes.

Passive-aggressive behavior: A type of manipulative behavior in which a client does not express hostile (angry, resentful) feelings directly but denies them and reveals them indirectly through behavior.

Personality disorder: Maladaptive traits or characteristics that involve behaviors manifested as a result of maladaptive coping mechanisms. These mechanisms are employed as a usual method of dealing with stress or problems and are often disturbing to others in terms of relationships, impulse control, and a sense of responsibility for one's behaviors.

Phobia: The persistent fear of an object or situation that presents no real threat, or in which the threat is magnified out of proportion to its actual severity.

Pick's disease: An organic mental disorder characterized by frontal and temporal lobe atrophy resulting in loss of speech, poor motor function, profound behavioral and personality changes, and death within 2 to 5 years.

Post-traumatic stress syndrome: Behavior that occurs as a response to experiencing an unusually traumatic event or situation, such as a violent crime, combat experience, or incest.

Precipitating factor: A factor or situation of importance to the client that is related to the development of an unhealthy response. It may be a major event (death in the family, loss of a job) or something that may seem minor to others (an argument with a friend). The client's perception of the magnitude of the event is the most significant factor to assess.

Presenile dementia: A general category of organic mental disorders involving progressive behavioral and personality changes due to primary degeneration and loss of brain neurons in people under age 65.

Problem-solving process: A logical, step-by-step approach to problem resolution that includes identifying the problem, identifying and evaluating possible solutions, choosing and implementing a possible solution, and evaluating its effectiveness.

Projection: A defense mechanism that employs unconscious transfer of blame or responsibility for unacceptable thoughts, feelings, or actions to someone else.

Psychogenic polydipsia: Excessive intake of water and/or other fluids commonly seen in clients with chronic mental illness.

Psychosomatic, psychophysiologic: Pertaining to physical symptoms, with accompanying organic pathology, that are caused by or influenced by psychological stress.

Psychotic: Refers to a dysfunctional state in which the individual is unable to recognize reality or communicate effectively with others, and/or the individual exhibits regressive or bizarre behavior.

Psychotic depression: An affective disorder involving extreme sadness, withdrawal, and a disruption in relatedness, characterized by delusions, hallucinations, and loss of reality contact.

Push of speech: Rapid verbalization that sounds forced from the person. Words are run together and spoken so rapidly that speech may be unintelligible.

Rationalization: A justification for an unreasonable, illogical, or destructive act or idea to make it appear reasonable or justified.

Reactive depression, depressive neurosis: An affective disorder, usually milder than major depression, often precipitated by an identifiable event, situation, or stressor.

Reinforcement: A response to behavior that may encourage or discourage that behavior. Reinforcement can be planned to be positive (giving a reward that has value to the client, designed to perpetuate certain behavior) or negative (a consequence that the client perceives as negative that is designed to eliminate or decrease certain behavior).

Relaxation techniques: Specific techniques to promote physical and mental relaxation, which can be taught by a nurse to a client. These may include breathing exercises (slow, deep, regular conscious breathing) and skeletal muscle tensing/relaxing exercises as well as suggestions for prebedtime measures, such as a warm bath or warm milk.

Ritualistic: Behavior that is automatic and repetitive in nature, frequently without reason or purpose; often elaborate and/or rigid.

Role modeling: The demonstration of a behavior as a teaching technique.

Rumination: Persistent meditation or pondering of thoughts. Carried to excess, rumination over past or present feelings (eg, worthlessness or guilt) can replace constructive problem solving.

Seclusion: A safe, controlled environment that has markedly decreased stimulation (no other people, no noise, minimal furnishings). It can be beneficial for individuals who are unable to tolerate stimulation or are exhibiting aggressive or self-destructive behavior to be confined in a seclusion room.

Secondary gains: Benefits that a client derives from exhibiting certain behaviors, or from illness or hospitalization, that are not the most direct logical consequences of those behaviors. For example, the client may be successfully avoiding certain responsibilities, receiving attention, or manipulating others as a result of destructive behaviors or illness.

Seizure precautions: Measures taken to ensure the client's safety when and if seizure activity occurs. They generally include padding the siderails of the client's bed, placing an airway or padded tongue blade at bedside, and alerting staff members to the potential for seizures.

Self-esteem: The degree to which a person feels valued and worthwhile.

Self-medicating behavior: Behavior in which a client attempts to alter moods, alleviate symptoms or distress, or manage his or her disease by using alcohol or illicit drugs, making changes in a prescribed medication regimen or obtaining prescription medications from others.

Senile dementia: A general category of organic mental disorders involving progressive behavioral and personality changes due to primary degeneration and loss of brain neurons in people over age 65.

Shaping: A procedure that rewards successive approximations of a behavior toward the successful performance of a target behavior.

Sheltered setting: An environment in which certain limits exist, some factors are controlled, and supportive elements are in place for the specific purpose of protecting clients who are unable to protect themselves adequately at a given time (eg, a hospital, a rehabilitation work environment, a group home, supervised apartments).

Significant other: A person who is important or valuable to another. This person may be a spouse or relative but could also be a partner, a friend, an employer, or a roommate.

Somatic: Physiologic in nature; pertaining to the body.

Stressor: Any stimulus that requires a response from the individual.

Substance abuse: See *Chemical dependence.*

Substance use: The ingestion of chemicals to alter mood, behavior, or feelings.

Suicidal gesture: A behavior that is self-destructive in nature but not lethal (eg, writing a suicide note, then taking 10 aspirin tablets). It is usually considered to be manipulative behavior, but it may be a result of the client's ignorance of the non-lethal nature of his or her behavior.

Suicidal ideation: Thoughts of committing suicide or thoughts of methods to commit suicide.

Suicide precautions: Specific actions taken by the nursing staff to protect a client from suicidal gestures and attempts and to ensure close observation of the client.

Support systems or groups: Persons, organizations, or institutions that provide help and assistance to a person in coping or dealing with problems or life situations (eg, family, friends, Alcoholics Anonymous, Weight Watchers, an outpatient program).

Systematic desensitization: A behavioral procedure using conscious relaxation to decrease the anxiety response to an identified phobic trigger.

Tangentiality: A pattern of thinking expressed by the individual's verbalization straying away from the central topic on to vaguely related details. The individual is unable to discuss a central idea due to thoughts evoked by a word or phrase in the idea.

Therapeutic milieu: See *Milieu; Milieu therapy.*

Time out: Retreat to a neutral environment to provide the opportunity to regain internal control.

Tolerance (drug): The need to increase the dose of a drug to achieve the same effect achieved in the past.

Volition: A conscious choice or decision.

Waxy flexibility: A condition in which the client's extremities are easily moved by another person but remain rigidly in the position in which they are placed, no matter how awkward or uncomfortable the position.

Withdraw attention: Ignoring a client or physically leaving a client alone for the purpose of reducing or eliminating an undesirable behavior or topic of interaction. This is effective only if attention is valuable to that client and if attention is given to the client for desired behaviors.

Withdrawal syndrome: Symptoms or behaviors that occur when use of a chemical substance is terminated abruptly.

Withdrawn behavior: Behavior manifested by emotional and physical distancing from the external world, resulting from a disruption in relatedness between the self and others and/or the environment.

Appendices

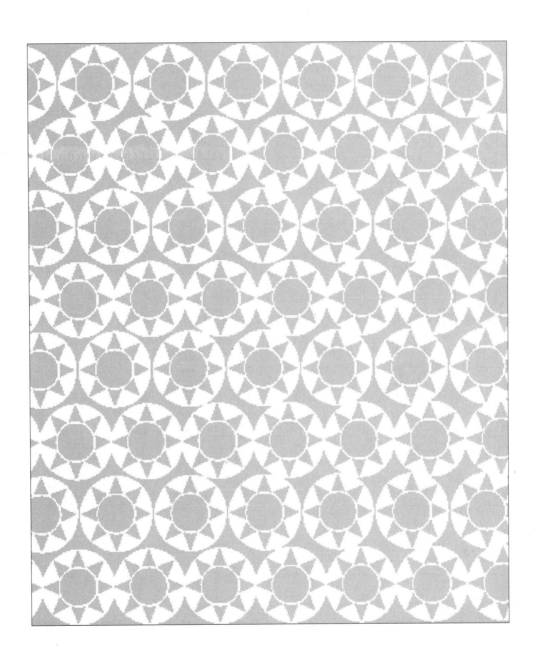

Appendix A:

DSM-III-R Classification: Axes I and II Categories and Codes

All official DSM-III-R codes are included in ICD-9-CM. Codes followed by a * are used for more than one DSM-III-R diagnosis or subtype in order to maintain compatibility with ICD-9-CM.

A long dash following a diagnostic term indicates the need for a fifth digit subtype or other qualifying term.

The term *specify* following the name of some diagnostic categories indicates qualifying terms that clinicians may wish to add in parentheses after the name of the disorder.

NOS = Not Otherwise Specified

The current severity of a disorder may be specified after the diagnosis as:

```
mild      ┐   currently
moderate  ├   meets
severe    ┘   diagnostic
              criteria
```

in partial remission
(or residual state)

in complete remission

Disorders Usually First Evident in Infancy, Childhood, or Adolescence

Developmental Disorders
Note: These are coded on Axis II.

Mental Retardation

317.00	Mild mental retardation
318.00	Moderate mental retardation
318.10	Several mental retardation
318.20	Profound mental retardation
319.00	Unspecified mental retardation

Pervasive Developmental Disorders

299.00	Autistic disorder
	Specify if childhood onset
299.80	Prevasive developmental disorders NOS

Specific Developmental Disorders

	Academic skills disorders
315.10	Developmental arithmetic disorder
315.80	Developmental expressive writing disorder
315.00	Developmental reading disorder
	Language and speech disorders
315.39	Developmental articulation disorder
315.31*	Developmental expressive language disorder
315.31*	Developmental receptive language disorder
	Motor skills disorder
315.40	Developmental coordination disorder
315.90*	Specific developmental disorder NOS

Other Developmental Disorders

315.90*	Developmental disorder NOS

Disruptive Behavior Disorders

314.01	Attention-deficit hyperactivity disorder
	Conduct disorder
312.20	group type
312.00	solitary aggressive type
312.90	undifferentiated type
313.81	Oppositional defiant disorder

Anxiety Disorders of Childhood or Adolescence

309.21	Separation anxiety disorder
313.21	Avoidant disorder of childhood or adolescence
313.00	Overanxious disorder

Eating Disorders

307.10	Anorexia nervosa
307.51	Bulimia nervosa
307.52	Pica
307.53	Rumination disorder of infancy
307.50	Eating disorder NOS

Gender Identity Disorders

302.60   Gender identity disorder of childhood
302.50   Transsexualism
         Specify sexual history: asexual, homosexual, heterosexual, unspecified
302.85* Gender identity disorder of adolescence or adulthood, nontranssexual type
         Specify sexual history: asexual, homosexual, heterosexual, unspecified
302.85* Gender identity disorder NOS

Tic Disorders

307.23   Tourette's disorder
307.22   Chronic motor or vocal tic disorder
307.21   Transient tic disorder
         Specify: single episode or recurrent
307.20   Tic disorders NOS

Elimination Disorders

307.70   Functional encopresis
         Specify: primary or secondary type
307.60   Functional enuresis
         Specify: primary or secondary type
         Specify: nocturnal only, diurnal only, nocturnal and diurnal

Speech Disorders Not Elsewhere Classified

307.00* Cluttering
307.00* Stuttering

Other Disorders of Infancy, Childhood, or Adolescence

313.23   Elective mutism
313.82   Identity disorder
313.89   Reactive attachment disorder of infancy or early childhood
307.30   Stereotypy/habit disorder
314.00   Undifferentiated attention-deficit disorder

Organic Mental Disorders

Dementias Arising in the Senium and Presenium

         Primary degenerative dementia of the Alzheimer type, senile onset,
290.30   with delirium
290.20   with delusions
290.21   with depression
290.00* uncomplicated
         (Note: code 331.00 Alzheimer's disease on Axis III)

Code in fifth digit:

1 = with delirium, 2 = with delusions,
3 = with depression, 0* = uncomplicated

290.1x   Primary degenerative dementia of the Alzheimer type, presenile onset, _____ (Note: code 331.00 Alzheimer's disease on Axis III)
290.4x   Multi-infarct dementia, _____
290.00* Senile dementia NOS
         Specify etiology on Axis III if known

290.10* Presenile dementia NOS
         Specify etiology on Axis III if known (eg, Pick's disease, Jakob-Creutzfeldt disease)

Psychoactive Substance-Induced Organic Mental Disorders

         Alcohol
303.00   intoxication
291.40   idiosyncratic intoxication
291.80   Uncomplicated alcohol withdrawal
291.00   withdrawal delirium
291.30   hallucinosis
291.10   amnestic disorder
291.20   Dementia associated with alcoholism
         Amphetamine or similarly acting sympathomimetic
305.70* intoxication
292.00* withdrawal
292.81* delirium
292.11* delusional disorder
         Caffeine
305.90* intoxication
         Cannabis
305.20* intoxication
292.11* delusional disorder
         Cocaine
305.60* intoxication
292.00* withdrawal
292.81* delirium
292.11* delusional disorder
         Hallucinogen
305.30* hallucinosis
292.11* delusional disorder
292.84* mood disorder
292.89* Posthallucinogen perception disorder
         Inhalant
305.90* intoxication
         Nicotine
292.00* withdrawal
         Opioid
305.50* intoxication
292.00* withdrawal
         Phencyclidine (PCP) or similarly acting arylcyclohexylamine
305.90* intoxication
292.81* delirium
292.11* delusional disorder
292.84* mood disorder
292.90* organic mental disorder NOS
         Sedative, hypnotic, or anxiolytic
305.40* intoxication
292.00* Uncomplicated sedative, hypnotic, or anxiolytic withdrawal
292.00* withdrawal delirium
292.83* amnestic disorder
         Other or unspecified psychoactive substance
305.90* intoxication
292.00* withdrawal
292.81* delirium
292.82* dementia
292.83* amnestic disorder
292.11* delusional disorder
292.12   hallucinosis
292.84* mood disorder
292.89* anxiety disorder

292.89*   personality disorder
292.90*   organic mental disorder NOS

Organic Mental Disorders associated with Axis III physical disorders or conditions, or whose etiology is unknown.

293.00   Delirium
294.10   Dementia
294.00   Amnestic disorder
293.81   Organic delusional disorder
293.82   Organic hallucinosis
293.83   Organic mood disorder
         Specify: manic, depressed, mixed
294.80* Organic anxiety disorder
310.10   Organic personality disorder
         Specify if explosive type
294.80* Organic mental disorder NOS

Psychoactive Substance Use Disorders

         Alcohol
303.90   dependence
305.00   abuse
         Amphetamine or similarly acting sympathomimetic
304.40   dependence
305.70*   abuse
         Cannabis
304.30   dependence
305.20*   abuse
         Cocaine
304.20   dependence
305.60*   abuse
         Hallucinogen
304.50*   dependence
305.30*   abuse
         Inhalant
304.60   dependence
305.90*   abuse
         Nicotine
305.10   dependence
         Opioid
304.00   dependence
305.50*   abuse
         Phencyclidine (PCP) or similarly acting arylcyclohexylamine
304.50*   dependence
305.90*   abuse
         Sedative, hypnotic, or anxiolytic
304.10   dependence
305.40*   abuse
304.90* Polysubstance dependence
304.90* Psychoactive substance dependence NOS
305.90* Psychoactive substance abuse NOS

Schizophrenia

Code in fifth digit: 1 = subchronic, 2 = chronic, 3 = subchronic with acute exacerbation, 4 = chronic with acute exacerbation, 5 = in remission, 0 = unspecified.

         Schizophrenia,
295.2x   catatonic, _____
295.1x   disorganized, _____
295.3x   paranoid, _____

         Specify if stable type
295.9x   undifferentiated, _____
295.6x   residual, _____
         Specify if late onset

Delusional (paranoid) Disorder

297.10   Delusional (Paranoid) disorder

         Specify type: erotomanic
                         grandiose
                         jealous
                         persecutory
                         somatic
                         unspecified

Psychotic Disorders Not Elsewhere Classified

298.80   Brief reactive psychosis
295.40   Schizophreniform disorder
         Specify: without good prognostic features or with good prognostic features
295.70   Schizoaffective disorder
         Specify: bipolar type or depressive type
297.30   Induced psychotic disorder
298.90   Psychotic disorder NOS (Atypical psychosis)

Mood Disorders

Code current state of Major Depression and Bipolar Disorder in fifth digit:

1 = mild
2 = moderate
3 = severe, without psychotic features
4 = with psychotic features (*specify* mood-congruent or mood-incongruent)
5 = in partial remission
6 = in full remission
0 = unspecified

For major depressive episodes, *specify* if chronic and *specify* if melancholic type.

For Bipolar Disorder, Bipolar Disorder NOS, Recurrent Major Depression, and Depressive Disorder NOS, *specify* if seasonal pattern.

Bipolar Disorders

         Bipolar disorder,
296.6x   mixed, _____
296.4x   manic, _____
296.5x   depressed, _____
301.13   Cyclothymia
296.70   Bipolar disorder NOS

Depressive Disorders

         Major Depression

296.2x   single episode, _____
296.3x   recurrent, _____

300.40   Dysthymia (or Depressive neurosis)
Specify: primary or secondary type
Specify: early or late onset
311.00   Depressive disorder NOS

Anxiety Disorders (or Anxiety and Phobic Neuroses)

Panic disorder
300.21   with agoraphobia
Specify current severity of agoraphobic avoidance
Specify current severity of panic attacks
300.01   without agoraphobia
Specify current severity of panic attacks
300.22   Agoraphobia without history of panic disorder
Specify with or without limited symptom attacks
300.23   Social phobia
Specify if genralized type
300.29   Simple phobia
300.30   Obsessive compulsive disorder (or Obsessive compulsive neurosis)
309.89   Post-traumatic stress disorder
Specify if delayed onset
300.02   Generalized anxiety disorder
300.00   Anxiety disorder NOS

Somatoform Disorders

300.70*   Body dysmorphic disorder
300.11   Conversion disorder (or Hysterical neurosis, conversion type)
Specify: single episode or recurrent
300.70*   Hypochondriasis (or Hypochondriacal neurosis)
300.81   Somatization disorder
307.80   Somatoform pain disorder
300.70*   Undifferentiated somatoform disorder
300.70*   Somatoform disorder NOS

Dissociative Disorders (or Hysterical Neuroses, Dissociative Type)

300.14   Multiple personality disorder
300.13   Psychogenic fugue
300.12   Psychogenic amnesia
300.60   Depersonalization disorder (or Depersonalization neurosis)
300.15   Dissociative disorder NOS

Sexual Disorders

Paraphilias

302.40   Exhibitionism
302.81   Fetishism
302.89   Frotteurism
302.20   Pedophilia
Specify: same sex, opposite sex, same and opposite sex
Specify if limited to incest
Specify: exclusive type or nonexclusive type
302.83   Sexual masochism
302.84   Sexual sadism
302.30   Transvestic fetishism
302.82   Voyeurism
302.90*   Paraphilia NOS

Sexual Dysfunctions

Specify: psychogenic only, or psychogenic and biogenic (Note: If biogenic only, code on Axis III)

Specify: lifelong or acquired

Specify: generalized or situational
Sexual desire disorders
302.71   Hypoactive sexual desire disorder
302.79   Sexual aversion disorder
Sexual arousal disorders
302.73*   Female sexual arousal disorder
302.72*   Male erectile disorder
Orgasm disorders
302.73   Inhibited female orgasm
302.74   Inhibited male orgasm
302.75   Premature ejaculation
Sexual pain disorders
302.76   Dyspareunia
306.51   Vaginismus
302.70   Sexual dysfunction NOS

Other Sexual Disorders

302.90*   Sexual disorder NOS

Sleep Disorders

Dyssomnias

Insomnia disorder
307.42*   related to another mental disorder (nonorganic)
780.50*   related to known organic factor
307.43*   Primary insomnia Hypersomnia disorder
307.44   related to another mental disorder (nonorganic)
780.50*   related to a known organic factor
780.54   Primary hypersomnia
307.45   Sleep-wake schedule disorder
Specify: advanced or delayed phase type, disorganized type, frequently changing type
Other dyssomnias
307.40*   Dyssomnia NOS

Parasomnias

307.47   Dream anxiety disorder (Nightmare disorder)
307.46*   Sleep terror disorder
307.46*   Sleepwalking disorder
307.40*   Parasomnia NOS

Factitious Disorders

Factitious disorder
301.51   with physical symptoms
300.16   with psychological symptoms
300.19   Factitious disorder NOS

Impulse Control Disorders Not Elsewhere Classified

312.34   Intermitten explosive disorder
312.32   Kleptomania

305.70	Amphetamine (or Related Substance) Intoxication
292.0	Amphetamine (or Related Substance) Withdrawal
292.81	Amphetamine (or Related Substance) Delirium
	Amphetamine (or Related Substance) Psychotic Disorder
291.11	with delusions
291.12	with hallucinations
292.84	Amphetamine (or Related Substance) Mood Disorder
292.89	Amphetamine (or Related Substance) Anxiety Disorder
292.89	Amphetamine (or Related Substance) Sexual Dysfunction
292.89	Amphetamine (or Related Substance) Sleep Disorder
292.9	Amphetamine (or Related Substance) Use Disorder NOS

Caffeine Use Disorders

305.90	Caffeine Intoxication
292.84	Caffeine Anxiety Disorder
292.89	Caffeine Sleep Disorder
292.9	Caffeine Use Disorder NOS

Cannabis Use Disorders

304.30	Cannabis Dependence
305.20	Cannabis Abuse
305.20	Cannabis Intoxication
292.81	Cannabis Delirium
	Cannabis Psychotic Disorder
291.11	with delusions
292.12	with hallucinations
292.89	Cannabis Anxiety Disorder
292.9	Cannabis Use Disorder NOS

Cocaine Use Disorders

304.20	Cocaine Dependence
305.60	Cocaine Abuse
305.60	Cocaine Intoxication
292.0	Cocaine Withdrawal
292.81	Cocaine Delirium
	Cocaine Psychotic Disorder
291.11	with delusions
291.12	with hallucinations
292.84	Cocaine Mood Disorder
292.89	Cocaine Anxiety Disorder
292.89	Cocaine Sexual Dysfunction
292.89	Cocaine Sleep Disorder
292.9	Cocaine Use Disorder NOS

Hallucinogen Use Disorders

304.50	Hallucinogen Dependence
305.30	Hallucinogen Abuse
305.30	Hallucinogen Intoxciation
292.89	Hallucinogen Persisting Perception Disorder
292.81	Hallucinogen Delirium
	Hallucinogen Psychotic Disorder
291.11	with delusions
291.12	with hallucinations
292.84	Hallucinogen Mood Disorder
292.89	Hallucinogen Anxiety Disorder
292.9	Hallucinogen Use Disorder NOS

Inhalant Use Disorders

304.60	Inhalant Dependence
305.90	Inhalant Abuse
305.90	Inhalant Intoxication
292.81	Inhalant Delirium
292.82	Inhalant Persisting Dementia
	Inhalant Psychotic Disorder
291.11	with delusions
291.12	with hallucinations
292.84	Inhalant Mood Disorder
292.89	Inhalant Anxiety Disorder
292.9	Inhalant Use Disorder NOS

Nicotine Use Disorders

305.10	Nicotine Dependence
292.0	Nicotine Withdrawal
292.9	Nicotine Use Disorder NOS

Opioid Use Disorders

304.00	Opioid Dependence
305.50	Opioid Abuse
305.50	Opioid Intoxication
292.0	Opioid Withdrawal
292.81	Opioid Delirium
	Opioid Psychotic Disorder
291.11	with delusions
291.12	with hallucinations
292.84	Opioid Mood Disorder
292.89	Opioid Sleep Disorder
292.89	Opioid Sexual Dysfunction
292.9	Opioid Use Disorder NOS

Phencyclidine (or Related Substance) Use Disorders

304.90	Phencyclidine (or Related Substance) Dependence
305.90	Phencyclidine (or Related Substance) Abuse
305.90	Phencyclidine (or Related Substance) Intoxication
292.81	Phencyclidine (or Related Substance) Delirium
	Phencyclidine (or Related Substance) Psychotic Disorder
291.11	with delusions
291.12	with hallucinations
292.84	Phencyclidine (or Related Substance) Mood Disorder
292.89	Phencyclidine (or Related Substance) Anxiety Disorder
292.9	Phencyclidine (or Related Substance) Use Disorder NOS

Sedative, Hypnotic, or Anxiolytic Substance Use Disorders

304.10	Sedative, Hypnotic, or Anxiolytic Dependence
305.40	Sedative, Hypnotic, or Anxiolytic Abuse
305.40	Sedative, Hypnotic, or Anxiolytic Intoxication
292.0	Sedative, Hypnotic, or Anxiolytic Withdrawal
292.81	Sedative, Hypnotic, or Anxiolytic Delirium
292.82	Sedative, Hypnotic, or Anxiolytic Persisting Dementia
292.83	Sedative, Hypnotic, or Anxiolytic Persisting Amnestic Disorder

Sedative, Hypnotic, or Anxiolytic Psychotic Disorder

291.11   with delusions
291.12   with hallucinations
292.84   Sedative, Hypnotic, or Anxiolytic Mood Disorder
292.89   Sedative, Hypnotic, or Anxiolytic Anxiety Disorder
292.89   Sedative, Hypnotic, or Anxiolytic Sleep Disorder
292.89   Sedative, Hypnotic, or Anxiolytic Sexual Dysfunction
292.9   Sedative, Hypnotic, or Anxiolytic Use Disorder NOS

Polysubstance Use Disorder

304.80   Polysubstance Dependence (E:27)

Other (or Unknown) Substance Use Disorders

304.90   Other (or Unknown) Substance Dependence
305.90   Other (or Unknown) Substance Abuse
305.90   Other (or Unknown) Substance Intoxication
292.0   Other (or Unknown) Substance Withdrawal
292.81   Other (or Unknown) Substance Delirium
292.82   Other (or Unknown) Substance Persisting Dementia
292.83   Other (or Unknown) Substance Persisting Amnestic Disorder
          Other (or Unknown) Substance Psychotic Disorder
291.11   with delusions
291.12   with hallucinations
292.84   Other (or Unknown) Substance Mood Disorder
292.89   Other (or Unknown) Substance Anxiety Disorder
292.89   Other (or Unknown) Substance Sexual Dysfunction
292.89   Other (or Unknown) Substance Sleep Disorder
292.9   Other (or Unknown) Substance Use Disorder NOS

Schizophrenia and Other Psychotic Disorders

          Schizophrenia
295.30   paranoid type
295.10   disorganized type
295.20   catatonic type
295.90   undifferentiated type
295.60   residual type
295.40   Schizophreniform Disorder
295.70   Schizoaffective Disorder
297.1   Delusional Disorder
298.8   Brief Psychotic Disorder
297.3   Shared Psychotic Disorder (Folie a Deux)
          Psychotic Disorder Due to a General Medical Condition
293.81   with delusions
293.82   with hallucinations
—.-   Substance-Induced Psychotic Disorder (refer to a specific substances for codes)
298.9   Psychotic Disorder NOS

Mood Disorders

Depressive Disorders

          Major Depressive Disorder
296.2x   single episode

296.3x   recurrent
300.4   Dysthymic Disorder
311   Depressive Disorder NOS

Bipolar Disorders

          Bipolar I Disorder
296.0x   single manic episode
296.4   most recent episode hypomanic
296.4x   most recent episode manic
296.6x   most recent episode mixed
296.5x   most recent episode depressed
296.7   most recent episode unspecified
296.89   Bipolar II Disorder (Recurrent major depressive episodes with hypomania)
301.13   Cyclothymic Disorder
296.80   Bipolar Disorder NOS
293.83   Mood Disorder Due to a General Medical Condition
—.-   Substance-Induced Mood Disorder (refer to specific substances for codes)
296.90   Mood Disorder NOS

Anxiety Disorders

          Panic Disorder
300.01   without agoraphobia
300.21   with agoraphobia
300.22   Agoraphobia Without History of Panic Disorder
300.29   Specific Phobia (Simple Phobia)
300.23   Social Phobia (Social Anxiety Disorder)
300.3   Obsessive-Compulsive Disorder
309.81   Posttraumatic Stress Disorder
300.3   Acute Stress Disorder
300.02   Generalized Anxiety Disorder (includes Overanxious Disorder of Childhood)
293.89   Anxiety Disorder Due to a General Medical Condition
—.-   Substance-Induced Anxiety Disorder (refer to specific substances for codes)
300.00   Anxiety Disorder NOS

Somatoform Disorders

300.81   Somatization Disorder
300.11   Conversion Disorder
300.7   Hypochondriasis
          Body Dysmorphic Disorder
300.71   Pain Disorder
307.80   associated with Psychological Factors
307.89   associated with Both Psychological Factors and a General Medical Condition
300.82   Undifferentiated Somatoform Disorder
300.89   Somatoform Disorder NOS

Factitious Disorders

          Factitious Disorder
300.16   with predominantly psychological signs and symptoms
300.17   with predominantly physical signs and symptoms

300.18	with combined psychological and physical signs and symptoms
300.19	Factitious Disorder NOS

Dissociative Disorders

300.12	Dissociative Amnesia
300.13	Dissociative Fugue
300.14	Dissociative Identity Disorder (Multiple Personality Disorder)
300.6	Depersonalization Disorder
300.15	Dissociative Disorder NOS

Sexual and Gender Identity Disorders

Sexual Dysfunctions

	Sexual Desire Disorders
302.71	Hypoactive Sexual Desire Disorder
?302.79	Sexual Aversion Disorder
	Sexual Arousal Disorders
302.72	Female Sexual Arousal Disorder
302.72	Male Erectile Disorder
	Orgasm Disorders
302.73	Female Orgasmic Disorder (Inhibited Female Orgasm)
302.74	Male Orgasmic Disorder (Inhibited Male Orgasm)
302.75	Premature Ejaculation
	Sexual Pain Disorders
302.76	Dyspareunia
306.51	Vaginismus
	Sexual Dysfunctions Due to a General Medical Condition
607.84	Male Erectile Disorder Due to a General Medical Condition
608.89	Male Dyspareunia Due to a General Medical Condition
625.0	Female Dyspareunia Due to a General Medical Condition
608.89	Male Hypoactive Sexual Desire Disorder Due to a General Medical Condition
625.8	Female Hypoactive Sexual Desire Disorder Due to a General Medical Condition
608.89	Other Male Sexual Dysfunction Due to a General Medical Condition
625.8	Other Female Sexual Dysfunction Due to a General Medical Condition
—.-	Substance-Induced Sexual Dysfunction (refer to specific substances for codes)
302.70	Sexual Dysfunction NOS
	Paraphilias
302.4	Exhibitionism
302.81	Fetishism
?302.85	Frotteurism
302.2	Pedophilia
302.83	Sexual Masochism
302.84	Sexual Sadism
302.82	Voyeurism
302.3	Transvestic Fetishism
302.9	Paraphilia NOS
S02.9	Sexual Disorder NOS

Gender Identity Disorders

	Gender Identity Disorder
302.5	In Children
302.85	In Adolescents and Adults
302.6	Gender Identity Disorder NOS

Eating Disorders

307.1	Anorexia Nervosa
307.51	Bulimia Nervosa
307.50	Eating Disorder NOS

Sleep Disorders

Primary Sleep Disorders

Dyssomnias

307.42	Primary Insomnia
307.44	Primary Hypersomnia
347	Narcolepsy
780.59	Breathing-Related Sleep Disorder
307.45	Circadian Rhythm Sleep Disorder (Sleep-Wake Schedule Disorder)
307.47	Dyasomnia NOS

Parasomnias

307.47	Nightmare Disorder (Dream Anxiety Disorder)
307.46	Sleep Terror Disorder
307.46	Sleepwalking Disorder
?307.47	Parasomnia NOS

Sleep Disorders Related to Another Mental Disorder

307.42	Insomnia related to [Axis I or Axis II Disorder]
307.44	Hypersomnia related to [Axis I or Axis II Disorder]

Other Sleep Disorders

	Sleep Disorder Due to a General Medical Condition
780.52	insomnia type
780.54	hypersomnia type
780.59	parasomnia type
780.59	mixed type
—.-	Substance-Induced Sleep Disorder (refer to specific substances for codes)

Impulse Control Disorders Not Elsewhere Classified

312.34	Intermittent Explosive Disorder
312.32	Kleptomania
312.33	Pyromania
312.31	Pathological Gambling
?312.39	Trichotillomania
312.30	Impulse Control NOS

Adjustment Disorders

Adjustment Disorder
309.24   With Anxiety
309.0   With Depressed Mood
309.3   With Disturbance of Conduct
309.4   With Mixed Disturbance of Emotions and Conduct
309.26   With Mixed Anxiety and Depressed Mood
309.9   Unspecified

Personality Disorders

301.0   Paranoid Personality Disorder
301.20   Schizoid Personality Disorder
301.22   Schizotypal Personality Disorder
301.7   Antisocial Personality Disorder
301.83   Borderline Personality Disorder
301.50   Histrionic Personality Disorder
301.81   Narcissistic Personality Disorder
301.82   Avoidant Personality Disorder
301.6   Dependent Personality Disorder
301.4   Obsessive-Compulsive Personality Disorder
301.9   Personality Disorder NOS

Other Conditions that May be a Focus of Clinical Attention

316   (Psychological Factors) Affecting Medical Condition
Choose name based on nature of factors:
Mental Disorder Affecting Medical Condition
Psychological Symptoms Affecting Medical Condition
Personality Traits or Coping Style Affecting Medical Condition
Maladaptive Health Behaviors Affecting Medical Condition
Unspecified Psychological Factors Affecting Medical Condition

Medication-Induced Movement Disorders

332.1   Neuroleptic-Induced Parkinsonism
333.92   Neuroleptic Malignant Syndrome
333.7   Neuroleptic-Induced Acute Dystonia
333.99   Neuroleptic-Induced Acute Akathisia
333.82   Neuroleptic-Induced Tardive Dyskinesia
333.1   Medication-Induced Postural Tremor
333.90   Medication-Induced Movement Disorder NOS
995.2   Adverse Effects of Medication NOS

Relational Problems

V61.9   Relational Problem Related to A Mental Disorder or General Medical Condition
V61.20   Parent-Child Relational Problem
V61.12   Partner Relational Problem
V61.8   Sibling Relational Problem
V62.81   Relational Problem NOS

Problems Related to Abuse or Neglect

V61.21   Physical Abuse of Child
V61.22   Sexual Abuse of Child
V61.21   Neglect of Child
V61.10   Physical Abuse of Adult
V51.11   Sexual Abuse of Adult

Additional Conditions that May be a Focus of Clinical Attention

V62.82   Bereavement
V40.0   Borderline Intellectual Functioning
V62.3   Academic Problem
V62.2   Occupational Problem
V71.02   Childhood or Adolescent Antisocial Behavior
V71.01   Adult Antisocial Behavior
V65.2   Malingering
V62.89   Phase of Life Problem
V15.81   Noncompliance with treatment for a mental disorder
313.82   Identity Problem
V62.61   Religious or Spiritual Problem
V62.4   Acculturation Problem
780.9   Age-Associated Memory Decline

Additional Codes

300.9   Unspecified Mental Disorder
V71.09   No Diagnosis or Condition on Axis I
799.9   Diagnosis or Condition Deferred on Axis I
V71.09   No Diagnosis on Axis II
799.9   Diagnosis Deferred on Axis II

Appendix C

Communication Techniques

Therapeutic Techniques	Definitions	Examples
Silence	Purposeful absence of verbal communication while continuing to focus on the client	Nodding; maintaining eye contact
Accepting	Indicating (verbally and nonverbally) that what is heard is acknowledged; does not necessarily indicate agreement with what was said	Nodding: Yes, um-hmm, I follow what you said.
Giving recognition	Acknowledgment; indicating awareness	I notice you've combed your hair. I see you're dressed this morning.
Giving information	Providing facts; answer questions	Visiting hours are from 2:00 PM to 4:00 PM. All clients are scheduled to attend the group meeting.
Offering self	Making yourself available without conditions or an expected response	I'll sit with you. I'll stay with you for 15 minutes.
Giving broad openings	Giving the initiative to the client	Where would you like to start? What is on your mind this morning?
Offering general leads	Encouraging the client to continue	And then? Go on.
Placing the event in time or sequence	Clarifying the time of an event or the relationship between events	Was that before or after . . . ? What happened just before that?
Making observations	Verbalizing and acknowledging what is observed or perceived about the client	I notice that you . . . I sense that you . . . You seem . . .
Encouraging description of perceptions	Asking the client to verbalize what is perceived	What is happening? Describe what you are hearing.
Encouraging comparison	Asking the client for similarities or differences	Has this happened before? Does this remind you of anything . . . ?
Reflecting	Directing back to the client's thoughts or feelings	Are you wondering if . . . ? Do you think that . . . ?
Exploring	Delving into an idea in more depth	Tell me more about that. Describe that to me.
Seeking clarification	Encouraging the client to make meaning more clear	I'm not sure I follow what you're saying. Do you mean to say that . . . ?
Presenting reality	Providing factual information in a nonthreatening manner	I don't hear anyone talking. I am your nurse, this is a hospital.
Voicing doubt	Interjecting the nurse's perception of reality	I find that hard to believe. That seems quite unusual.

Therapeutic Techniques	Definitions	Examples
Verbalizing the implied	Putting into words what the client is hinting at or suggesting	*Client*: My wife pushes me around just like my mother and sister do. *Nurse*: Is it your impression that women are domineering?
Attempting to translate into feelings	Assisting the client to identify feelings associated with events or statements	*Client*: I might as well be dead. *Nurse*: Is it your feeling that no one cares?
Encouraging formulation of a plan of action	Giving the client the opportunity to anticipate alternative courses of action for the future	How might you handle this next time? What are some safe ways you could express your anger?
Summarizing	Clarifying main points of discussion and providing closure	Today I have understood you to say . . .

Nontherapeutic Techniques	Definitions	Examples
Reassuring	Indicating that there is no cause for concern	You're going to be fine. I wouldn't even worry about that if I were you.
Approving	Personally sanctioning the client's thoughts, behavior, or feelings	Oh yes, that's what I'd do. That's good.
Disapproving	Denouncing the client's thoughts, behavior, or feelings	That's bad. It's wrong for you to feel that way about your mother.
Rejecting	Refusing to listen to the client's ideas or feelings	I don't want to hear about that. Let's not discuss depressing subjects.
Advising	Telling the client what to do	I think you should . . . Why don't you . . . ?
Probing	Asking persistent questions	Tell me your psychiatric history.
Challenging	Demanding proof from the client	*Client*: I was sacrificed by demons. *Nurse*: If that's true, how can you be here talking to me?
Defending	Attempting to dispute the client's negative statements	All the staff here are caring people. Your doctor is the best in this city.
Requesting an explanation	Asking for reasons (usually "why" questions) that are unanswerable	Why would you say a thing like that? Why do you feel that way?
Indicating the existence of an external source	Attributing the basis for the client's statements, thoughts, feelings, or behavior to others or outside influences	What made you do that? What makes you say that?
Belittling feelings	Dismissing or minimizing the importance of the client's feelings, usually an attempt to be cheerful	*Client*: I have no reason to live. *Nurse*: You have a wife that loves you. *or* I've felt like that before.
Making stereotypical comments	Offering platitudes or trite expressions	Tomorrow will be a better day. This, too, shall pass.
Giving literal responses	Responding to the content of figurative comments, rather than the meaning	*Client*: My heart is made of stone. *Nurse*: If that were true, I couldn't hear it beating.
Introducing an unrelated topic	Changing the subject, usually because of the nurse's discomfort	*Client*: I wish my sister was dead. *Nurse*: Is she older or younger than you?

Adapted from Hays, J. H., & Larson, K. H. (1965). Interacting with patients. *New York: MacMillan Company.*

Appendix D

Defense Mechanisms

Defense mechanisms are processes by which the self deals with unacceptable or unpleasant thoughts, feelings, or actions. These mechanisms are not inherently bad or good but are often seen in everyday life and are an acceptable way of coping. However, when the prolonged or exclusive use of defense mechanisms precludes other effective ways of coping with stress and/or anxiety, the individual begins to experience difficulties in meeting the demands of life.

Name	Definition	Example
Compensation	Overachievement in one area to offset real or perceived deficiencies in another area	A student with little interest in sports works hard to be on the honor roll
Conversion	Expression of an emotional conflict through the development of a physical symptom, usually sensorimotor in nature	A child who is expected to go to college develops blindness, but is unconcerned about it
Denial	Failure to acknowledge obvious ideas, conflicts, or situations that are emotionally painful or anxiety-provoking	A person with a newly diagnosed terminal illness is cheerful and makes no mention of the illness
Displacement	Ventilation of intense feelings toward persons less threatening than the one(s) who aroused those feelings	A person who is mad at the boss yells at his or her spouse
Dissociation	Dealing with emotional conflict by a temporary alteration in consciousness or identity	An adult remembers nothing of childhood abuse
Identification	Unconscious modeling of the behaviors, attitudes, and values of another person	A teenager espouses the beliefs and behavior of an admired relative, although he or she is unaware of doing so
Intellectualization	Separation of the emotion of a painful event or situation from the facts involved; acknowledging the facts but not the emotion	A person involved in a serious car accident discusses what happened with no emotional expression
Introjection	Acceptance of another person's values, beliefs, and attitudes as one's own	A person who dislikes guns becomes an avid hunter, just like a best friend
Projection	Attributing unacceptable thoughts, feelings, or actions to someone else	A person with many prejudices loudly identifies others as bigots
Rationalization	Justification of unacceptable thoughts, feelings, or behavior with logical-sounding reasons	A student who cheats on a test claims everyone does it, therefore it is necessary to cheat to be able to get passing grades

Name	Definition	Example
Reaction Formation	Unacceptable thoughts and feelings are handled by exhibiting the opposite behavior	A person with sexist ideas does volunteer work for a women's organization
Repression	Exclusion of emotionally painful or anxiety-provoking thoughts and feelings from conscious awareness	A student who is jealous of another's student's scholarship award is unaware of those feelings
Sublimation	Substitution of socially acceptable behavior for impulses or desires that are unacceptable to the person	A person who is trying to stop smoking cigarettes chews gum constantly
Suppression	Conscious exclusion of unacceptable thoughts and feelings from conscious awareness	A student decides not to think about a parent's illness in order to study for a test
Undoing	Exhibiting acceptable behavior to make up for or negate previous unacceptable behavior	A person who has been cheating on a spouse sends the spouse a bouquet of roses

Appendix E

Psychopharmacology

ANTIDEPRESSANT MEDICATIONS

Antidepressant medications are used to alleviate the discomfort of clients with moderate to severe symptoms of depressed mood and affect.

Tricyclic and tetracyclic antidepressants often require 1 to 2 weeks to reach the full therapeutic effect.

Generic Name	Trade names
Amitriptyline hydrochloride	Elavil, Amitid, Amitril, Endep
Desipramine hydrochloride	Norpramin, Pertofrane
Doxepin hydrochloride	Adapin, Sinequan
Imipramine hydrochloride	Tofranil
Nortriptyline hydrochloride	Aventyl
Protriptyline hydrochloride	Vivactil
Trimipramine maleate	Surmontil
Maprotiline hydrochloride	Asendin

Common side effects of tricyclic and tetracyclic antidepressants include dry mouth, constipation, orthostatic hypotension, anxiety, agitation, disorientation, drowsiness, ataxia, gastric upset, altered blood sugar, and altered hepatic function.

Monoamine Oxidase Inhibitors (MAO Inhibitors) are long-acting, often requiring 2 to 4 weeks to achieve full therapeutic effect. In addition, clients must avoid tyramine-rich foods since the interaction of MAO Inhibitors and tyramine produces hypertensive crisis.

Generic Name	Trade Name
Isocarboxazid	Marplan
Phenelzine sulfate	Nardil
Tranylcypromine sulfate	Parnate

Common side effects of monoamine oxidase inhibitors include orthostatic hypotension, dizziness, insomnia, GI upsets, headache, tremors, anorexia, dry mouth, blurred vision, dysuria, palpitations, weight gain, sodium retention, photosensitivity reactions, edema, and impotence.

Other antidepressant medications include Fluoxetine (Prozac), Sertraline (201ft), Trazadone (Desyrel), and Amoxapine (Asendin). Common side effects of these antidepressants include dry mouth, blurred vision, constipation, anorexia, nausea, diarrhea, headache, and weakness.

ANTIPSYCHOTIC MEDICATIONS

Antipsychotic medications, also known as neuroleptics, ataractics, or major tranquilizers, are used to decrease the severity of hallucinations, delusions, and related behaviors.

Phenothiazine antipsychotics

Generic Name	Trade Names
Chlorpromazine hydrochloride	Chlor-PZ, Promachel, Promapar, Sonazine, Thorazine
Acetophenazine maleat	Tindal
Butaperazine maleat	Repoise
Carphenazine maleate	Proketazine
Fluphenazine enanthate, Fluphenazine decanoate	Prolixin
Mesoridazine besylate	Serentil
Perphenazine	Trilafon
Trifluoperazine hydrochloride	Stelazine
Thioridazine hydrochloride	Mellaril

Common side effects of phenothiazines include: drowsiness, hypotension, extrapyramidal symptoms (uncoordinated spasmodic movements, involuntary motor restlessness, Parkinsonism), dry mouth, blurred vision, weight gain, decreased libido, delayed ovulation, phototoxicity, and jaundice. Tardive dyskinesia, characterized by involuntary tongue movements, lip-smacking, and chewing motions, and for which there is no effective treatment, may appear after long-term use.

Butyrophenones

Generic Name	Trade Name
Haloperidol	Haldol

Common side effects of butyrophenones are similar to phenothiazines with a higher incidence of extrapyramidal symptoms, but less sedation, hypotension. Severe depression leading to suicidal tendencies may develop.

Thioxanthenes

Generic Name	Trade Name
Chlorprothixene	Taractan
Thiothixene	Navane

Common side effects of thioxanthenes include frequent drowsiness, orthostatic hypotension, and dry mouth. Extrapyramidal symptoms are less frequent than with other antipsychotics.

Dibenzoxepines

Generic Name	Trade Name
Loxipine	Loxitane

Dihydroindolones

Generic Name	Trade Names
Molindone	Lidone, Moban

Side effects for dihydroindolones and dibenzoxepines are similar to other antipsychotic agents.

ANTIANXIETY MEDICATIONS

Antianxiety medications, also called minor tranquilizers, are used to reduce high anxiety levels and treat alcohol withdrawal.

Benzodiazepines

Generic Name	Trade Names
Diazepam	Valium
Chlordiazepoxide	Librium, Libritabs
Clorazepate dipotassium	Tranxene
Oxazepam	Serax
Alprazolam	Xanax

Common side effects of benzodiazepines include drowsiness, lethargy, ataxia, confusion, headache, syncope, dry mouth, constipation, urinary retention, hypotension, weight gain, and depression.

Propanediols

Generic Name	Trade Names
Meprobamate	Equanil, Miltown

Side effects of propanediols are similar to those of the benzodiazepines.

Antimanic medications are used to control acute manic and hypomanis behaviors, such as hyperactivity, flight of ideas, and aggressiveness.

ANTIMANIC MEDICATIONS

Antimanic

Generic Name	Trade Names
Lithium carbonate	Eskalith, Lithane, Lithonate

Common side effects include dry mouth, metallic taste, thyroid enlargement, glycosuria, hyperglycemia, weight gain, and edema. Toxic symptoms are nausea, diarrhea, tremors, blurred vision, and slurred speech.

Anticonvulsant

Generic Name	Trade Name
Carbamazepine	Tegretol

Although Tegretol is an anticonvulsant, it is also used for its effects in controlling mania, particularly when Lithium is not effective. Common side effects include nausea, vomiting, nystagmus, urinary retention, and changes in blood pressure. Toxic symptoms are dizziness, ataxia, drowsiness, restlessness, disorientation, confusion, agitation, tremor, and coma.

ANTIPARKINSONIAN MEDICATIONS

Antiparkinsonian medications are used to treat drug-induced extrapyramidal symptoms that may result from use of major tranquilizers.

Anticholinergic agents

Generic Name	Trade Names
Trihexyphenidyl hydrochloride	Artane, Hexyphen, Pipanol, Tremin, Trihexidyl
Benztropine mesylate	Cogentin

Generic Name	Trade Names
Beperiden hydrochloride	Akineton
Chlorphenoxamine hydrochloride	Phenoxene
Procyclidine hydrochloride	Kemadrin

Common side effects of anticholinergics include dry mouth, blurred vision, dizziness, nausea, and nervousness. In the elderly, confusion and drowsiness also may occur.

Antihistamines

Generic Name	Trade Names
Diphenhydramine hydrochloride	Benadryl, Phenamine
Orphenadrine hydrochloride	Disipal

Common side effects of antihistamines include dry mouth, urinary hesitancy, constipation, and drowsiness.

Antiparkinsonian agents

Generic Name	Trade name
Levodopa, carbidopa	Sinemet
Amantadine hydrochloride	Symmetrel

Common side effects include nausea, vomiting, dystonia, depression, psychosis, confusion, and irritability.

SYMPATHOMIMETIC MEDICATIONS

Sympathomimetic stimulants are used to treat hyperactivity, minimal brain dysfunctions, and attention deficit disorders.

Generic Name	Trade Names
Methylphenidate hydrochloride	Methidate, Ritalin
Pemoline	Cylert

Common side effects include insomnia, anorexia, transitory weight loss, headaches, tachycardia, dry mouth, and alterations in blood pressure.

Index

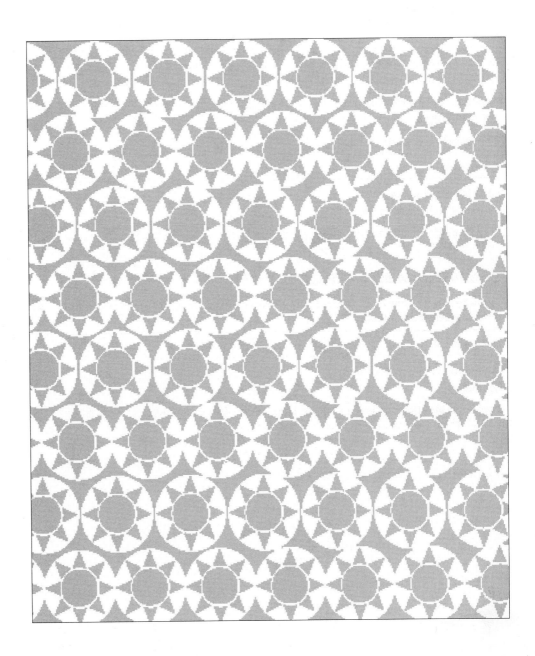

Psychotic behavior, 101–124
Psychotic depression, 191
PTSD. *See* Post-traumatic stress disorder (PTSD)
Purge behavior, 261

Rape, 415
Rape trauma syndrome, 361, 362
Rapid eye movement (REM) sleep, 375
Reality orientation, 17
Recognition, of client, 22
Recreational activities, client teaching, 22
Relationships, 10, 114. *See also* Therapeutic relationship;
     Trust relationship
Religious delusions, 103
REM cycle. *See* Rapid eye movement (REM) sleep
Renal failure, in delirium tremens, 273
Residual schizophrenia, 114
Resources, community, 22
Respect
   of beliefs, 13
   of sexuality, 12
Response, emotional, of staff, 23–24
Responsibility(ies)
   caregiver, 22
   client, 20, 22, 25
   psychiatric nurse, 20, 22–23
Restriction. *See* Limit-setting
Revision, and evaluation, 19
Rights, clients', 24–25
Ritalin. *See* Methylphenidate (Ritalin)
Rituals, 355
Role(s)
   caregiver, 56
   client, 25
   professional, 22–25, 23
Role modeling, 22
Role-play, 22

Safe environment, 9–10, 22
Schizoaffective disorders, schizophrenia versus, 114
Schizoid personality disorder, 339–342
   diagnosis
      Impaired Adjustment, 340
   versus schizotypal personality disorder, 339
Schizophrenia, 113–120
   chemical dependence treatment program and, 291
   diagnoses
      Personal Identity Disturbance, 115
      Self-Care Deficit, 119
      Social Isolation, 118
   hallucinations in, 107
   negative signs in, 71
Schizotypal personality disorder, 339–342
   diagnosis
      Impaired Adjustment, 340
   versus schizoid personality disorder, 339
Secondary gain, 223

Seductive behavior. *See* Histrionic behavior
Seizures, in alcohol detoxification, 273
Self, sense of, 10–11, 114
Self-blame, in chronic/terminal illness, 171
Self Care Deficit, 119, 128, 197
Self-care, responsibility for, 22
Self-destructive behavior, direct and indirect, 201
Self-esteem, building of, 10–11
Self-Esteem Disturbance, 98, 169, 211, 423
Self-help groups, adult children of alcoholics, 297
Self-medication, 291, 375
Senile dementia, 127
Sense of self, loss of, 114
Sensory deprivation, 107
Sensory/Perceptual Alterations (Specify) (Visual, Auditory, Kinesthetic, Gustatory, Tactile, Olfactory) 108, 122
Sexual abuse, 415–424
Sexual behavior, adolescent, 93
Sexual behavior. *See* Histrionic behavior
Sexuality. *See also* Homosexuality
   beliefs and, 12
   client, 17
   feelings and, 11–12
Significant others, 16
Skill(s)
   communication, 20–21, 22
   daily living, 72
   interaction, 3–4
   nursing, 3
   social, 3, 22, 72
   stress management, 13
   therapeutic vs. vocational, 22
Sleep deprivation, 107, 121
Sleep disturbances, 375–378
   diagnosis
      Sleep Pattern Disturbance, 376
Social Isolation, 58, 118
Social phobia, 351
Social skills, 22, 72
Somatic delusions, 103, 335
Spirituality, 13, 17
Staff, clinical nursing, 4–6
Staff-splitting behaviors, 321
Standards, personal, 17
Stereotyped movements, 114
Stimulants, withdrawal from, 279
Strategies, barriers and, 4–5
Strengths, client, 16
Stress, 12–13. *See also* Anxiety
   and anxiety, 343–372
   management of, 22
   in psychosomatic illness, 215
   staff, 24
Stress management, client teaching, 22
Stressors, 93, 369
Substance abuse, 17, 93, 191, 285. *See also* Chemical dependence
Sudden death, from drug withdrawal, 280